Interventions in Infectious Disease Emergencies

Editor

NANCY MISRI KHARDORI

MEDICAL CLINICS
OF NORTH AMERICA

www.medical.theclinics.com

November 2012 • Volume 96 • Number 6

ELSEVIER

1600 John F. Kennedy Boulevard • Suite 1800 • Philadelphia, Pennsylvania 19103-2899

http://www.theclinics.com

MEDICAL CLINICS OF NORTH AMERICA Volume 96, Number 6
November 2012 ISSN 0025-7125, ISBN-13: 978-1-4557-5094-8

Editor: Pamela Hetherington

Medical Clinics of North America (ISSN 0025-7125) is published bimonthly by Elsevier Inc., 360 Park Avenue South, New York, NY 10010-1710. Months of issue are January, March, May, July, September, and November. Periodicals postage paid at New York, NY, and additional mailing offices. Subscription prices are USD 232 per year for US individuals, USD 424 per year for US institutions, USD 117 per year for US students, USD 295 per year for Canadian individuals, USD 551 per year for Canadian institutions, USD 184 per year for Canadian students, USD 358 per year for international individuals, USD 551 per year for international institutions and USD 184 per year for international students. To receive student/resident rate, orders must be accompanied by name of affiliated institution, date of term, and the *signature* of program/residency coordinator on institution letterhead. Orders will be billed at individual rate until proof of status is received. Foreign air speed delivery is included in all *Clinics* subscription prices. All prices are subject to change without notice. **POSTMASTER:** Send address changes to *Medical Clinics of North America*, Elsevier Health Sciences Division, Subscription Customer Service, 3251 Riverport Lane, Maryland Heights, MO 63043. **Customer Service: Telephone: 1-800-654-2452** (U.S. and Canada); **1-314-447-8871** (outside U.S. and Canada). **Fax: 1-314-447-8029. E-mail: journalscustomerservice-usa@elsevier.com** (for print support); **journalsonlinesupport-usa@elsevier.com** (for online support).

Reprints. For copies of 100 or more of articles in this publication, please contact the Commercial Reprints Department, Elsevier Inc., 360 Park Avenue South, New York, NY 10010-1710. Tel.: 212-633-3812; Fax: 212-462-1935; E-mail: reprints@elsevier.com.

Medical Clinics of North America is also published in Spanish by McGraw-Hill Interamericana Editores S. A., P.O. Box 5-237, 06500 Mexico, D.F., Mexico.

Medical Clinics of North America is covered in *MEDLINE/PubMed (Index Medicus), Current Contents, ASCA, Excerpta Medica, Science Citation Index, and ISI/BIOMED.*

Printed in the United States of America.

MEDICAL CLINICS OF NORTH AMERICA

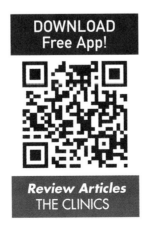

NOW AVAILABLE FOR YOUR iPhone and iPad

GOAL STATEMENT

The goal of *Medical Clinics of North America* is to keep practicing physicians up to date with current clinical practice by providing timely articles reviewing the state of the art in patient care.

ACCREDITATION

The *Medical Clinics of North America* is planned and implemented in accordance with the Essential Areas and Policies of the Accreditation Council for Continuing Medical Education (ACCME) through the joint sponsorship of the University of Virginia School of Medicine and Elsevier. The University of Virginia School of Medicine is accredited by the ACCME to provide continuing medical education for physicians.

The University of Virginia School of Medicine designates this enduring material activity for a maximum of 15 *AMA PRA Category 1 Credit*(s)™ for each issue, 90 credits per year. Physicians should only claim credit commensurate with the extent of their participation in the activity.

The American Medical Association has determined that physicians not licensed in the US who participate in this CME enduring material activity are eligible for a maximum of 15 *AMA PRA Category 1 Credit*(s)™ for each issue, 90 credits per year.

Credit can be earned by reading the text material, taking the CME examination online at http://www.theclinics.com/home/cme, and completing the evaluation. After taking the test, you will be required to review any and all incorrect answers. Following completion of the test and evaluation, your credit will be awarded and you may print your certificate.

FACULTY DISCLOSURE/CONFLICT OF INTEREST

The University of Virginia School of Medicine, as an ACCME accredited provider, endorses and strives to comply with the Accreditation Council for Continuing Medical Education (ACCME) Standards of Commercial Support, Commonwealth of Virginia statutes, University of Virginia policies and procedures, and associated federal and private regulations and guidelines on the need for disclosure and monitoring of proprietary and financial interests that may affect the scientific integrity and balance of content delivered in continuing medical education activities under our auspices.

The University of Virginia School of Medicine requires that all CME activities accredited through this institution be developed independently and be scientifically rigorous, balanced and objective in the presentation/discussion of its content, theories and practices.

All authors/editors participating in an accredited CME activity are expected to disclose to the readers relevant financial relationships with commercial entities occurring within the past 12 months (such as grants or research support, employee, consultant, stock holder, member of speakers bureau, etc.). The University of Virginia School of Medicine will employ appropriate mechanisms to resolve potential conflicts of interest to maintain the standards of fair and balanced education to the reader. Questions about specific strategies can be directed to the Office of Continuing Medical Education, University of Virginia School of Medicine, Charlottesville, Virginia.

The faculty and staff of the University of Virginia Office of Continuing Medical Education have no financial affiliations to disclose.

The authors/editors listed below have identified no professional or financial affiliations for themselves or their spouse/partner:

Aarti Agrawal, MD; Jody P. Boggs, MD; Danielle Castillo, MD; Ian A. Chen, MD; Kenji M. Cunnion, MD, MPH; Catherine J. Derber, MD; Himanshu Desai, MD; Neeraj Goel, MBBS, MD; B. Mitchell Goodman III, MD; Pamela Hetherington, (Acquisitions Editor); Tin Han Htwe, MD; Nancy Misri Khardori, MD, PhD (Guest Editor); Romesh Khardori, MD, PhD; Neel K. Krishna, PhD; Thomas J. Lynch, PharmD; Mayar Al Mohajer, MD; Praveen K. Mullangi, MD; Jennifer L. Ryal, MD; Sushma Singh, MD; Sami G. Tahhan, MD; Stephanie B. Troy, MD; Chand Wattal, BSc, MBBS, MD; and Andrew Wolf, MD (Test Author).

The authors/editors listed below identified the following professional or financial affiliations for themselves or their spouse/partner:

Rabih O. Darouiche, MD is a consultant and holds a patent for Cook, Inc.

Disclosure of Discussion of Non-FDA Approved Uses for Pharmaceutical Products and/or Medical Devices.

The University of Virginia School of Medicine, as an ACCME provider, requires that all faculty presenters identify and disclose any off-label uses for pharmaceutical and medical device products. The University of Virginia School of Medicine recommends that each physician fully review all the available data on new products or procedures prior to clinical use.

TO ENROLL

To enroll in the Medical Clinics of North America Continuing Medical Education program, call customer service at 1-800-654-2452 or visit us online at http://www.theclinics.com/home/cme. The CME program is available to subscribers for an additional fee of USD 228.

Contributors

GUEST EDITOR

NANCY MISRI KHARDORI, MD, PhD, FACP, FIDSA
Professor of Internal Medicine, Division of Infectious Diseases, Professor of Microbiology and Molecular Cell Biology, Eastern Virginia Medical School, Norfolk Virginia

AUTHORS

AARTI AGRAWAL, MD
Infectious Disease Consultants of Hampton Roads, Norfolk, Virginia

MAYAR AL MOHAJER, MD
Infectious Disease Fellow, Michael E. DeBakey VA Medical Center, Baylor College of Medicine, Houston, Texas

JODY P. BOGGS, MD, MPH
Assistant Professor of Medicine, Department of Internal Medicine, Eastern Virginia Medical School, Norfolk, Virginia

DANIELLE CASTILLO, MD
Fellow in Endocrinology, Division of Endocrinology and Metabolism, Department of Internal Medicine, Strelitz Diabetes Institute for Endocrine and Metabolic Disorders, Eastern Virginia Medical School, Norfolk, Virginia

IAN A. CHEN, MD, MPH
Associate Professor of Medicine, Department of Internal Medicine, Eastern Virginia Medical School, Norfolk, Virginia

KENJI M. CUNNION, MD, MPH
Associate Professor, Department of Microbiology and Molecular Cell Biology; Department of Pediatrics, Eastern Virginia Medical School; Division of Infectious Diseases, Children's Specialty Group, Norfolk, Virginia

RABIH O. DAROUICHE, MD
Michael E. DeBakey VA Medical Center; VA Distinguished Service Professor, Departments of Medicine, Surgery and PM&R, Director of the Center of Prostheses Infection, Baylor College of Medicine, Houston, Texas

CATHERINE J. DERBER, MD
Assistant Professor, Department of Internal Medicine, Division of Infectious Diseases, Eastern Virginia Medical School, Norfolk, Virginia

HIMANSHU DESAI, MD
Assistant Professor of Medicine, Division of Pulmonary and Critical Care Medicine, Eastern Virginia Medical School, Norfolk, Virginia

NEERAJ GOEL, MBBS, MD
Associate Professor, Consultant, Department of Clinical Microbiology and Immunology, Sir Ganga Ram Hospital, New Delhi, India

B. MITCHELL GOODMAN III, MD
Assistant Professor of Medicine, Department of Internal Medicine, Eastern Virginia Medical School, Norfolk, Virginia

TIN HAN HTWE, MD
Division of Infectious Diseases, Sentara Medical Group, Norfolk, Virginia

NANCY MISRI KHARDORI, MD, PhD, FACP, FIDSA
Professor, Division of Infectious Diseases, Department of Internal Medicine; Department of Microbiology and Molecular Cell Biology, Eastern Virginia Medical School, Norfolk, Virginia; Division of Infectious Diseases, Springfield Clinic, Springfield, Illinois

ROMESH KHARDORI, MD, PhD, FACP
Professor of Medicine/Endocrinology, Professor and Director, Endocrinology Fellowship Training Program, Division of Endocrinology and Metabolism, Department of Internal Medicine, Strelitz Diabetes Center for Endocrine and Metabolic Disorders, Eastern Virginia Medical School, Norfolk, Virginia

NEEL K. KRISHNA, PhD
Associate Professor, Department of Microbiology and Molecular Cell Biology; Department of Pediatrics, Eastern Virginia Medical School, Norfolk, Virginia

THOMAS J. LYNCH, PharmD
Associate Professor, Department of Family and Community Medicine, Eastern Virginia Medical School, Norfolk, Virginia

PRAVEEN K. MULLANGI, MD
Division of Infectious Diseases, Springfield Clinic, Springfield, Illinois

JENNIFER L. RYAL, MD
Assistant Professor of Medicine, Eastern Virginia Medical School, Norfolk, Virginia

SUSHMA SINGH, MD
Division of Infectious Diseases, Department of Internal Medicine and Microbiology and Molecular Cell Biology, Eastern Virginia Medical School, Norfolk, Virginia

SAMI G. TAHHAN, MD
Assistant Professor of Medicine, Department of Internal Medicine, Eastern Virginia Medical School, Norfolk, Virginia

STEPHANIE B. TROY, MD
Division of Infectious Diseases, Assistant Professor, Department of Internal Medicine, Assistant Professor (Dual Appointment), Department of Microbiology and Molecular Cell Biology, Eastern Virginia Medical School, Norfolk, Virginia

CHAND WATTAL, BSc, MBBS, MD
Professor, Senior Consultant and Chairman, Department of Clinical Microbiology and Immunology, Sir Ganga Ram Hospital, New Delhi, India

Contents

goal has been somewhat relaxed based on evidence that very tight glucose control may be undesirable. Relative adrenal insufficiency has receded into the background, and the unconditional love for steroids is no longer justified. Instead, glucocorticoids need to be used in special cases, and testing for adrenal reserve is no longer necessary or justifiable. Thyroid dysfunction, and hypogonadism, both often noted with sepsis, do not require any treatment. Abnormalities in growth hormone, prolactin, and vasopressin secretion similarly require no treatment.

infections. The common causes include penetrating abdominal trauma, abdominal surgery, diverticulitis, appendicitis, pancreatitis, biliary disease, perforated viscus, and primary peritonitis. Intra-abdominal infections can masquerade as fever of obscure origin or as dysfunction of neighboring organs, such as lower lobe pneumonia related to a subphrenic abscess or an abscess causing small bowel obstruction. An urgent surgical intervention is the mainstay of the management of serious intra-abdominal infections.

Soft-tissue infections encompass a wide spectrum of presentations ranging from superficial skin infection (cellulitis) to deep-seated infection (myositis and fasciitis), based on the depth and the area of involvement. Although less frequent, necrotizing soft-tissue infections (NSTIs) occur based on the interactions between the host factors and the causative pathogens. NSTIs are rapidly progressing and aggressive infections that can be lethal, with high morbidity and mortality. This article reviews some of the causative agents of NSTIs, clinical features, and the need for high index of suspicion for early recognition and prompt surgical and medical management.

The diagnosis of sepsis is challenging given the lack of appropriate diagnostic methods and the inaccuracy of diagnostic criteria. Early resuscitation, intravenous antibiotics, and source control are crucial in the management of septic patients. The treatment of catheter-related bloodstream infection (CRBSI) often comprises 1 to 2 weeks of intravenous antibiotics plus catheter removal. Infections related to surgical devices are more difficult to manage because they require longer duration of therapy and possibly multiple surgical procedures. This review represents an update on the diagnosis and management of sepsis, catheter-related blood stream infections and some clinically important device-related infections.

This review article discusses important infectious illnesses, namely malaria, dengue, and chikungunya, in travelers returning from endemic areas. Malaria and dengue are two of the most common systemic illnesses reported in returning travelers. Because chikungunya is gaining importance, it is also briefly discussed. The clinical significance of these diseases is mainly due to the possibility of sudden deterioration with high mortality in clinically healthy looking patients. The key clinical features, their diagnosis, and treatment algorithms are discussed in detail to help in early diagnosis and appropriate clinical management of such travelers presenting in emergency departments.

Preface

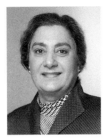

Nancy Misri Khardori, MD, PhD, FACP, FIDSA
Guest Editor

The most significant aspect of infectious diseases is that a majority of serious emergencies are curable if diagnosed early and managed appropriately rather than just treatable, contrary to most other emergent disease processes. Unfortunately, serious infectious disease manifestations are often not seen by patients, families, and health care providers in the same light as other emergencies. Delay in seeking medical attention and recognizing the urgency for intervention often result in a worse prognosis.

Like other medical emergencies, the initial encounter for infectious disease emergencies is in the emergency department or outpatient setting. Noninfectious disease physicians, particularly general internists, are often the front-line providers for diagnostic workup and initial management. The reader should keep that in mind, as the first article in this issue has been compiled by 5 of my general internal medicine colleagues. Each section starts with a case vignette and is followed by articulation of questions about diagnosis and management at the very outset. They have very skillfully abstracted a few clinical pearls for each of the serious clinical presentations in their respective sections. The next 10 articles review in detail epidemiology, microbiology, clinical presentations, diagnostic workup, and management, including presumptive and definitive antimicrobial therapy for infectious disease emergencies involving various organ systems. They include articles on the role of molecular diagnosis and pharmacotherapy of infectious disease emergencies.

It seems very appropriate to use one of the many quotes from Sir William Oster, "The whole life of the profession, whether moving in the units or expressed in its great institutions, is controlled to-day, as it ever has been controlled, by what we think of the nature of disease. Why is a right judgment on this one point the aim of medical education and of research—the be-all and the end-all of our efforts? Because upon correct knowledge depends the possibility of the control of disease, and upon our views of its nature the measures for its prevention or cure."[1]

Clearly, this issue of *Medical Clinics of North America* was made possible by the effort and experience of the contributing authors. Although acknowledging their

Med Clin N Am 96 (2012) xi–xii
http://dx.doi.org/10.1016/j.mcna.2012.09.004
0025-7125/12/$ – see front matter © 2012 Elsevier Inc. All rights reserved.

medical.theclinics.com

contributions, I would like to dedicate this issue to all those patients who did or did not see the light of the next day battling infectious disease emergencies.

Nancy Misri Khardori, MD, PhD, FACP, FIDSA
Division of Infectious Diseases
Eastern Virginia Medical School
825 Fairfax Avenue
Norfolk, VA 23507

E-mail address:
nkhardori@gmail.com

REFERENCE

1. Silverman ME, Murray TJ, Bryan CS, editors. The quotable osler, quote. 317. Philadelphia: American College of Physicians; 2003.

Infectious Disease Emergencies
Frontline Clinical Pearls

B. Mitchell Goodman III, MD*, Jody P. Boggs, MD, MPH,
Sami G. Tahhan, MD, Jennifer L. Ryal, MD, Ian A. Chen, MD, MPH

KEYWORDS

- Antibiotic resistance • *Staphylococcus aureus* • Necrotizing fasciitis • Meningitis
- Sepsis

KEY POINTS

- General internists are often the first practitioners to evaluate and manage hospitalized patients who have developed a severe, life-threatening infection.
- Early recognition of infectious disease emergencies is essential to guide appropriate initial therapy and avert avoidable morbidity and mortality.
- Many diseases have certain hallmarks which, if recognized, may dictate specific life-saving intervention.
- In an era of antibiotic resistance, the primary care practitioner must have a high index of suspicion for resistant pathogens and be familiar with appropriate broad and organism-specific therapies.
- The armamentarium of therapies in infectious disease emergencies includes not only anti-microbial drugs, but also such diverse modalities as surgical inintervention and immuno-logic agents.

INTRODUCTION

Infectious diseases in the mild to moderate form represent a bulk of office visits for internists and general practitioners. Often, when one of their patients develops a serious life-threatening infection, they are the first ones to manage the patients in the hospital. The hallmark of infectious disease emergencies is that with early and appropriate diagnosis and management, most of them are not just treatable, but curable. It is the first 48 hours of initial management that determines the further course and prognosis. Even when infectious disease specialists are available for consultation, the immediate management is rendered by the admitting physician. It is with this in mind that the editor of this issue requested our team to write the first article as a gener-alists' view of infectious disease emergencies. We chose to start each organ system

Department of Internal Medicine, Eastern Virginia Medical School, 825 Fairfax Avenue, Norfolk, VA 23507, USA
* Corresponding author.
E-mail address: goodmabm@evms.edu

Med Clin N Am 96 (2012) 1033–1066
http://dx.doi.org/10.1016/j.mcna.2012.09.001
0025-7125/12/$ – see front matter © 2012 Elsevier Inc. All rights reserved.

with relevant clinical vignettes. Our goal is to provide a case-based learning tool for the generalist aimed at providing help in rationalizing differential diagnosis followed by presumptive antimicrobial therapy and diagnostic workup. Each discussion offers a few frontline clinical pearls.

HEAD AND NECK INFECTIONS
Meningitis

An 18-year-old previously healthy college freshman presents with about 24 hours of fever, nausea, vomiting, headache, and decreased ability to concentrate. He is also complaining of severe myalgias and a rash. On physical exam, he is febrile, tachycardic, tachypneic, and hypotensive. He has positive Brudzinski and Kernig signs but no focal neurologic signs. He has a petechial rash, which is worsening. Laboratory data show a leukocytosis accompanied by thrombocytopenia, as well as a coagulopathy. A lumbar puncture is done emergently by the emergency department (ED) physician and cerebrospinal fluid (CSF) is sent for a cell count, glucose, protein level, Gram stain, culture, and sensitivity. The ED calls you to admit the patient.

While awaiting the results on the CSF, you are trying to decide on the best presumptive antibiotic therapy for this patient. You decide the best course of action is the following:

A. Ceftriaxone 1 g intravenous (IV) daily
B. Ceftriaxone 2 g IV daily
C. Zosyn 3.375 IV every 6 hours
D. Vancomycin 1 g IV every 12 hours
E. Ceftriaxone 2 g IV every 12 hours plus vancomycin 15 mg/kg IV every 12 hours

The patient will be going to the intensive care unit (ICU) and the ED nurse would like to know how to prevent transmission of his infection in the hospital setting. The patient has been heard coughing.

You order the following status:

A. Contact precautions
B. Airborne precautions with a negative-pressure room
C. Droplet precautions
D. Standard hygiene precautions with good hand-washing practices

The patient is now in the ICU and is on aggressive volume repletion and has already received the antibiotics you had ordered. You take a further look at his laboratory data and realize he is hypoglycemic, hyponatremic, and mildly hyperkalemic. The ICU team is having difficulties maintaining his blood pressure and have had to start him on vasopressors.

You decide to order the following laboratory studies:

A. A disseminated intravascular coagulation (DIC) panel
B. A cortisol level
C. A peripheral smear
D. A cosyntropin stimulation test
E. All of the above

Discussion

Meningitis caused by *Neisseria meningitidis* tends to strike young, previously healthy individuals, and can be devastating, progressing to death over a few hours. *N meningitidis* is the most common cause of bacterial meningitis in children and young adults in the United States, with an overall mortality rate of 14%.[1] It has replaced *Haemophilus influenzae* as the second most common cause of community-acquired adult bacterial meningitis.

The typical triad of fever, neck stiffness, and altered mental status is seen less commonly than with *Streptococcus pneumoniae* meningitis but those findings are more common when a petechial rash is present. The myalgia associated with *N meningitidis* infection is more severe than that seen with influenza virus infection and can be an alerting symptom as to the possibility of meningococcemia. Other signs and symptoms of sepsis and shock, such as leg pain, cold hands and feet, and pale or mottled skin, should be sought out, as they correlate with severity of disease.

Physical examination should include special attention to vascular instability, such as hypotension and tachycardia. Meningeal irritation should be explored with Brudzinski and Kernig testing. A thorough examination for a petechial rash should be done, including areas of pressure on the body where it is most commonly found, such as belt lines and elastic straps regions.

The severity of the petechial rash correlates with the severity of DIC and thrombocytopenia in these patients. Progression of the rash from a petechial rash to ecchymoses, to painful indurated areas with erythematous borders can be prevented with early antibiotic therapy. The areas can form bullae and vesicles with ensuing gangrenous necrosis called purpura fulminans.

Diagnosis is made with culture and Gram stain from a sterile site. CSF, blood in patients with meningitis and meningococcemia, or skin biopsy can all yield a diagnosis.

The yield of these studies will depend on the scope of meningococcal disease, whether it is meningitis with or without meningococcemia.

Lumbar puncture should be performed and typically shows low glucose, less than 45 mg/dL, protein higher than 500 mg/dL and a white cell count higher than 1000 with neutrophilic predominance. Latex agglutination testing on the CSF can be useful but has limitations, as the sensitivity for serogroup B, which is the most common serogroup in the United States, is low.

Thrombocytopenia and coagulopathy should prompt an evaluation for DIC, and in the presence of DIC, poor response to treatment with shock should alert to the possibility of adrenal infarction leading to adrenal insufficiency (the Waterhouse-Friderichsen syndrome).

Presumptive treatment for *N meningitidis* meningitis is a third-generation cephalosporin, such as cefotaxime, or high-dose ceftriaxone at 2 mg IV every 12 hours to achieve ideal CSF levels. Vancomycin is not effective but is rather used for *S pneumoniae* meningitis at hospitals with high resistance rates to ceftriaxone. It is added to ceftriaxone for initial therapy of meningitis while a microbiological diagnosis is being sought. Antibiotic administration should not be delayed until a lumbar puncture is done, as *N meningitis* infection can be lethal in a matter of hours.

Droplet precautions should be instituted because the organism is a respiratory pathogen and spread is most likely by the aerosol route, especially in patients who are actively coughing. The organism is larger than other organisms, such as *Mycobacterium tuberculosis,* and therefore airborne precautions with a negative-pressure room are not needed.

Persistent shock with thrombocytopenia and a coagulopathy should trigger a search for DIC with a DIC panel, a peripheral smear looking for fragmented red blood cells secondary to DIC, as well as a workup for adrenal insufficiency with a cortisol level and a cosyntropin stimulation test.

Morbidity and mortality rates have changed little since the 1960s because endotoxin-induced vascular damage has been difficult to treat. In addition, because of its lower incidence, practitioners often do not have enough exposure to the disease to be able to diagnose it quickly enough.

Clinical Pearls

1. Consider *N meningitidis* meningitis in a young healthy patient with a sepsis syndrome, meningitis symptoms, and a rash.
2. Treat as soon as the diagnosis is considered with a third-generation cephalosporin, such as high-dose ceftriaxone 2 g IV every 12 hours.
3. Patients should be placed on droplet precautions immediately to prevent respiratory spread in the hospital.
4. Look for the Waterhouse-Friderichsen syndrome in patients who have persistent shock and features of DIC.

Encephalitis

A 40-year-old previously healthy man is brought in to the ED by emergency medical services (EMS), as his family was concerned over a 3-day history of fevers and an altered mental status. It is winter and he has not had any insect or animal exposures. His family has not noticed any rashes. He has not had any recent travel or sick contacts.

In the ED, the patient is confused, febrile, and tachycardic but has a normal blood pressure and oxygen saturation. He does not have signs of meningeal irritation or a rash and any focal neurologic signs. At the end of the physical examination, the patient experiences tonic clonic activity on the left side of his body followed by generalized tonic clonic activity bilaterally with loss of consciousness.

His laboratory studies show leukocytosis and a normal creatinine. The patient appears postictal and is going to be wheeled away for a magnetic resonance image (MRI) scan of the head.

Based on the patient's presentation your most likely diagnosis is

A. Septic bacterial meningitis
B. Aseptic viral meningitis
C. West Nile virus encephalitis
D. Eastern equine encephalitis
E. Herpes simplex virus encephalitis

You recognize that the patient needs a lumbar puncture and an MRI of the head but you would like to start presumptive treatment for the patient's condition. The most important therapeutic intervention in this case would be the initiation of:

A. Ceftriaxone 2 g IV every 12 hours
B. Ampicillin IV
C. Vancomycin 1 g IV every 12 hours
D. Acyclovir 10 mg/kg IV every 8 hours

The patient has been started on antimicrobial therapy and gets a lumbar puncture, which shows 200 white blood cells (WBCs) with lymphocytic pleocytosis with mildly elevated protein of 100 mg/dL and normal CSF glucose. His MRI shows necrosis in the right temporal lobe and the neurologist was able to perform an electroencephalogram (EEG) and read it at once with the comment that there were PLEDS (periodic lateralizing epileptiform discharges).

The best diagnostic test you would like to make sure was done is

A. Herpes simplex viral culture from the CSF
B. Paired antibody test on the CSF and serum for West Nile virus

C. Herpes simplex virus polymerase chain reaction (PCR) from the CSF
D. Herpes simplex CSF antibody
E. Paired antibody test on the CSF and serum for St Louis encephalitis virus

Discussion

Herpes simplex virus type 1 (HSV-1) is the most common cause of fatal sporadic encephalitis worldwide. Herpes simplex virus type 2 (HSV-2) encephalitis is usually not seen in adults but is seen in neonates. Disease can occur in any season as opposed to West Nile virus, eastern equine encephalitis virus, and St Louis encephalitis virus, which tend to occur in summer and fall and require an insect/animal exposure.

The virus can cause infection following an acute episode of HSV-1, during an episode of HSV-1 reactivation with invasion into the central nervous system (CNS), or by reactivation of latent HSV-1 into the CNS without apparent skin lesions or rash.

Clinical symptoms include fever, headache, altered mental status, focal symptoms, and focal seizures with or without secondary generalization. Mental status changes and abnormal brain activity, such as focal deficits and seizures, are seen in herpetic encephalitis and are absent in meningitis. Signs of meningeal irritation may or may not be present on examination, and a herpetic rash is not seen when the virus is latent and directly reactivates into the CNS.

CSF laboratory abnormalities include a high WBC count but usually less than 250, as opposed to meningitis in which the WBC count is often in the thousands. There is lymphocytic pleocytosis as opposed to neutrophil predominance in septic meningitis. Protein levels may be elevated but usually are less than 150 mg/dL, whereas protein levels are higher than that threshold in septic meningitis. Glucose levels in the CSF are usually normal in herpes encephalitis, whereas they are often low in meningitis.

Abnormal MRI findings in the temporal region are suggestive of herpes encephalitis, as are EEG findings, such as PLEDS, which indicate focality in the lateral lobe regions[2]

The standard diagnostic test for herpes encephalitis in adults is herpes simplex PCR testing from the CSF. It has a sensitivity of 98% and a specificity of 94%. CSF PCR for HSV-2 is more useful in neonates, in whom it is more likely to cause herpes encephalitis.

CSF viral culture for herpes has a sensitivity of less than 10% and has been abandoned for diagnosing herpes encephalitis. CSF antibody testing for herpes simplex yields better results than HSV CSF cultures with a sensitivity of 8% and specificity of 90%.

Brain biopsy had been the gold standard but has the drawback of being invasive. There are often delays in obtaining results from the tissue and there is a possibility of a false-negative result owing to errors in sampling and culturing. It has been replaced by PCR testing and is reserved for patients who are deteriorating and a clear diagnosis has not been made.

Patients who are untreated have significant morbidity and mortality. Mortality approaches 70% without treatment and is reduced to 20% to 30% with treatment. Early therapy with acyclovir 10 mg/kg IV every 8 hours reduces mortality and morbidity such as cognitive deficits.

Clinical Pearls

1. Consider herpes encephalitis in patients with fever, headache, and altered mental status.
2. Herpes encephalitis has a propensity to localize to the temporal lobes, causing seizures and temporal lobe abnormalities on EEG, such as PLEDS.
3. Temporal lobe abnormalities on MRI, such as necrosis, are suggestive of herpes encephalitis.

4. The diagnostic test of choice is HSV PCR from the CSF.
5. Early treatment with IV acyclovir should be instituted as soon as possible and reduces morbidity and mortality.

Brain Abscess

A 55-year-old male with a past medical history of poorly controlled diabetes is brought into the ED by EMS. His family called EMS, as he had tonic clonic activity on his right side with subsequent generalization and loss of consciousness. He was postictal when EMS arrived. You meet the family and learn that he has had extensive dental disease and had extensive dental work in the past 2 to 3 weeks.

He had a left frontal headache, which was not responding to acetaminophen or nonsteroidal anti-inflammatory drugs (NSAIDs). They had also noticed that he was growing increasingly inattentive in the past few days and his judgment was impaired. The day of admission, he was getting drowsier before he had seizure activity.

On physical examination, the patient is febrile and postictal and he has papilledema. The next diagnostic step is

A. You obtain consent from the family and proceed to do a lumbar puncture
B. You send the patient for an MRI of the brain
C. You obtain an EEG at once
D. You start the patient on aspirin for stroke prevention

The patient has had diagnostic imaging and laboratory work is back showing a leukocytosis and pre-renal azotemia. He has received some medications through EMS and is now awake. You proceed to examine him and he does have difficulty focusing his attention. He also has extensive dental caries and periodontal disease with evidence of abscesses, as well as a right-sided hemiparesis. He does not have neck stiffness. Grasp, suck, and snout reflexes are present.

You find out that he received decadron 10 mg IV with an order for 4 mg IV every 6 hours thereafter. The MRI is showing a large left frontal abscess with substantial surrounding edema and mass effect. You decide to call neurosurgery to evaluate the patient for potential aspiration of the abscess to identify the causative organism. Meanwhile, you are contemplating starting antibiotic therapy. The best option at this point for what you suspect to be an odontogenic source of the brain abscess is

A. IV metronidazole with the addition of IV ceftriaxone or cefotaxime
B. IV erythromycin
C. IV doxycycline
D. IV cefazolin

Discussion

Brain abscess can occur by direct spread or through the hematogenous route. Direct spread tends to cause solitary abscesses, whereas hematogenous spread usually results in multiple abscesses.

Otogenic infections tend to spread to the temporal lobe and cerebellum.

Sinus and odontogenic infections tend to spread to the frontal lobes.

Headache is the most common symptom and localizes to the area of the abscess. Symptoms are also representative of the part of cerebral cortex involved. Frontal abscesses are most common and can present with drowsiness, impaired judgment and attention, seizures, and if the abscess is large enough, contralateral hemiparesis.

In the setting of unilateral symptoms (headache) or signs (hemiparesis or cranial palsy), or evidence of elevated intracranial pressure, such as papilledema, a lumbar puncture (LP) is contraindicated because of the risk of herniation. MRI is the study of choice to identify brain abscesses and should be performed before an LP if there is risk for herniation.

Microorganisms involved in causing brain abscesses from odontogenic sources include aerobic and anaerobic streptococci and *Haemophilus* species and anaerobes *Bacteroides*, *Prevotella,* and *Fusobacterium* species.

Penicillin G covers most oral microorganisms, including both aerobic and anaerobic streptococci. Metronidazole has excellent penetration into brain abscesses and has excellent bactericidal activity against anaerobes. The combination of IV ceftriaxone or cefotaxime and IV metronidazole[3] is the preferred empiric treatment for a brain abscess from an odontogenic source. Tetracycline, erythromycin, and cefazolin do not cross the blood brain barrier effectively and should not be used for treatment of brain abscesses.

IV glucocorticoids should be added if there is significant mass effect on imaging, as seen in our patient.

Neurosurgical consultation should be pursued with the hope of aspirating the abscess to guide antimicrobial therapy and decreasing the size of the abscess.

Clinical Pearls

1. Brain abscesses can occur by direct spread or through hematogenous spread.
2. Direct spread results in a solitary abscess, whereas hematogenous spread tends to result in multiple abscesses.
3. LP should not be performed if focal signs, symptoms, or papilledema are present because of the risk of herniation.
4. MRI is the modality of choice to detect brain abscesses.
5. IV glucocorticoids should be given to patients with evidence of mass effect from a brain abscess.
6. Odontogenic brain abscesses are best treated with a combination of IV ceftriaxone and IV metronidazole.

Sinusitis

A 30-year-old man with type 1 diabetes presents to his primary care physician. He is complaining of polyuria, polydipsia, and polyphagia and has had poor blood sugar control in the past few days. His blood sugar was in the 200 to 300 mg/dL range originally but today is reading in the critical range (above 500) on his machine. In the past 24 to 48 hours he has had complaints of chills, facial swelling, headache, and purulent nasal discharge.

On physical examination the patient is febrile and appears uncomfortable, toxic, and has facial swelling and sinus pain on palpation. Quick nasal examination shows nasal ulceration with a black eschar. His blood glucose in the office is critically high.

You call 911 and have the patient transferred emergently to the ED for treatment.

You call the ED attending and ask him to administer the following antifungal as you are worried that the patient has mucormycosis:

A. IV amphotericin B
B. IV fluconazole
C. Oral ketoconazole
D. Oral posaconazole

The patient arrives to the ED and testing shows that he has a high anion gap metabolic acidosis. Antifungal therapy is started and emergent infectious disease consultation and ear, nose, and throat (ENT) consultation for debridement are obtained.

Discussion

Life-threatening rhinosinusitis and pulmonary infections are the most common presentations of mucormycoses. Infection occurs through inhalation of spores and inability to clear them. Mucor has a ketone reductase, which allows it to thrive in an acidic environment. As a consequence, a patient with diabetes and acidosis is at risk for mucormycosis.

Signs and symptoms of rhinosinusitis include fever, nasal ulceration or necrosis, periorbital or facial swelling, and headache.

Diagnosis is made by identification of organisms through histopathology, which is confirmed by culture. Endoscopic evaluation by an ENT should be performed early to look for necrosis/ulceration and to obtain tissue for histopathology.

IV amphotericin B is the first-line antifungal agent, whereas posaconazole is used as step-down therapy or in patients who do not respond or cannot tolerate amphotericin B.[4]

Correction of hyperglycemia and metabolic acidosis is critical, as is early surgical consultation for aggressive surgical debridement.

Clinical Pearls

1. Patients with diabetes and acidosis are at risk for fungal rhinosinusitis attributable to mucor.
2. Mucor has a ketone reductase, which allows it to thrive in an acidic environment.
3. IV amphotericin B is first-line treatment.
4. Posaconazole is used as step-down therapy or in amphotericin-intolerant nonresponding patients.
5. Early surgical consultation is needed for aggressive debridement and to help make the diagnosis through histopathology and culture.

Septic Thrombophlebitis

A 20-year-old previously healthy male presents to the ED with a 7-day history of fevers, sore throat, and right-sided neck pain. He has also started to have coughing and feels short of breath. He had not seen a physician for his symptoms. In the ED, he is febrile and has an erythematous pharynx with exudates. He has tenderness and swelling along the right jaw over the sternocleidomastoid muscle and has scattered rhonchi on examination.

Blood cultures are drawn and a chest radiograph demonstrates multiple nodules consistent with septic emboli. Before sending the patient for a computed tomography (CT) scan of the neck and chest, you would like to give him empiric antibiotics for what you think is Lemierre syndrome (suppurative thrombophlebitis of the jugular vein following pharyngitis).

All of the following are good first-line choices for this infection except

A. An IV carbapenem
B. IV ampicillin-sulbactam
C. IV piperacillin-tazobactam
D. IV ticarcillin-clavulanate
E. IV vancomycin

Discussion

Lemierre syndrome is a condition frequently associated with a previous pharyngeal infection. Patients tend to be young and healthy before their pharyngitis.[5] It can also be seen in the setting of an IV catheter coursing through the jugular vein.

Patients typically present with fevers, rigors, and pharyngeal erythema or exudates. Tenderness, erythema, and induration along the course of the vein can be present on examination.

In patients with an oral cause of Lemierre syndrome, the most common pathogens are anaerobic *Fusobacterium* species. Other causative organisms include *Eikenella corrodens, Porphyromonas asaccharolytica*, streptococci including *Streptococcus pyogenes*, and *Bacteroides*.

In patients with a catheter-related Lemierre syndrome, skin flora and nosocomial pathogens cause the disease.

Diagnosis can be made through blood cultures or by culture of purulent material. CT scanning of the neck may demonstrate filling defects in the internal jugular vein. CT scanning of the chest may show septic pulmonary emboli.

Fusobacterium necrophorum produces beta lactamases, so a beta lactamase–resistant antibiotic should be used when the nidus of infection is oral to begin with.

Appropriate choices include an IV carbapenem, IV ampicillin-sulbactam, IV piperacillin-tazobactam, and IV ticarcillin-clavulanate.

When the infection is caused by an intravascular catheter, IV vancomycin should be used for good skin flora coverage and the catheter should be removed.

Surgical intervention is needed if the patient does not respond to antibiotics.

Anticoagulation should be considered if the thrombus is extending.

Clinical Pearls

1. Lemierre syndrome represents suppurative jugular vein thrombosis.
2. It can be caused by an oral infection or an intravascular catheter.
3. A beta lactamase–resistant antibiotic or carbapenem is needed if the infection arises from the oral region.
4. IV vancomycin for good skin flora coverage is needed if an intravascular catheter is the nidus of the infection.
5. Surgery is indicated in case of lack of response to antibiotics.
6. Intravascular catheter removal is necessary to remove the nidus of infection.
7. Anticoagulation should be considered if the thrombus is expanding.

Upper Airway Obstruction

An 18-year-old male presents to the ED complaining of sore throat with odynophagia, difficulties clearing secretions, and fevers. He is also complaining of hoarseness. The patient is febrile and appears toxic. He has labored breathing and on quick examination has erythema in the oropharynx with tenderness in the neck, as well as pooled secretions. He has intercostal retractions and stridor. The patient is turning cyanotic and is emergently intubated by the ED physician. The ED physician does notice significant erythema in the oropharynx and inflammation and erythema of the epiglottitis.

You happen to be in the ED admitting another patient and the ED physician approaches you about the this patient, whom you have been taking care of in an outpatient setting.

You recognize the patient and tell the ED physician that his family does not believe in immunizations and the patient has not had *Haemophilus influenzae* serotype b (Hib) immunization and he has several younger siblings who have not had childhood immunizations either.

The ED physician would like your help in making antibiotic selection. There is a high incidence of community-associated methicillin-resistant *Staphylococcus aureus* (MRSA) in the area.

You ask him to administer the following antibiotics:

A. Ceftriaxone only
B. Cefotaxime only
C. Clindamycin only

D. Vancomycin only

E. Ceftriaxone and vancomycin

Discussion

Epiglottitis is inflammation of the epiglottis and surrounding structures. It can progress rapidly and cause fatal airway protection.

Symptoms of epiglottitis in adults include sore throat, odynophagia, fever, drooling, and hoarseness. Signs on physical examination include fever, stridor, pooled secretions, inflammation, and edema of the epiglottis, as well as varying degrees of upper airway obstruction. More severe disease is associated with cyanosis and intercostal retractions.

Laboratory findings include leukocytosis. Bacteremia can be detected in some cases.

Radiologic findings include a thumb sign (enlarged protruding epiglottis).

Visualizing the airway in a secure setting, such as the ED, the operating room, or ICU, is recommended and in patients with respiratory difficulties securing the airway is paramount.

Laboratory and radiographic studies should be deferred until airway patency is secured.[6]

Empiric antibiotic therapy should be directed at *Haemophilus influenzae* b, especially in patients who are not immunized, beta hemolytic streptococci, and *S aureus*, including MRSA in areas of high incidence.

Ceftriaxone or cefotaxime plus clindamycin or vancomycin depending on local resistance patterns are recommended as first-line empiric treatment.

Clinical Pearls

1. Epiglottitis is inflammation of the epiglottis and surrounding structures and can result in rapidly lethal upper airway obstruction.
2. Maintenance of an airway is the primary objective.
3. Empiric antibiotic therapy includes ceftriaxone or cefotaxime plus clindamycin or vancomycin, depending on local resistance patterns.

CHEST INFECTIONS
Pneumonia

A 76-year-old woman with recurrent chronic obstructive pulmonary disease exacerbations, requiring frequent oral steroids, presents with 2 days of cough with productive sputum, shortness of breath, chills, and fatigue. A chest radiograph shows a right lower lobe infiltrate.

Which of the following is not a clinical predictor of severity?

A. Age

B. Sex

C. Confusion

D. Tachypnea

E. Infiltrate on chest radiograph

F. All of the above are clinical predictors of severity

The patient's sputum Gram stain is positive for gram-negative bacilli. Which is the best initial antibiotic regimen?

A. Moxifloxacin

B. Ceftriaxone and azithromycin

C. Piperacillin-tazobactam and ciprofloxacin
D. Piperacillin-tazobactam and vancomycin

This patient responds rapidly to parenteral antibiotics. Further hospital management includes which of the following?

A. Counseling on smoking cessation
B. Repeat chest radiograph
C. Influenza and pneumococcal vaccines
D. Transition to oral antibiotics

Discussion

Clinical predictors of severity can help identify patients who do not need hospital admission for treatment of pneumonia. Two common prediction calculators include the Pneumonia Severity Index (PSI) and CURB 65. The PSI is calculated based on age, sex, comorbid diseases, physical examination, and laboratory and chest x-ray findings.[7] CURB65 is the pneumonic for confusion, urea (BUN) higher than 20 mg/dL (7 mmol/L), respiratory rate of 30 breaths per minute or more, blood pressure higher than 90 mm Hg systolic or higher than 60 mm Hg diastolic, and age older than 65 years. It is a simpler predictor and can be used in the absence of a urea measurement in the office setting.[8] An infiltrate on chest imaging is a diagnostic requirement for pneumonia according to guidelines from the Infectious Diseases Society of America and the American Thoracic Society (IDSA/ATS).[9] In addition, multilobar pneumonia is a risk factor for treatment failure.

Patients with gram-negative bacilli in the sputum should receive empiric treatment for *Pseudomonas aeruginosa* pneumonia. Treatment guidelines recommend coverage with 2 antipseudomonal antibiotics, which would include a combination of an antipseudomonal beta-lactam, antipseudomonal quinolone (ciprofloxacin or levofloxacin), and an aminoglycoside. The most common cause of community-acquired pneumonia remains *S pneumoniae*. Other common causes include *Mycoplasma pneumoniae*, *H influenzae*, *Chlamydia pneumoniae*, *Legionella*, and respiratory viruses, such as influenza. Community-acquired MRSA can cause a necrotizing pneumonia and empiric coverage should be considered in all patients who present with severe community-acquired pneumonia.[9]

An infiltrate on chest radiograph may take several weeks to clear. Similarly, patients may have persistent cough for several weeks following a lower respiratory tract infection. A chest radiograph should be repeated after several weeks in patients older than 50 years to document resolution of the infiltrate and screen for underlying disease or malignancy.

Parapneumonic Effusion/Empyema

A 67-year-old man presents with cough, shortness of breath, and fever. His chest radiograph shows a left lower lobe infiltrate with left-sided pleural effusion, which layers to 1.5 cm on decubitus view.

In addition to IV antibiotics for pneumonia, what is the next best step in this patient's management?

A. IV diuretics
B. Echocardiogram
C. Repeat chest radiograph in 24 to 48 hours to reassess effusion
D. Thoracentesis
E. Chest tube

For this patient, which of the following pleural fluid values is not indicative of empyema?

A. pH lower than 7.20
B. Glucose higher than 60 mg/dL
C. Pleural fluid lactate dehydrogenase (LDH)/serum LDH ratio higher than 0.6
D. Nucleated white blood cells of more than 50,000 cells/μL
E. Negative culture

Which of the following is not appropriate surgical management of loculated empyema?

A. Thoracentesis
B. Chest tube
C. Video-assisted thoracoscopic surgery (VATS)
D. Open thoracostomy

Discussion

All parapneumonic effusions that are greater than or equal to 10 mm and free flowing must be differentiated from empyema. Uncomplicated effusions are usually sterile and resolve with treatment of pneumonia. They should be followed with serial chest radiographs. Complicated parapneumonic effusions may or may not respond to antibiotics alone. Empyema should always be drained, in addition to antibiotic therapy.[10]

Although the bacterial infiltration of pleural fluid causes neutrophil invasion, decrease in pleural fluid pH, and decrease in glucose through anaerobic metabolism, bacteria may not always grow on culture. Pleural effusions with pH lower than 7.20 and glucose less than 60 mg/dL are not likely to resolve on their own and need drainage. Empyemas are associated with a high number of neutrophils, which lyse and cause elevated fluid LDH.[10]

In addition to a prolonged course of antibiotics for sterilization of the pleural space, empyemas must be completely drained.[10] Although thoracentesis can be both a diagnostic and therapeutic treatment of pleural effusion, it is ineffective in removing loculated empyemas.

Drainage options for loculated effusions include chest tube placement under ultrasound or CT guidance, VATS, and open thoracostomy. Pleural fibrosis may restrict lung reexpansion and maintain a cavity from an empyema. Decortication or pleurectomy may be needed to remove the pleural peel. Decortication can be done with thorascopy or thoracotomy.

Myocarditis

A 28-year-old man presents with 3 days of worsening dyspnea and sudden-onset sharp left-sided chest pain. On physical examination he is febrile and tachycardic. An electrocardiogram (ECG) shows diffuse P-R depression and ST elevation. An ST-segment elevation myocardial infarction (STEMI) alert is called.

What is the best initial management?

A. Tissue plasminogen activator
B. Cardiac catheterization
C. Ibuprofen
D. Methylprednisolone
E. Colchicine

Subsequent workup reveals an elevated brain natriuretic peptide and creatinine kinase MB. An echocardiogram shows a small pericardial effusion and ejection fraction of 25%.

Which is the most common cause of his presentation?

A. Ischemia
B. Viral infection
C. Bacterial infection
D. Drug hypersensitivity
E. Collagen vascular disease

Which of the following is the most definitive diagnostic test?

A. Endomyocardial biopsy
B. Radionucleotide angiography
C. Cardiac catheterization
D. Gallium scan
E. Cardiovascular magnetic resonance

Discussion

Myopericarditis can present with acute ST segment elevations, which are usually diffuse. Initial management is with nonsteroidal anti-inflammatories. Steroids may exacerbate an acute infectious process. Colchicine is helpful for recurrent pericardial effusions that can be associated with myocarditis.

Viral infection is the most common cause of myocarditis in developed countries.[11]

Endomyocardial biopsy is the gold standard for diagnosing myocarditis; however, the biopsy sample may not always include affected myocardial tissue.[12] Most patients will respond to supportive management and do not need a biopsy.[13,14] Workup for cardiomyopathy, including investigations for ischemic heart disease, collagen vascular disease, hemachromatosis, and amyloidosis, should be completed before proceeding to endomyocardial biopsy. With time, ventricular dysfunction attributable to acute myocarditis often returns to normal.[14]

Infective Endocarditis

A 78-year-old man develops fever following a dental procedure. On physical examination he has a soft holosystolic murmur at the apex. His ECG is unchanged, and chest radiograph is normal.

His initial blood cultures come back positive from both samples; however, subsequent cultures on antibiotics show no growth.

Which is the next best step in diagnosis?

A. Await speciation of blood cultures
B. CT angiogram chest
C. Transthoracic echocardiogram
D. Transesophageal echocardiogram

Which complication of infective endocarditis is from an immune-mediated process?

A. Stroke
B. Perivalvular abscess
C. Pulmonary embolism
D. Osteomyelitis
E. Glomerulonephritis

Which of the following is NOT an indication for surgery in infective endocarditis?

A. Heart failure
B. Stroke

C. Perivalvular abscess

D. A large vegetation

E. All of the above are indications for surgery

Discussion

Transthoracic echocardiogram is a noninvasive initial test of choice for investigating suspected endocarditis. Although vegetations might not be visible early in the course of the disease, a new regurgitant murmur is evidence of endocardial involvement. Totally normal valve structure and function on transthoracic echocardiogram has a very high negative predictive value for infective endocarditis.[15]

Transesophageal echocardiogram has much better resolution and is therefore better for imaging valves for vegetations and perivalvular abscesses. It is the test of choice for prosthetic valves.

Vascular phenomena associated with endocarditis include mycotic aneurysm, arterial emboli, septic pulmonary infarcts, intracranial hemorrhage, conjunctival hemorrhages, and Janeway lesions (painless erythematous macules on palms and soles). The immunologic sequelae are glomerulonephritis, Osler nodes (violaceous painful nodules in the pulp of fingers and toes), Roth spots (retinal hemorrhagic exudates), and positive rheumatoid factor. These findings, along with fever, nondiagnostic positive blood cultures, structural heart lesions, and IV drug use, make up the minor criteria for diagnosing infective endocarditis.[16,17]

American College of Cardiology/American Heart Association guidelines suggest surgical management for patients with valvular dysfunction leading to heart failure, difficult-to-treat pathogens, severe regurgitant murmurs with elevated left ventricular end-diastolic or left atrial pressures, perivalvular abscess, and embolic events. Vegetation size alone is not an indication for surgery.

Aortitis and Mycotic Aneurysm

A 69-year-old man with hypertension, diabetes, and hyperlipidemia presents with a 2-week history of fever, and abdominal and back pain associated with malaise, weakness, and weight loss after an episode of gastroenteritis. He has leukocytosis (WBC = 16,000/mL) and the laboratory reports that his blood culture is growing a gram-negative rod.

Questions:

1. What are the common clinical manifestations of aortitis caused by *Salmonella* sp, and how is it diagnosed?
2. How is *Salmonella* aortitis managed?

Discussion

Nontyphoidal *Salmonella* are an important cause of food-borne illnesses and gastroenteritis. In some patients, especially those with risk factors for atherosclerotic disease, salmonellae are able to invade the arterial intima causing endothelial infection. Consequently, aortitis can develop in these patients, which can then lead to mycotic aneurysms that can rupture. Patients often present with a subacute course of fever and abdominal or back pain. Mortality is high if the disease is unrecognized. CT scan with contrast enhancement is the diagnostic test of choice, but arteriography can also be considered. Blood cultures are usually positive (85% of patients) and stool cultures can also be positive (64% of patients).

Surgical intervention along with antimicrobial therapy is the treatment of choice. Medical therapy alone is insufficient and carries a high mortality rate (96%). Bactericidal antibiotics, such as ampicillin/gentamicin, fluoroquinolones, or third-generation cephalosporins, are recommended. Long-term suppression with antibiotics has also been suggested to improve survival.[18]

Clinical Pearls

1. Aortitis secondary to *Salmonella* should be considered in patients with subacute fever and abdominal/back pain in the setting of atherosclerotic risk factors and gastroenteritis.
2. CT scan with contrast is the imaging modality of choice.
3. Surgical intervention combined with antibiotic therapy is the treatment of choice.

INTRA-ABDOMINAL AND PELVIC INFECTIONS
Clostridium difficile Colitis

Your patient who is being treated for cellulitis develops fever, abdominal pain, and diarrhea, with tachycardia and hypotension. A dilated colon and ileus is seen on radiograph. His laboratory tests reveal an elevated WBC count of 28,000 and *Clostridium difficile* infection is suspected.

Questions
1. What are the common clinical manifestations of *C difficile*–associated diarrhea (CDAD)?
2. What is the treatment of choice for severe *C difficile* infection (CDI), and how is recurrent CDI treated?

Discussion

CDI of the colon is a common cause of antibiotic-associated diarrhea, often referred to as CDAD. CDI is often seen after recent antibiotic use, in the elderly or severely ill, in the hospitalized, and in the long-term care setting. CDI refers to a patient with diarrhea who has tested positive for the *C difficile* toxin and/or has a positive stool culture. *C difficile* colitis refers to signs of mucosal inflammation, whereas pseudomembranous colitis refers to the presence of pseudomembranes, seen on endoscopy. The term CDAD is often used to refer to all forms of *C difficile* infection that are symptomatic.

Clinical manifestations of CDI may vary, from mild symptoms, such as abdominal pain and diarrhea, to severe symptoms related to fulminant colitis with resultant fever, shock, acidosis, or ileus (which can progress to toxic megacolon or bowel perforation). Leukocytosis is often present in CDI, and a high, unexplained WBC count (higher than 15,000–20,000/mL) in hospitalized patients may be the only clue to this infection. Cytotoxin assay is the gold standard, with high sensitivity and specificity, but is costly and has a long turnaround. Enzyme immunoassay is often used for rapid screening because of its rapid turnaround (<24 hours) and high specificity, but the test has only moderate and variable sensitivity (leading to some false negatives). Clinical suspicion for CDI should play a strong role in treatment decisions.

In treating CDI, the inciting antimicrobial agent should be discontinued, if possible. Metronidazole and oral vancomycin have been the leading agents used to treat CDI, although other agents have been under development and investigation. Although there is no consensus definition for "severe" CDI, the literature has suggested that older age (>60), leukocytosis (WBC >15,000/mL), fever higher than 38.3°C, elevated creatinine, presence of pseudomembranes, or location in the ICU should all be considered. Peritoneal signs, severe ileus, or toxic megacolon should all be considered a surgical emergency requiring an urgent surgical evaluation The 2010 Infectious Disease Society of America (IDSA) guidelines suggest that, for nonsevere *C difficile* infection, metronidazole is preferred over oral vancomycin because of similar efficacy and lower cost, whereas for severe *C difficile* infection, oral vancomycin should be used as first-line treatment.[19] Treatment of the first reoccurrence is usually with the same initial regimen, but second or later reoccurrence should be with vancomycin, using a tapered or pulse regimen.

Clinical Pearls

1. Unexplained leukocytosis may be the presenting clue for *C difficile* infection.
2. Oral vancomycin should be used as the antibiotic treatment of choice for severe *C difficile* infection.
3. Treatment of reoccurrence should involved a prolonged tapered or pulse regimen.

Acute Cholangitis

Your patient presents with fever and confusion. Clinically, she has tachycardia, jaundice, and marked upper abdominal pain and tenderness. The family notes that she is scheduled for a cholecystectomy for symptomatic gallstones next week.

Questions
1. What are the common clinical manifestations of ascending cholangitis?
2. What are the treatment measures that should be considered, including antibiotic choice, biliary drainage, or surgery?

Discussion

Biliary stones often predispose a patient to biliary obstruction and stasis. These factors, in turn, can cause migration of bacteria into the biliary system, resulting in septicemia. The most common bacteria are of colonic origin with the most common gram-negative organisms being *Escherichia coli* (25%–50%), *Klebsiella* (15%–20%), and *Enterobacter* (5%–10%). *Enterococcus* (10%–20%) is the most common gram-positive organism, whereas anaerobic bacteria (*Bacteroides* or *Clostridium*) are usually present only when there is a mixed infection. The classic Charcot triad of fever, right upper quadrant pain, and jaundice is seen in about 50% of patients with acute cholangitis. The additional presence of neurologic changes and hypotension (Reynold pentad), portends a worse prognosis with significant morbidity and mortality (approximately 50%). Leukocytosis and a cholestatic pattern of liver function tests (high alkaline phosphatase, bilirubin, and gamma-glutamyl transpeptidase) are often seen. Ultrasound is the first study recommended to noninvasively look for common bile duct dilatation and stones; however, false negatives with ultrasound may occur (10%–20%) because of the presence of small stones or a delay in common bile duct dilation, so magnetic resonance cholangiopancreatography is another option. Endoscopic retrograde cholangiopancreatography (ERCP) can be used to confirm the diagnosis, as well as intervene therapeutically.

Treatment for cholangitis should begin with appropriate antibiotic coverage and then establishment of biliary drainage within 24 hours. Common antibiotic regimens include extended-spectrum beta-lactam–based therapy, including carbapenems, or third-generation cephalosporins with metronidazole. Alternative therapies include fluoroquinolones with metronidazole. ERCP has the benefit of visualizing the biliary system as well as being able to perform sphincterotomy, stone extraction, or stent insertion, and is the preferred treatment. Percutaneous drainage by interventional radiology may be considered when ERCP is not an option. Emergent surgery is often avoided, as the nonoperative options, ERCP and percutaneous drainage, have lower morbidity and mortality.[20]

Clinical Pearls:

1. Ultrasound should be considered as the first test, to noninvasively look for common bile duct dilatation and stones.

2. Coverage for cholangitis should involve broad-spectrum (gram-positive, gram-negative, anaerobic) coverage until culture results are available.
3. Biliary drainage within 24 hours is best accomplished by ERCP, with percutaneous drainage being an option.

Spontaneous Bacterial Peritonitis

Your patient with hepatitis C–induced cirrhosis presents with fever and abdominal pain. On examination, you note a distended abdomen with shifting dullness consistent with ascites, and generalized abdominal pain. A diagnostic paracentesis is performed.

Questions
1. How is spontaneous bacterial peritonitis (SBP) diagnosed?
2. What are the suggested antibiotic classes for treatment of SBP?

Discussion

SBP is commonly seen in patients with cirrhosis. It should be differentiated from secondary peritonitis, in which there is usually an evident intra-abdominal source. Common clinical manifestations include fever, diffuse abdominal pain, and altered mental status in patients with known ascites. If left untreated, ileus, shock, and multi-system organ failure can develop. Patients with signs or symptoms suggestive of infection should undergo a diagnostic paracentesis. SBP is diagnosed with a positive ascitic fluid culture and an elevated fluid polymorphonuclear neutrophil (PMN) count (>250 cells/mm^3). Empiric treatment with antibiotics is recommended as soon as possible if the cell count is elevated, as culture results may be delayed.

The most common bacteria seen in SBP are *Escherichia coli*, *Streptococcus* species, and *Klebsiella pneumoniae*. Most antibiotic regimens use a third-generation cephalosporin (eg, cefotaxime) or a fluoroquinolone. Because of resistance issues, however, if a patient has already been on a fluoroquinolone for prophylaxis, this antibiotic class should not be used for treatment.

In patients with SBP who develop renal insufficiency, the expansion of plasma volume by IV albumin has been suggested to reduce morbidity and mortality. Additionally, the incidence of SBP in patients with cirrhosis who are hospitalized for gastrointestinal bleeding is fairly high (7%–23%); therefore, empiric treatment with antibiotics is recommended.[21]

Clinical Pearls

1. Empiric therapy for SBP is suggested in the presence of fever, abdominal pain, change in mental status, and ascitic fluid PMN higher than 250 cells/mm^3.
2. Cefotaxime (or similar third-generation cephalosporin) is the treatment of choice for suspected SBP.
3. Patients with cirrhosis who have gastrointestinal bleeding should be empirically treated with antibiotics.

Secondary Peritonitis

Your patient with multiple medical problems is transferred to the hospital after developing severe, acute right lower quadrant pain. She is febrile and hypotensive with diffuse rebound abdominal tenderness. CT scan of the abdomen shows free air in the peritoneum.

Questions
1. What are the treatment considerations in an "acute abdomen" and sepsis syndrome?
2. What are the common antibiotic regimens for treatment of secondary peritonitis?

Discussion

Secondary peritonitis usually refers to an infection after a serious disease or injury of the abdominal cavity. Most patients present with rapid-onset abdominal pain, gastrointestinal dysfunction (anorexia, nausea, vomiting, obstipation), and systemic inflammatory response syndrome criteria (hypothermia/hyperthermia, tachycardia, tachypnea, and leukopenia/cytosis). Most episodes of secondary peritonitis can be related to bowel (ie, appendicitis, diverticulitis, gastric ulcer, inflammatory bowel disease) perforation or genitourinary issues (ie, perinephric abscess). CT scan is the preferred imaging modality. Untreated, peritonitis often can lead to intraperitoneal abscesses and sepsis syndrome with significant morbidity and mortality. Intra-abdominal infections are predominantly (>80%) polymicrobial, as noted in **Table 1**, and empiric broad-spectrum antibiotics should be considered.

Common antibiotic regimens that may be used empirically to treat intra-abdominal infections are listed in **Table 2**. The 2010 guidelines suggest that patients are in the "high risk" group if the following factors are met: Delay in initial intervention (>24 hours), high severity of illness (Acute Physiology and Chronic Health Evaluation score >15), advanced age, comorbid organ dysfunction, low albumin or poor nutritional status, diffuse peritonitis, presence of malignancy, or inability to achieve adequate debridement or source control. Even though initiation of antibiotics is important, definitive treatment involves surgical exploration, and in selected cases, percutaneous drainage.[20]

Clinical Pearls

1. Intra-abdominal infections are polymicrobial and broad-spectrum antibiotics should be administered as soon as possible (within 8 hours, and within 1 hour if septic shock is present).
2. Early source control improves morbidity and mortality.

Table 1
Common organisms in secondary peritonitis/abdominal abscesses

Gram Positive	Gram Negative	Anaerobes
Enterococcus sp	*Escherichia coli*	*Bacteroides* sp
Streptococcus sp	*Enterobacter* sp	*Clostridium* sp
Staphylococcus aureus	*Klebsiella* sp	*Peptostreptococcus* sp
	Proteus sp	*Fusobacterium* sp
	Pseudomonas aeruginosa	

Table 2
Empiric treatment of extrabiliary intra-abdominal infections

	Mild-Moderate Severity	High Risk or Severity
Single agents	Ertapenem, moxifloxacin, tigecycline, and ticarcillin-clavulanic	Imipenem-cilastatin, meropenem, doripenem, and piperacillin-tazobactam
Combination	Cefuroxime, ceftriaxone, cefotaxime, ciprofloxacin, or levofloxacin in combination with metronidazole	Cefepime, ceftazidime, ciprofloxacin, or levofloxacin in combination with metronidazole

URINARY TRACT INFECTIONS

A 60-year-old diabetic woman presents to the ED with urinary urgency, dysuria, and flank pain. Her symptoms started 3 days ago but have intensified over the past

24 hours. She is febrile at 101°F, and her heart rate is 100, respiratory rate 18, and blood pressure 135/80. She is moderately distressed because of pain in her flank. Examination shows tachycardia and tenderness to palpation of the costovertebral angle on the right.

1. You initially suspect acute pyelonephritis. What imaging is necessary to establish this diagnosis?
   a. Magnetic resonance imaging of the abdomen
   b. Contrast-enhanced CT of the abdomen and pelvis
   c. Abdominal radiograph
   d. Abdominal ultrasound
   e. No imaging is required
2. Emphysematous pyelonephritis is a possible complication of upper urinary tract infection. It is almost exclusively diagnosed in patients with what comorbidity?
   a. Prior urinary tract instrumentation
   b. Diabetes mellitus
   c. Endocarditis
   d. Prostatitis

Pyelonephritis is a common infection in women of all ages, with a predominance in the second and third decades of life. It most often results from ascending infection originating in the lower urinary tract. Diagnosis is largely made clinically in a patient with dysuria and flank pain. Imaging is not necessary unless to exclude obstruction or other structural abnormalities of the urinary tract.[22] Although most often readily treated with appropriate antibiotic therapy, it can progress to serious, life-threatening disease in various clinical scenarios. These include emphysematous and xanthogranulomatous pyelonephritis, and renal abscess.

Although treatment of uncomplicated cystitis does not require urine culture, 2010 IDSA guidelines highlight the importance of local resistance patterns in selecting therapy for cystitis and acute pyelonephritis. A 5-day regimen of nitrofurantoin (Macrobid) is recommended as first-line therapy for acute uncomplicated cystitis, with efficacy near 93%. Impaired renal function is a relative contraindication because of concern for increased toxicity and decreased efficacy. Use in patients with a glomerular filtration rate less than 60 is contraindicated. Pulmonary injury and severe peripheral neuropathy are among the major toxicities. Three days of trimethoprim-sulfamethoxazole (Bactrim) is an acceptable alternative if resistance of typical infecting organisms, such as E coli, is less than 20% in the area. Use of trimethoprim-sulfamethoxazole in the previous 3 months is considered a contraindication to its use for acute cystitis. To avoid development of resistance, fluoroquinolones are not recommended as first-line agents despite their efficacy. In addition, resistance of E coli to fluoroquinolones can exceed 20% in some areas.[23] Moreover, extended-spectrum beta-lactamase (ESBL)-producing E coli are increasingly common even in community settings. Effective oral therapy is limited, but fosfomycin appears to be a reasonable first-line choice.[24]

In contrast to cystitis, urine culture and sensitivity should be performed in all patients with suspected acute pyelonephritis. Further, first-line therapy in acute uncomplicated pyelonephritis is a fluoroquinolone, such as ciprofloxacin (Cipro), whether or not a patient is to be hospitalized. Initial IV therapy is recommended in patients requiring hospitalization. In every instance, if local resistance to fluoroquinolones exceeds 10%, alternative therapy should be considered, at least initially. For most patients, 1 g of ceftriaxone daily is an acceptable replacement. Once again ESBL-producing organisms are a consideration in pyelonephritis and should be treated with a carbapenem.[24] Treatment duration is related to choice of agent and ranges from 5 to 14 days.[23]

Urinary tract infections are considered complicated when associated with pregnancy, diabetes, immunosuppression, and functional or structural derangement of the genitourinary system, including presence of a urinary catheter. Infections in males are also generally considered complicated. Treatment of complicated infections requires urine culture, initial IV broad-spectrum antibiotic therapy, and 7 to 14 days of antibiotic.[24]

When symptoms of pyelonephritis fail to improve after 2 to 3 days of appropriate antibiotic therapy, development of one of the aforementioned complications should be considered. Imaging, such as CT or ultrasound, not required for most cases of acute pyelonephritis, should be performed. Dilation of the renal collecting system, discrete fluid collection, or gas in the renal parenchyma may be revealed, suggesting obstruction, abscess, or emphysematous pyelonephritis, respectively. Renal calculi are the most common source of obstruction and can contribute to any of these processes. Emphysematous pyelonephritis occurs almost exclusively in diabetic individuals (80%). Nephrolithiasis represents a significant predisposing factor, and women are afflicted 6 times as often as men.[24,25] Patients are typically quite ill and hemodynamically unstable. Mortality approaches 20% to 40%.[24] Xanthogranulomatous pyelonephritis is also strongly associated with renal calculi and is typically a chronic inflammatory and infectious process. Necrosis can lead to large abscess formation, affecting overall renal function.

In each of these complications, consideration for prompt intervention by interventional radiology or urology is indicated. Options include percutaneous nephrostomy and nephrectomy in severe cases. Broad-spectrum antibiotics are essential, pending cultures of urine, blood, and abscess fluid.[24]

Clinical Pearls

- Nitrofurantoin is IDSA recommended as first-line therapy for acute uncomplicated cystitis.
- Fosfomycin is reasonable oral therapy for uncomplicated cystitis caused by ESBL-producing organisms.
- Imaging is not necessary in most cases of acute uncomplicated pyelonephritis.
- Carbapenems are the mainstay of therapy in pyelonephritis caused by ESBL-producing organisms.
- Diabetes and renal calculi are common entities that confer substantial increased risk of serious complications from urinary tract infections.
- Emphysematous pyelonephritis, although rare, has substantial mortality and should be suspected in patients with gas in the renal parenchyma.
- Prompt urologic intervention for percutaneous drainage is indicated in cases of infection in the setting of obstruction.

SKIN AND SOFT TISSUE INFECTIONS

A 40-year-old man with diabetes presents to the ED with exquisite pain of the left forearm. He reports 2 days of increasing pain and swelling. He recalls no trauma. Examination reveals low-grade fever at 100.8°F and heart rate of 92 beats per minute. Blood pressure is 140/90 and respiratory rate is 16 breath per minute. He is in mild distress because of pain. His left arm is swollen compared with his right and is mildly erythematous at the forearm with ill-defined borders. It is very tender to palpation.

1. You suspect a soft tissue infection and are considering empiric antibiotic therapy. Were he to provide a history of salt water exposure, in addition to usual

gram-positive, gram-negative, and anaerobic coverage, you would consider which of the following?
   a. Azithromycin
   b. Doxycycline
   c. Metronidazole
   d. Vancomycin
2. You suspect necrotizing fasciitis (NF) and have ordered empiric antibiotics and blood cultures. The appropriate next step in management is
   a. Await Gram stain from blood cultures and tailor antibiotics appropriately
   b. Order soft tissue imaging with MRI and await results to guide further therapy
   c. Consult surgery for immediate evaluation and consideration of tissue exploration
   d. Culture the skin overlying the erythema
3. The role of clindamycin in initial antibiotic therapy in cases of NF suspected to be caused by *Streptococcus pyogenes* or *S aureus* is related to
   a. Anaerobic coverage
   b. Gram-negative coverage
   c. Antipseudomonal coverage
   d. Antitoxigenic effect in cases of suspected toxin-producing staphylococcal or streptococcal infection

NF describes a soft tissue infection involving the subcutaneous tissues from the skin to the underlying musculature. Although precise incidence is elusive, the Centers for Disease Control and Prevention report approximately 650 to 800 cases of NF caused by Group A Streptococcal (GAS) infection annually in the United States. This rate has remained stable over the past several years but likely underestimates true incidence, as many cases are not caused by GAS.[26] Mortality rates have fallen in recent years, but remain near 25% or greater in most series.[27] Mortality is far greater in cases with hemodynamic compromise, as in toxic shock syndrome. NF is often classified as Type I (polymicrobial), accounting for up to 80% of infections, or Type II (usually *S pyogenes*, *S aureus*, or a combination of the two). Some investigators describe a Type III, which denotes infection resulting from deep penetrating trauma and typically involves clostridial species.[28]

In any patient presenting with erythema, pain, and swelling of an extremity or of a site of recent injury, a diagnosis of NF should be considered. Several underlying diseases or conditions may predispose to necrotizing infections, including diabetes, IV drug use, peripheral vascular disease, chronic kidney disease, liver disease, and decubitus ulcers. Some inciting event or injury is present in up to 80% of cases. Exposure history is very important, as salt water, fresh water, and human and animal bites may suggest particular bacteriologic characteristics.

Examination may reveal erythema and edema with ill-defined margins. Blistering or bullae may be present and erythema may progress to bluish-gray discoloration or necrosis in a matter of 1 to 2 days. Pain is usually out of proportion to examination findings. Additionally, marked tenderness and a firm, woody feel to the subcutaneous tissues should prompt further investigation. Although imaging, including plain films, may help to identify depth of infection and gas in tissues, there is no substitute for prompt surgical exploration. If there is suspicion for NF, a small incision can be made at the bedside and a probe inserted into the wound. In the patient with NF, there will be little to no resistance of dissection down to muscle. Further, a classic "dishwater" exudate may be identified.[28,29] Gram stain of this fluid may help to tailor antibiotic therapy in the early stages of treatment, although blood cultures and tissue culture obtained at surgery are superior. If initial exploration at the bedside supports a diagnosis of NF, further debridement should occur promptly in the operating room and continued until only viable tissue remains. Patients should be reexplored in the operating room within 24 hours. Although NF usually presents and progresses rapidly, it may occur more insidiously and present first as cellulitis. Clues to development of NF and therefore indications for surgical exploration and debridement in a patient being treated for cellulitis include failure to respond to antibiotics, hemodynamic compromise, and skin necrosis or subcutaneous gas.

As aforementioned, NF may be polymicrobial or monomicrobial. Clues to polymicrobial or Type I infection include involvement of a decubitus ulcer, recent bowel surgery, infection at the injection site in IV drug users, and spread from a perineal lesion. Fournier gangrene describes such an infection of the perineum, classically in males, typically arising from a genitourinary source. Ludwig angina refers to NF in the neck and mediastinum, which typically originates from oral flora. Organisms may be numerous, with an average of 5 isolates, and typically include aerobes and anaerobes. Because of their respective locations and the marked morbidity and mortality associated with local spread, these infections can be particularly severe. In all cases of suspected Type I NF, initial antibiotic therapy should include agents directed at gram-positive bacteria, anaerobes, and enteric gram negatives. Additional therapy targeting resistant gram positives and gram negatives should also be considered (**Box 1**).

Type II infection should be suspected when disease presents in the extremities in patients with some predisposing condition or recent superficial injury. Such injuries may range from scratches to insect bites to recent varicella infection. Group A streptococcus (*S pyogenes*) and *S aureus* are the most common isolates; however, in patients with saltwater exposure, especially those with underlying liver disease or a history of alcohol abuse, *Vibrio vulnificus* should be suspected. Similarly, in patients with freshwater exposure, *Aeromonus hydrophila* should be considered. Tetracyclines are shown to be effective against both of these water-borne bacteria and should be added in patients with a suggestive history. Because of the prevalence of resistant *S aureus* species, strong consideration should be given to gram-positive coverage directed at MRSA.[5] In addition to its activity against gram-positive bacteria, clindamycin is a mainstay of therapy in both type I and type II infection because of its antitoxigenic effects.[29,30] **Box 1** presents a summary of antibiotic recommendations.

There is growing literature on the role of IV immune globulin (IVIG) in the treatment of hemodynamically unstable patients with NF.[28,30] The mechanism of action centers around antibody neutralization of exotoxins and resultant modification of the inflammatory response seen in toxic shock syndrome. It is reasonable to consider early initiation of IVIG in patients who are hypotensive with suspected staphylococcal or streptococcal infection. Hyperbaric oxygen therapy has been suggested, based on similar antitoxigenic effects and the role of high oxygen tensions in combating anaerobic organisms. True benefit to morbidity and mortality requires further study.

Clinical Pearls

- Early surgical intervention is mandatory and should not be delayed.
- Clindamycin has significant benefit not only related to its antimicrobial spectrum, but also to its antitoxigenic effects.
- Water exposure should prompt consideration of *Vibrio vulnificus* (salt water) or *Aeromonus Hydrophila* (fresh water) infection and addition of doxycycline therapy.
- IVIG may be an important tenet of therapy in patients with hemodynamic compromise or organ failure.

Box 1
Initial intravenous antibiotic selection by disease type

Type I Infections

    Piperacillin-tazobactam[a,b] (Zosyn) 3.375 g every 6 hours plus

    Clindamycin 600–900 mg every 6–8 hours plus

    Ciprofloxacin (Cipro) 400 mg every 12 hours

Type II infections

    Clindamycin 600–900 mg every 6–8 hours plus

    Vancomycin[c] 30 mg/kg/d divided into 2 doses or

    Linezolid (Zyvox) 600 mg every 12 hours

    If *Vibrio vulnificus* or *Aeromonus hydrophila* suspected, add –

    Doxycycline 1 g every 12 hours

[a] Some authorities advocate antibiotic coverage directed against MRSA in all patients. In this case, vancomycin can replace piperacillin-tazobactam.
[b] Patients who are allergic to penicillin may also be treated with vancomycin in lieu of piperacillin-tazobactam.
[c] Some authorities advocate penicillin, nafcillin, or cefazolin as first-line therapy, but current concerns favor initial coverage for MRSA.
    Data from Refs.[28–30]

A 65-year-old man with history of hypertension presents within 2 hours after suffering a fall in his garden. He had been preparing stakes for tomato plants when he fell onto the sharp point of one of the stakes. He suffered a penetrating wound to the right shoulder and complains of pain in that area. At initial examination, he is afebrile and hemodynamically stable. He has a deep wound to the right deltoid area. He is given a tetanus immunization. The wound is irrigated and sutures applied. He is discharged from the ED. One day later, he returns with erythema and edema in the area of the wound and feeling weak. He is febrile to 101.4°F with a heart rate of 110 per minute and blood pressure of 110/60 mm Hg. Blisters now overlie the area and it is very tender to palpation.

1. Given the deep penetrating wound and soil exposure, you consider which of the following organisms?
    a. *Pseudomonas aeruginosa*
    b. *Enterococcus*
    c. *Clostridium perfringens*
    d. *Escherichia coli*
2. Infection with which of the following organisms should prompt investigation for occult gastrointestinal malignancy?
    a. *Pseudomonas aeruginosa*
    b. *Clostridium septicum*
    c. *Clostridium perfringens*
    d. *Escherichia coli*

Clostridial myonecrosis is a subset of necrotizing soft tissue infections responsible for fewer than 5% of cases. Some authorities refer to is as type III NF.[27] More than half of cases can be traced to some type of deep penetrating trauma or a crush injury, whereas approximately one-third are related to surgery (usually gastrointestinal). The remainder are spontaneous.[31] Causal organisms include several clostridial species, including *perfringens, septicum, histolyticum,* and *novyi*. Predisposing conditions are similar to other causes of NF, although isolation of *C septicum*, particularly in patients without antecedent injury or surgery, should prompt investigation for colonic or hematologic malignancy, as these have been found in up to 80% of cases.[28]

Hallmarks of clostridial infection include extremely rapid progression, bullae on the skin, gas in the tissues, and early onset of hemodynamic compromise and organ failure. Hemodynamic instability is related largely to multiple toxins produced by the organism. Although classically described as gram-positive bacteria, clostridia may appear gram positive or gram negative when stained from infected tissue.[30]

Treatment is once again early surgical debridement and antibiotic therapy. First-line therapy is clindamycin (for antimicrobial and antitoxigenic effects) with the addition of penicillin, primarily because 5% of isolates are clindamycin resistant. IVIG and hyperbaric oxygen therapies are additional therapeutic modalities. Evidence for hyperbaric oxygen is stronger for clostridial species than some other bacteria because they are strict anaerobes.

Clinical Pearls

- *Clostridium* infection may be marked by extremely rapid progression of local infection (up to 2 cm/h)[28] and hemodynamic compromise.
- Gas in tissues is a diagnostic clue, although not exclusive to *Clostridium*.
- Clindamycin is a vital part of effective antibiotic therapy.
- Spontaneous infection with *C septicum* is associated with gastrointestinal or hematologic malignancy in 80% of cases.

A 24-year-old man presents several hours after suffering a wound to his right hand. He was in an altercation at a bar and suffered the wound when he punched another patron in the mouth. He reports moderate pain in the right hand. He is afebrile with stable vital signs. There are abrasions along the metacarpal phalangeal joints (MCPs) of his right hand and a 0.5-mm laceration over the third MCP. There is minor swelling and pain with active motion.

1. Which of the following represents appropriate initial management?
   a. Cleanse and suture the wound.
   b. Cleanse the wound and discharge the patient without further therapy. Tell him to return if he develops fevers or drainage from the wound.
   c. Consult general surgery to evaluate the wound.
   d. Begin empiric antibiotic therapy.

Human bite wounds may result from actual bites or from trauma involving one person's body part striking the teeth of another. Physical altercations are often involved. Common isolates include streptococci (present in 80% of cases), *S aureus, Eikenella corrodens* (10% to 29% of cases), and *Fusobacterium* species.[29,32] Typical infections include 5 or more isolates and include anaerobes in more than 60% of cases. Many anaerobic isolates are beta-lactamase producers.[29]

No matter the time interval from injury to presentation, copious irrigation and local wound disinfection should be performed on all human bite wounds. Wounds should not be sutured.[32] All patients should be assessed for appropriateness of tetanus toxoid administration. Prophylactic antibiotics are mandatory in even the most superficial wounds. For hand wounds, as in the patient described in the question, consultation with a surgeon with expertise in hand injuries should be sought. Exploration to evaluate for involvement of the joint and/or tendon is often necessary in puncture wounds.[29] Imaging, including plain films, can help uncover fractures, gas in the tissues, and osteomyelitis.

Optimal antibiotic therapy must consider the common organisms and their particular resistance patterns. Amoxicillin/clavulanate (Augmentin) is an acceptable prophylactic agent but will not cover MRSA or some of the gram-negative rods common in infected bite wounds. Patients should be reassessed with short-term follow-up. In actively infected wounds, hospital admission and IV antibiotic therapy in addition to hand surgeon consultation are appropriate.[4] In these cases, broad-spectrum antibiotic therapy, often with more than one agent, is required. IDSA guidelines, currently in revision, are noncommittal but are summarized in **Box 2**.

Animal bite wounds are more common than human bites, but tend to be less severe from an infectious disease standpoint. Dogs and cats are the most common culprits and again the wounds typically involve several microbes, including aerobes and anaerobes. *Bacteroides*, propionobacteria, and fusobacteria are common anaerobes. In 40% or more cases, staphylococci and streptococci are present. *Pasteurella* species are present in 75% and 50% of cat and dog bites respectively. Mild cases can often be treated effectively with amoxicillin-clavulanate. More severe cases require IV therapy. Typical duration of therapy is 5 to 10 days but is guided by severity.[29]

Box 2
Suggested antibiotics for infected human and animal bite wounds requiring hospitalization

Human

- Cefoxitin[a] 1 g IV every 6–8 hours OR
- Ampicillin-sulbactam[a] 1.5–3.0 g IV every 6–8 hours OR
- Moxifloxacin[b] 400 mg IV every 24 hours

Animal

- Ampicillin-sulbactam OR
- Piperacillin-tazobactam 3.375 g every 6–8 hours OR
- Meropenem 1 g every 8 hours OR
- Moxifloxacin plus clindamycin

[a] Additional therapy targeting MRSA and/or resistant *Eikenella* may include trimethoprim-sulfamethoxazole and doxycycline.
[b] Additional therapy targeting MRSA and some anaerobes may include clindamycin.
   Data from Nolan CM, Beaty HN. *Staphylococcus aureus* bacteremia. Current clinical patterns. Am J Med 1976;60(4):495.

Clinical Pearls

- Dog and cat bites commonly involve *Pasteurella* species.
- Human bites often involve *Eikenella* species, which may be resistant.
- Both bites may also include staphylococci and streptococci.
- Augmentin is often sufficient treatment for animal bites and for prophylaxis after human bites.

- Antimicrobial prophylaxis is a necessity following human bites.
- Human bites, particularly those in the hand, often require specialized surgical evaluation.
- Most human bite wounds should not be sutured early on.
- More severe infections require IV antibiotics, with careful consideration for likely resistant organisms.

SEPSIS SYNDROMES

A 32-year-old male IV drug user presents to the ED complaining of fevers and fatigue for the past 2 weeks with rapidly worsening dyspnea over the past 4 days. On arrival, the patient is in respiratory distress, with a heart rate of 100 beats per minute, and a WBC count of 14,000/μL. His chest radiograph reveals widespread round opacities. What is the most likely diagnosis?

This patient meets the definition of sepsis in this scenario: systemic inflammatory response syndrome (SIRS) with a suspected microbial etiology (right-sided endocarditis in this case given his history of IV drug use) (**Box 3**).

S aureus is the most common cause of infective endocarditis among injection drug users[33] and about a third of patients with S aureus bacteremia have infective endocarditis.[34] Septic pulmonary emboli (as demonstrated here) are common, specifically in patients with tricuspid involvement.[35]

What is the Next Step in Management?

The mortality rate for S aureus bacteremia is around 20%, with MRSA carrying a higher mortality.[36] Therefore, MRSA must be empirically treated with vancomycin, and changed to nafcillin or oxacillin if methicillin-susceptible S aureus (MSSA) is grown. Parenteral therapy is the preferred route of treatment; however, oral therapy can be used to complete a full course of therapy if IV is not an option or to provide a longer course of therapy in selected patients. Dicloxacillin and cephalexin are the preferred oral alternatives for MSSA. For MRSA, the choices include trimethoprim-sulfamethoxazole, doxycycline, and linezolid (see **Table 3**).

The emergence of S aureus with diminished vancomycin susceptibility has been fully anticipated. Vancomycin-intermediate S aureus (VISA) is defined as having a minimal inhibitory concentration (MIC) of 4 to 8 μg/mL. Vancomycin-resistant S aureus (VRSA) is defined as having a MIC higher than 16 μg/mL. In these cases, an alternative antimicrobial (eg, daptomycin, linezolid) should be chosen (**Table 3**).

Box 3
SIRS

SIRS (2 or more)

1. Temperature >38.3°C or <36°C

2. Heart rate >90 beats per minute

3. Respiratory rate >20 breaths per minute or $Paco_2$ <32 mm Hg

4. WBC >12,000 cells/mm³, <4000 cell/mm³, or >10% band forms

Data from Annane D, Bellissant E, Cavaillon JM. Septic shock. Lancet 2005;365(9453):63.

Table 3
Treatment for *Staphylococcus aureus* bacteremia

Empiric Treatment	
Vancomycin (30 mg/kg per 24 h in 2 equally divided doses)	
Continue if *S aureus* is resistant to methicillin and sensitive to vancomycin	
Prove methicillin-susceptible *S aureus*, change to nafcillin or oxacillin (2 g every 4 h)	
OR	
Cefazolin (2 g every 8 h)	
Alternative Agents	
Daptomycin (6 mg/kg once daily)	For *S aureus* bacteremia and right-sided endocarditis, monitor weekly creatine phosphokinase levels.
Linezolid (Zyvox)	Monitor for side effects (thrombocytopenia, anemia, neuropathy). Beware of resistance.
Quinupristin-dalfopristin	Requires central venous administration due to risk of severe infusion-associated phlebitis. Monitor for side effects (hyperbilirubinemia, myalgias). Beware of resistance.
Trimethoprim-sulfamethoxazole (Bactrim)	
Clindamycin (600 mg every 8 h)	D test should be performed to ensure they are D-zone negative.
Minocycline (100 mg every 12 h)	
Levofloxacin/Levaquin (500 mg daily)	

Is a Transesophageal Echocardiogram Necessary in all Patient with S aureus Bacteremia?

Not always. Transesophageal echocardiogram (TEE) may not be necessary if the following criteria are not met: (1) prolonged bacteremia longer than 4 days, (2) presence of a permanent intracardiac device, (3) hemodialysis dependency, (4) spinal infection or nonvertebral osteomyelitis.[37]

Clinical Pearls

1. About a third of patients with *S aureus* bacteremia have infective endocarditis.
2. Recognize the emergence of VISA and VRSA strains.
3. TEE is not always necessary in *S aureus* bacteremia.

A 72-year-old man on chronic hemodialysis was admitted 1 week ago to the ICU for volume overload and acute respiratory failure requiring mechanical ventilation. Over the past 2 days, the patient has become febrile to 102°F. He is now requiring vasopressors, and has developed worsening respiratory alkalosis and an oval 1-cm ecthymic lesion with a halo of erythema on his chest. What is the most likely diagnosis?

Given that this patient is hospitalized in a critical care unit, nosocomial infection is high on the differential. Manifestations of gram-negative bacilli infections include fevers/chills, disorientation, hypotension, respiratory alkalosis, and respiratory failure in 25% of cases.[38]

Pathogenesis involves release of endotoxins. Ecthyma gangrenosum (seen in this patient) results from perivascular bacterial invasion with secondary ischemic necrosis, and are more common in *P aeruginosa* infections.[39]

Infections caused by gram-negative bacilli have decreased overall; however, emergence of multidrug resistance continues to be a rising problem.[40] Risk factors include chronic comorbidities, hypoalbuminemia, organ transplantation, HIV infection, gluco-corticoid use, being elderly, recent urogenital surgery, or injury during a natural disaster involving water.

Although most gram-negative infections arise from the urinary tract, the most common source in patients in the ICU is the respiratory tract.[41] In these patients, the common species isolated include *Enterobacter* species, *K pneumoniae*, and *P aeruginosa*. *E coli* is the most common species isolated in the community.

What is the Next Step in Management?

See **Box 4** for empiric treatment of gram-negative bacteremia in immunocompetent patients; however, antibiotic resistance must be considered, as it contributes to an increase in mortality. ESBL-producing organisms (*E coli, K pneumoniae*) inactivate and confer resistance to most beta-lactam agents (including penicillins, cephalosporins, and aztreonam). There has been emergence and dissemination of new ESBLs, particularly CTX-M beta lactamases and more carbapenemases.

Should I Provide Double Coverage for P aeruginosa?

Whether to use 1 or 2 drugs for *P aeruginosa* is controversial; however, a broad-spectrum antibiotic combination is recommended for patients with severe sepsis or septic shock or when the level of resistance among the most common gram-negative pathogens in a hospital is more than 20% to 25%.[42] Vancomycin should be added if culture results are not yet available.

Definitive antibiotic therapy should be based on culture and susceptibility results; however, if the isolate is an *Enterobacter* sp, treat with cefepime or a carbapenem even if the isolate appears to be sensitive to a third-generation cephalosporin or a beta-lactam/beta-lactamase inhibitor. This is because of the high rate of resistance that may develop during treatment.

Clinical Pearls

1. Although gram-negative bacilli infections have decreased, multidrug resistance continues to cause difficulties in empiric antibiotic selection.
2. Consider combination broad-spectrum antibiotics in patients with severe sepsis or septic shock, or when the level of resistance among the most common gram-negative pathogens in a hospital is more than 20% to 25% (see **Box 5**).

Box 4
Empiric antibiotic choices for gram-negative sepsis

Immunocompetent Patients

Antipseudomonal cephalosporin (ceftazidime 2 g every 8 hours or cefepime 2 g every 12 hours)

OR

Beta-lactam/beta-lactamase inhibitor (piperacillin-tazobactam/Zosyn 4.5 g every 6 hours, ticarcillin-clavulanate/Timentin 3.1 g every 4 hours)

OR

Carbapenem (eg, imipenem 500 mg every 6 hours, meropenem 1 g every 8 hours, doripenem 500 mg every 8 hours, or ertapenem 1 g once daily)

If patient grows a multiresistant gram-negative bacteria not susceptible to the above agents, consider Colistin (100–200 mg every 8–12 hours).

> **Box 5**
> **Combination broad-spectrum therapy for antibiotic regimens**
>
> Amikacin (7.5 mg/kg every 12 hours) PLUS 1 of the following:
>
> Antipseudomonal cephalosporin (eg, cefepime 2 g every 12 hours or ceftazidime 2 g every 8 hours)
>
> OR
>
> Antipseudomonal beta-lactam/beta-lactamase inhibitor (piperacillin-tazobactam 4.5 g every 6 hours or ticarcillin-clavulanate 3.1 g every 4 hours)
>
> OR
>
> Carbapenem (eg, imipenem 500 mg every 6 hours or meropenem 1 g every 8 hours, or Doripenem 500 mg every 8 hours)

A 36-year-old previously healthy woman presents to the ED complaining of severe lethargy and fevers. Per family, the patient developed a diffuse red rash followed by some sloughing of the palms and soles. She had a recent motor vehicle accident resulting in some lacerations along her arms and legs. On arrival to the ED, she requires intubation because of acute respiratory failure. Blood pressure is 90/60 mm Hg. She is found to have a profound transaminitis as well as acute renal failure.

What is the Most Likely Diagnosis?

Toxic shock syndrome (TSS) can be caused by either *S aureus* or group A streptococcus (GAS). Staphylococcal toxic shock must be considered in association with recent surgery, any localized staphylococcal abscess, osteomyelitis, or respiratory infection following influenza. *S aureus* strains that produce exotoxins result in 3 syndromes: food poisoning resulting from ingestion of *S aureus* enterotoxin, scalded skin syndrome (caused by exfoliative toxin), and toxic shock syndrome, caused by toxic shock syndrome toxin-1.

Severe invasive GAS infections can manifest as bacteremia, pneumonia, or necrotizing fasciitis. Toxins activate the immune system, resulting in a release of large quantities of inflammatory cytokines causing capillary leak and tissue damage, which leads to shock and multiorgan failure. Risk factors for developing TSS include minor trauma, surgical procedures, use of tampons, viral infections (varicella, influenza), and the prior use of NSAIDs.[43]

How is the Diagnosis Made?

Diagnosis of TSS is made clinically (see **Box 6**).[44,45]

What is the Next Step of Management?

Management includes hemodynamic support, aggressive surgical debridement, and empiric antibiotics (which includes clindamycin to inhibit toxin production).

- Initial empiric antibiotics should include clindamycin (900 mg IV every 8 hours) PLUS a carbapenem OR a penicillin plus beta-lactamase inhibitor combination drug (ticarcillin- clavulanate or piperacillin-tazobactam) PLUS vancomycin.
- Once microbiologic diagnosis is established, antibiotics can be tailored to include clindamycin (900 mg IV every 8 hours) PLUS vancomycin/linezolid for *S aureus* OR penicillin G for GAS.
- IVIG may be considered in severe cases.

> **Box 6**
> **Clinical criteria for the diagnosis of TSS**
>
> *Clinical criteria for staphylococcal TSS:*
>
> Fever (temperature >38.9°C)
>
> PLUS
>
> Hypotension
>
> PLUS
>
> Diffuse macular erythroderma ± desquamation
>
> PLUS
>
> Multisystem involvement (3 or more of the following: gastrointestinal, muscular, mucous membranes, renal hepatic, or hematologic, CNS)
>
> *Clinical criteria for diagnosis of GAS TSS:*
>
> Isolation of GAS from a normally sterile site
>
> PLUS
>
> Hypotension
>
> PLUS
>
> Two or more of the following: renal impairment, coagulopathy, liver involvement, adult respiratory distress syndrome, erythematous macular rash (which may desquamate) or soft tissue necrosis.

Clinical Pearls

1. In a patient with a local wound or other risk factors discussed previously with fever, hypotension, and skin manifestations, consider TSS.
2. Clindamycin is useful in mitigating toxin effects.
3. IVIG may have some role in severe cases.

A 24-year-old man with a history of sickle cell disease sees his primary care physician for headache and purulent nasal drainage. He is diagnosed with acute bacterial sinusitis and given a course of amoxicillin. Three days later, he presents to a local ED complaining of intractable rigors, disorientation, and a sudden rise in temperature to 102.6°F. He is found to be hypotensive on arrival. What is the most likely diagnosis?

The spleen filters blood through a series of capillaries. Mononuclear phagocytes within this system ingest circulating bacteria and process foreign material to stimulate the production of opsonizing antibody, which is imperative in clearing encapsulated organisms.

Asplenic patients (such as patients with sickle cell disease) are at increased risk for postsplenectomy sepsis (PSS). PSS is a fulminant and rapidly fatal complication of bacteremic infections caused by encapsulated organisms such as *S pneumoniae*, *N meningitidis*, and *H influenzae*. They are also at risk for parasitic infections, such as malaria and babesiosis. In a review of 349 episodes of sepsis in patients with anatomic or functional asplenia, *S pneumoniae* accounted for 57% of infections and 59% of deaths.[46]

How do These Patients Typically Present?

PSS may follow minor upper or lower respiratory tract symptoms; however, it can develop rather precipitously, presenting with complications of high-grade bacteremia with petechiae, purpura, meningitis, and hypotension.

Laboratory results reveal an elevated or markedly depressed WBC count with a marked left shift and bandemia. Earlier myeloid forms with toxic granulations and Dohle bodies can also be seen. Howell-Jolly bodies may be present, revealing evidence of asplenia. Other findings may include thrombocytopenia and DIC, along with evidence of multiorgan dysfunction. Spinal fluid may not have significant abnormalities during the early course; however, culture may be positive. Chest radiography may reveal cardiomegaly and a primary pneumonitis. Blood cultures often turn positive within hours of inoculation.

Is Antigen Testing Helpful to me?

The pneumococcal antigen test is a rapid immunochromatographic membrane assay that detects the presence of capsular polysaccharide common to all serotypes of S pneumoniae. The test is approved for the diagnosis of invasive pneumococcal disease using urine samples and, because most patients with pneumococcal meningitis are also bacteremic, it can also be used for the diagnosis of pneumococcal meningitis (by testing CSF or urine). Its sensitivity is 75%, whereas its specificity nears 95% compared with traditional microbiology.[47]

What is the Next Step in Management?

Appropriate broad-spectrum antibiotic therapy and supportive measures (including mechanical ventilation) must be rapidly instituted. Patients tend to have minimal response to fluid resuscitation, therefore inotropic agents are generally necessary (**Table 4**).

Splenectomy or asplenia was a risk factor for penicillin nonsusceptibility of S pneumoniae in a prospective international observational study of 844 patients with pneumococcal bacteremia.[48,49]

Even with appropriate antimicrobial treatment, pneumococcal meningitis has a mortality rate of 20% to 30%.

Clinical Pearls

1. Asplenic patients are at increased risk for PSS.
2. The pneumococcal antigen test in urine is a highly specific diagnostic test, and useful for the diagnosis of invasive pneumococcal disease.
3. Always consider penicillin-resistant pneumococcal infections and beta-lactamase producing H influenzae when choosing initial empiric therapy in patients who are postsplenectomy/asplenic.

Table 4 Empiric therapy for postsplenectomy sepsis	
Initial Empiric Therapy	**If Meningitis is Suspected**
Vancomycin 1 g IV every 12 h	Vancomycin 30–60 mg/kg IV/d in divided doses
PLUS	PLUS
Ceftriaxone (2 g IV daily)[a]	Ceftriaxone (2 g IV twice daily) Dexamethasone - in patients with suspected pneumococcal meningitis (15–20 min before or at the time of first dose of antibiotic administration).

Abbreviation: IV, intravenous.
[a] If patient has a beta-lactam allergy, may substitute levofloxacin 750 mg for ceftriaxone.

REFERENCES

1. Thigpen MC, Whitney CG, Messonnier NE. Bacterial meningitis in the United States, 1998–2007. N Engl J Med 2011;364(21):2016.
2. Misra UK, Kalita J. Neurophysiological studies in herpes simplex encephalitis. Electromyogr Clin Neurophysiol 1998;38(3):177.
3. Jansson AK, Enblad P, Sjölin J. Efficacy and safety of cefotaxime in combination with metronidazole for empirical treatment of brain abscess in clinical practice. Eur J Clin Microbiol Infect Dis 2004;23(1):7.
4. van Burik JA, Hare RS, Solomon HF, et al. Posaconazole is effective as salvage therapy in zygomycosis: a retrospective summary of 91 cases. Clin Infect Dis 2006;42(7):e61.
5. Riordan T, Wilson M. Lemierre's syndrome: more than a historical curiosa. Postgrad Med J 2004;80(944):328.
6. Glynn F, Fenton JE. Diagnosis and management of supraglottitis (epiglottitis). Curr Infect Dis Rep 2008;10(3):200.
7. Fine MJ, Auble TE, Yealy DM, et al. A prediction rule to identify low-risk patients with community-acquired pneumonia. N Engl J Med 1997;336(4):243.
8. Lim WS, Van der Eerden MM, Laing R, et al. Defining community acquired pneumonia severity on presentation to hospital: an international derivation and validation study. Thorax 2003;58(5):377.
9. Mandell LA, Wunderink RG, Anzueto A, et al, Infectious Diseases Society of America, American Thoracic Society. Infectious Diseases Society of America/American Thoracic Society consensus guidelines on the management of community-acquired pneumonia in adults. Clin Infect Dis 2007;44(Suppl 2):S27.
10. Colice GL, Curtis A, Deslauriers J, et al. Medical and surgical treatment of parapneumonic effusions: an evidence-based guideline. Chest 2000;118(4):1158.
11. Mahrholdt H, Wagner A, Deluigi CC, et al. Presentation, patterns of myocardial damage, and clinical course of viral myocarditis. Circulation 2006;114(15):1581.
12. Aretz HT, Billingham ME, Edwards WD, et al. Myocarditis. A histopathologic definition and classification. Am J Cardiovasc Pathol 1987;1(1):3.
13. McCarthy RE 3rd, Boehmer JP, Hruban RH, et al. Long-term outcome of fulminant myocarditis as compared with acute (nonfulminant) myocarditis. N Engl J Med 2000;342(10):690.
14. Cooper LT, Baughman KL, Feldman AM, et al. The role of endomyocardial biopsy in the management of cardiovascular disease: a scientific statement from the American Heart Association, the American College of Cardiology, and the European Society of Cardiology. Circulation 2007;116(19):2216.
15. Irani WN, Grayburn PA, Afridi I. A negative transthoracic echocardiogram obviates the need for transesophageal echocardiography in patients with suspected native valve active infective endocarditis. Am J Cardiol 1996;78(1):101.
16. Baddour LM, Wilson WR, Bayer AS, et al. Infective endocarditis: diagnosis, antimicrobial therapy, and management of complications: a statement for healthcare professionals from the Committee on Rheumatic Fever, Endocarditis, and Kawasaki Disease, Council on Cardiovascular Disease in the Young, and the Councils on Clinical Cardiology, Stroke, and Cardiovascular Surgery and Anesthesia, American Heart Association: endorsed by the Infectious Diseases Society of America. Circulation 2005;111(23):e394.
17. Bonow RO, Carabello BA, Chatterjee K, et al. ACC/AHA 2006 guidelines for the management of patients with valvular heart disease: a report of the American

College of Cardiology/American Heart Association Task Force on Practice Guidelines (writing Committee to Revise the 1998 guidelines for the management of patients with valvular heart disease) developed in collaboration with the Society of Cardiovascular Anesthesiologists endorsed by the Society for Cardiovascular Angiography and Interventions and the Society of Thoracic Surgeons. J Am Coll Cardiol 2006;48(3):e1.

18. Soravia-Dunand VA, Loo VG, Salit IE. Aortitis due to Salmonella: report of 10 cases and comprehensive review of the literature. Clin Infect Dis 1999;29: 862–8.

19. Cohen SH, Gerding DN, Johnson S, et al. Clinical practice guidelines for *Clostridium difficile* infection in adults: 2010 update by the Society of Healthcare Epidemiology of America (SHEA) and the Infectious Disease Society of America (IDSA). Infect Control Hosp Epidemiol 2010;31(No 5):431–55.

20. Solomkin JS, Mazuski JE, Bradley JS, et al. Diagnosis and management of complicated intra-abdominal infection in adults and children: guidelines by the Surgical Infection Society and the Infectious Diseases Society of America. Clin Infect Dis 2010;50:133–64.

21. Runyon BA, AASLD Practice Guidelines Committee. Management of adult patients with ascites due to cirrhosis: an update. Hepatology 2009;49(6):2087–107.

22. Colgan R, Williams M. Diagnosis and treatment of acute pyelonephritis in women. Am Fam Physician 2011;84(5):519–26.

23. Gupta K, Hooton T, Naber K, et al, Infectious Disease Society of America. International clinical practice guidelines for the treatment of acute uncomplicated cystitis and pyelonephritis in women: a 2010 update by the Infectious Diseases Society of America and the European Society for Microbiology and Infectious Diseases. Clin Infect Dis 2011;52(5):e103–20.

24. Lane DR, Takhar SS. Diagnosis and management of urinary tract infection and pyelonephritis. Emerg Med Clin North Am 2011;29(3):539–52.

25. Ubee SS, McGlynn L, Fordham M. Emphysematous pyelonephritis. BJU Int 2011; 107(9):1474–8.

26. Available at: http://www.cdc.gov/features/NecrotizingFasciitis/. Accessed August 11, 2012.

27. Available at: http://www.cdc.gov/ncidod/dbmd/diseaseinfo/groupastreptococcal_g. htm How common is invasive. Accessed August 11, 2012.

28. Uslin JS, Malangoni MA. Necrotizing soft-tissue infections. Crit Care Med 2011; 39(9):2156–62.

29. Stevens DL, Bisno AL, Chambers HF, et al, Infectious Disease Society of America. Practice guidelines for the diagnosis and management of skin and soft-tissue infections. Clin Infect Dis 2005;41(10):1373–406.

30. Ahmed MS, Khardori NM. Spreading soft tissue infection. In: Khardori NM, Wattal C, editors. Emergencies in infectious diseases from head to toe. Delhi (India): Byword Books; 2010. p. 215–38.

31. Abella BS, Kuchinic P, Hiraoka T, et al. Atraumatic clostridial myonecrosis: a case report and literature review. J Emerg Med 2003;24(4):401–5.

32. Clark DC. Common acute hand infections. Am Fam Physician 2003;68(11): 2167–76.

33. Matthew J, Addai T, Anand A, et al. Clinical features, site of involvement, bacteriologic findings, and outcome of infective endocarditis in intravenous drug users. Arch Intern Med 1995;155(15):1641.

34. Abraham J, Mansour C, Veledar E, et al. *Staphylococcus aureus* bacteremia and endocarditis: the Grady Memorial Hospital experience with methicillin-sensitive

S aureus and methicillin-resistant *S aureus* bacteremia. Am Heart J 2004;147(3): 536.

35. Steckelberg JM, Murphy JG, Ballard D, et al. Emboli in infective endocarditis: the prognostic value of echocardiography. Ann Intern Med 1991;114(8):635.

36. Nolan CM, Beaty HN. *Staphylococcus aureus* bacteremia. Current clinical patterns. Am J Med 1976;60(4):495.

37. Kaasch AJ, Fowler VG Jr, Rieg S, et al. Use of a simple criteria set for guiding echocardiography in nosocomial *Staphylococcus aureus* bacteremia. Clin Infect Dis 2011;53(1):1.

38. Kang CL, Kim SH, Park WB, et al. Bloodstream infections caused by antibiotic-resistant gram-negative bacilli: risk factors for mortality and impact of inappropriate initial antimicrobial therapy on outcome. Antimicrob Agents Chemother 2005;49(2):760.

39. Roberts R, Tarpay MM, Marks ML, et al. Erysipelaslike lesions and hyperesthesia as manifestations of *Pseudomonas aeruginosa* sepsis. JAMA 1982;248(17):2156.

40. Suarez CJ, Lolans K, Villegas MV, et al. Mechanisms of resistance to beta-lactams in some common gram-negative bacteria causing nosocomial infections. Expert Rev Anti Infect Ther 2005;3(6):915.

41. Sligl W, Taylor G, Brindley PG. Five years of nosocomial gram-negative bacteremia in a general intensive care unit: epidemiology, antimicrobial susceptibility patterns, and outcomes. Int J Infect Dis 2006;10(4):320.

42. Micek ST, Lloyd AE, Ritchie DJ, et al. *Pseudomonas aeruginosa* bloodstream infection: importance of appropriate initial antimicrobial treatment. Antimicrob Agents Chemother 2005;49(4):1306.

43. Stevens DL, Tanner MH, Winship J, et al. Severe group A streptococcal infections associated with a toxic shock-like syndrome and scarlet fever toxin A. N Engl J Med 1989;321(1):1.

44. Case definitions for infectious conditions under public health surveillance. Centers for Disease Control and Prevention. MMWR Morb Mortal Wkly Rep 1997;46(RR–10):39.

45. Defining the group A streptococcal toxic shock syndrome. Rationale and consensus definition. The Working Group on Severe Streptococcal Infections. JAMA 1993;269(3):390.

46. Holdsworth RJ, Irving AD, Cuschieri A. Postsplenectomy sepsis and its mortality rate: actual versus perceived risks. Br J Surg 1991;78(9):1031.

47. Boulware DR, Daley CL, Merrifield C, et al. Rapid diagnosis of pneumococcal pneumonia among HIV-infected adults with urine antigen detection. J Infect 2007;55:300–9.

48. Yu VL, Chiou CC, Feldman C, et al. An international prospective study of pneumococcal bacteremia: correlation with in vitro resistance, antibiotics administered, and clinical outcome. Clin Infect Dis 2003;37(2):230.

49. Aronin SI, Peduzzi P, Quagliarello VJ. Community-acquired bacterial meningitis: risk stratification for adverse clinical outcome and effect of antibiotic timing. Ann Intern Med 1998;129(11):862.

Role of Molecular Diagnostics in the Management of Infectious Disease Emergencies

Neel K. Krishna, PhD[a,b,*], Kenji M. Cunnion, MD, MPH[a,b,c]

KEYWORDS

- Real-time polymerase chain reaction • Molecular diagnosis • Infectious disease
- Microbiology • Normal vs immune compromised

KEY POINTS

- Clinical laboratories have traditionally relied on time-consuming phenotypic methods such as culture, serology, and biochemical tests for detection, identification, and characterization of microbial pathogens.
- Real-time polymerase chain reaction (PCR) technology is now available to identify many of the pathogenic organisms that constitute infectious disease emergencies in normal and immune-compromised hosts.
- Use of this molecular technology for the accurate diagnosis of infectious disease agents by clinical laboratories reduces the time to diagnosis for many pathogens.

INTRODUCTION

The role of molecular diagnostic tests in the evaluation of infectious etiology is rapidly evolving, with new tests becoming available each year.[1] This article discusses the various real-time polymerase chain reaction (PCR)-based assays and antigen detection assays currently available for use in emergency settings for making a specific microbiological diagnosis. Serologic assays, cultures, and stains are not covered in this article.

In the emergency setting, molecular diagnostic methods yield several advantages over serologic methods. Molecular methods directly assay for the presence of the microorganism at the time the specimen is obtained, which is ideal for the acutely ill patient. Serologic methods assay for an antibody response to the microorganism,

Funding sources: The authors have nothing to disclose.

Conflict of interest: The authors have nothing to disclose.

[a] Department of Microbiology and Molecular Cell Biology, Eastern Virginia Medical School, 700 West Olney Road, Norfolk, VA 23507, USA; [b] Department of Pediatrics, Eastern Virginia Medical School, 855 West Brambleton Avenue, Norfolk, VA 23510, USA; [c] Division of Infectious Diseases, Children's Specialty Group, 601 Children's Lane, Norfolk, VA 23507, USA

* Corresponding author. Department of Microbiology and Molecular Cell Biology, Eastern Virginia Medical School, 700 West Olney Road, Norfolk, VA 23507.

E-mail address: krishnnk@evms.edu

Med Clin N Am 96 (2012) 1067–1078

http://dx.doi.org/10.1016/j.mcna.2012.08.005

0025-7125/12/$ – see front matter © 2012 Elsevier Inc. All rights reserved.

typically requiring at least a week of symptoms even for immunoglobulin M tests. Immune-compromised and immune-suppressed patients frequently will not mount an appropriate antibody response. Thus for serologic assays, evaluation of the patient early in the course of the disease or testing a patient with immune dysregulation will often yield false-negative results. Patients who have been treated with intravenous immunoglobulin in the preceding year will typically have immunoglobulin G present against a wide array of infectious agents that they have never seen, which can lead to false-positive serologic tests. Optimal serologic evaluation typically requires retesting at 4 to 6 weeks after infection (ie, convalescent titers) to demonstrate an increase in titer associated temporally with the recent illness, further delaying a definitive diagnosis.

Molecular methods can also provide a more rapid diagnosis of etiology than is possible with culture, with results available within hours if the assay can be performed locally. Many infectious agents cannot be grown by standard culture methodologies (eg, *Mycoplasma pneumoniae*) or are fastidious (eg, *Bordetella pertussis*), leading to frequent false-negative results. Other organisms grow very slowly (eg, *Mycobacterium tuberculosis*) such that culture results are not available for weeks. Most clinical microbiology laboratories cannot afford to offer virology services owing to the high expense of performing tissue culture because it is labor intensive, requiring highly skilled laboratory personnel and the purchase of tissue culture cell lines every week that may not be used. Even when available, virus culture typically requires 3 to 10 days for results, depending on the particular virus. However, for the vast majority of bacterial pathogens culture still remains the gold standard of diagnosis, typically yielding a microbiological diagnosis in 1 to 3 days followed by antibiotic susceptibility results. Molecular methods to assay for resistance genes are being developed for some organisms, but are generally not available at this time.

The sections of this article have been organized by organ systems most likely to be affected in emergency settings, designed such that the clinician evaluating a patient with severe acute illness can reference the most relevant molecular diagnostics available pertinent to the predominant organ system involved. There is considerable overlap for the various tests among the organ systems, and some tests will be present under multiple organ systems headings. Each section is further divided between diagnostics most appropriate for normal hosts, then additional diagnostics pertinent to immune-compromised hosts. Thus, diagnostics for the normal host will usually also be relevant to immune-compromised hosts. Before addressing infections of the various organs systems, a brief overview is provided of the principle behind the most common molecular assay currently in use in diagnostic laboratories for pathogen detection, real-time PCR. Antigen tests for specific organisms are addressed as they appear.

REAL-TIME PCR

While a variety of molecular methods exist in diagnostic microbiology, PCR is by far the most universal methodology used for pathogen detection.[2] In recent years real-time PCR, also known as quantitative PCR (qPCR), has become the "go-to" technique in the clinical laboratory (reviewed in Ref.[1]). In contrast to conventional PCR, which simply amplifies a targeted DNA molecule, real-time PCR can detect, amplify, and quantify a targeted DNA molecule in real time. In real-time PCR, fluorescent dyes are used to label PCR products during thermal cycling. Real-time PCR instruments then measure the accumulation of fluorescent signal during the exponential phase of the reaction for rapid and precise quantitation of PCR products. Quantitation can yield absolute numbers of copies of a given sequence or a relative amount when standardized to a known amount of DNA. Clinically this is particularly useful, for example, in determining viral load from plasma or serum of an individual infected with human immunodeficiency virus (HIV).[3] Fluorescence-based diagnostic real-time PCR assays are now available in-house as well as commercially (approved by the Food and Drug Administration [FDA]) for many human pathogens (reviewed in Ref.[1]). By virtue of its ability to simultaneously detect and quantify in a sealed PCR plate with no post-PCR processing steps, real-time PCR lends itself to automation and rapid turnaround time while reducing human error. In addition, multiplex real-time PCR assays on the same automated instrument to simultaneously detect and screen for a variety of pathogens are currently under development and are expected in time to replace stand-alone assays for specific pathogens.[4] Despite these exciting possibilities, the cost of such multiplex instrumentation is a significant limitation for many smaller clinical laboratories. This review focuses on the individual real-time PCR assays that are currently widely available in the diagnosis of infectious disease emergencies.

In the following sections, pathogenic organisms that affect each major organ system (Central Nervous System, Pulmonary, Cardiac, Gastrointestinal, and Bloodstream/Systematic) are accompanied by a table listing the following information: host (normal or compromised), microorganism (viral, bacterial, fungal, or parasitic), method of detection (antigen or real-time PCR), specimen type, and representative commercial test from national reference laboratories, Mayo Medical Laboratories (http://www.mayomedicallaboratories.com) and Quest Diagnostics (www.questdiagnostics.com). Regarding the nomenclature of the PCR methodology, PCR as denoted in the tables refers to real-time PCR. qPCR refers to real-time PCR that is truly quantitative. The authors have purposely avoided using the term RT-PCR, as this can refer to real-time PCR or reverse-transcriptase PCR in the literature (real-time, reverse-transcriptase PCR is used for viruses containing a plus-sense or minus-sense RNA genome [influenza virus, West Nile virus, and so forth]).

CENTRAL NERVOUS SYSTEM (MENINGITIS AND ENCEPHALITIS)
Clinical Perspective and Molecular Diagnosis

This section focuses on molecular diagnostics pertinent in the evaluation of infectious causes of encephalitis and meningitis (**Table 1**). Bacterial meningitis remains the most dangerous and treatable form, such that cerebral spinal fluid (CSF) should always be tested for bacterial culture.[5] These molecular diagnostic tests will be most informative for testing CSF to identify the presence of genetic or antigenic material of microorganisms. However, if CSF cannot be obtained, many of these tests can also be performed on blood. For meningoencephalitis in the normal host, herpes simplex virus (HSV)[6] and enterovirus[7] testing have become routine tests on CSF in many centers. Bacterial antigen testing has been available for decades, but the accuracy of this test remains poor, resulting in limited clinical utility. Molecular diagnostic tests are unlikely to yield an origin in the setting of postinfectious encephalitis because the inciting microorganism is no longer present.

Molecular diagnostic tests likely have their greatest utility for immune-compromised hosts with central nervous system infection because of the ability to make an accurate diagnosis via lumbar puncture. This clinical setting is an exceptionally challenging one whereby there are many microbial pathogens that can cause similar-appearing disease, and the need for a rapid diagnosis is urgent. Many of these diagnostics have become available fairly recently, aiding the diagnostician in meeting these challenges.

Table 1
Molecular diagnostics for central nervous system infections: encephalitis and meningitis

Normal Host	Microorganism	Methods	Specimens	Diagnostic Test
	HSV	PCR	CSF, other	MAYO: VDER
	Enterovirus	PCR	CSF, blood, other	MAYO: LENT
	West Nile virus	PCR	CSF, blood	MAYO: WNVP
	Treponema pallidum	PCR	CSF, blood, other	QUEST: 87798
	Mycoplasma pneumoniae	PCR	CSF, other	QUEST: 87581
	Bacterial meningitis	Antigens	CSF, blood, urine	Becton Dickinson: Directigen
Compromised	EBV	qPCR	CSF	MAYO: QEBV
	CMV	qPCR	CSF, other	MAYO: QCMV
	Cryptococcus neoformans	Antigen	CSF, blood	MAYO: CCRYR/SCRYP
	Toxoplasma gondii	PCR	CSF, blood	MAYO: PTOX
	JC virus	PCR	CSF, blood, urine	MAYO: LCJC
	HHV 6	PCR	CSF, blood, other	MAYO: HHV6V

Abbreviations: CMV, cytomegalovirus; EBV, Epstein-Barr virus; HHV 6, human herpesvirus 6; HSV, herpes simplex virus; MAYO, Mayo Medical laboratories test identifier; QUEST, Quest Diagnostics test identifier.

As illustrated in **Table 1**, real-time PCR tests are commercially available for many of the listed viruses and bacteria. Unfortunately, in the case of bacterial meningitis molecular techniques to identify the etiologic agent are currently lacking. In the absence of reliable CSF cultures (eg, antibiotic therapy before lumbar puncture), identification of suspected pathogens has traditionally depended on the use of assays such as the latex agglutination or related immunochromatographic membrane assays for the direct qualitative detection of antigens to common bacterial pathogens causing meningitis (eg, *Haemophilus influenzae* B, *Neisseria meningitides*, Group B *Streptococcus, Escherichia coli*, and *Streptococcus pneumoniae*). In the latex agglutination assay, for example, specific antibodies are bound to the surface of the latex particles on a slide. On addition of the specimen, visible agglutination occurs when the specimen containing any of these bacterial antigens reacts with its respective antibody-coated latex bead. As this assay is completely dependent on accumulation of polysaccharide antigen in the specimen, many false negatives can occur and sensitivity remains a critical issue. In addition, antigen in the sample can come from organism colonization of mucosal surfaces, leading to false-positive results.[8]

For the immune-compromised category, a quantitative assay for Epstein-Barr virus (EBV) and cytomegalovirus (CMV) exists and is in extensive use. The quantitative assay for these pathogens and HIV are discussed in the Bloodstream and Systemic Infections section. For *Cryptococcus neoformans*, identification in CSF relies on antigen identification through latex agglutination assay or enzyme immunosorbent assays; however, as opposed to bacterial antigen testing, the cryptococcal antigen test has proved itself to be very accurate and reliable.[9,10] For the other pathogens listed here, qualitative real-time PCR assays exist to identify these pathogens in CSF and blood.

PULMONARY (PNEUMONIA)
Clinical Perspective and Molecular Diagnosis

The diagnostic tests in this section focus on the evaluation of pneumonia (**Table 2**). A variety of rapid influenza diagnostic tests (RIDTs) have been available for several

Table 2
Molecular diagnostics for pulmonary infections: pneumonia and pneumonitis

Normal Host	Microorganism	Methods	Specimens	Diagnostic Test
	Influenza A, B	Antigen, PCR	Swab	MAYO: 800167
	RSV	Antigen, PCR	Swab	MAYO: RSVP
	Parainfluenza 1,2,3	PCR	Swab	QUEST: 87798 (×3)
	Adenovirus	PCR	Swab, other	MAYO: LADV
	Human metapneumovirus	PCR	Swab	QUEST: 87798
	Rhinovirus	PCR	Swab	QUEST: 87798
	Mycobacterium tuberculosis	PCR	Sputum, BAL, other	MAYO: MTBRP
	Mycoplasma pneumoniae	PCR	Swab, sputum, other	QUEST: 87581
	Chlamydophila pneumoniae	PCR	Swab, sputum, BAL	QUEST: 87486
	Legionella pneumophila	PCR	Swab, sputum, BAL	MAYO: LEGRP
	Bordetella pertussis	PCR	Swab	MAYO: BPRP
	Histoplasma capsulatum	Antigen, PCR	Urine, blood, BAL	MAYO: HBRPB
Compromised	*Pneumocystis jirovecii*	PCR	BAL, sputum	MAYO: PNRP
	Aspergillus spp	Antigen	Blood	MAYO: ASPBA
	Aspergillus spp	PCR	BAL, sputum, blood	QUEST: 87798 (×3)
	CMV	PCR	BAL, blood, other	MAYO: QCMV
	Adenovirus	PCR	BAL, sputum, blood	MAYO: LADV

Abbreviations: BAL, bronchoalveolar lavage; CMV, cytomegalovirus; MAYO, Mayo Medical laboratories test identifier; QUEST, Quest Diagnostics test identifier; RSV, respiratory syncytial virus.

years, providing a very useful tool in the emergency, urgent care, and outpatient settings for detection of influenza virus A and B.[11] The RIDTs are immunoassays that identify the presence of influenza A or B nucleoprotein antigens from clinical specimens in a qualitative fashion. These tests are popular in that they can provide a result within 15 minutes or less, and many such commercially available tests are approved for office/bedside use. Disadvantages of the test include suboptimal test sensitivity, resulting in false negative results, especially in periods when influenza activity is high. In addition, although specificity is high, false-positive results may also occur when influenza activity, and therefore pretest probability, is low.[12] The H1N1 2009 pandemic strain was poorly detected by standard RIDT at the time, leading to development of reverse-transcription PCR technology to identify this strain.[13] The reference standards for laboratory confirmation of influenza virus infection are currently viral culture or real-time PCR.

Rapid respiratory syncytial virus (RSV) antigen detection has become a standard diagnostic tool in the evaluation of children with bronchiolitis or pneumonia.[14] The development of PCR diagnostics for fastidious organisms such as *Legionella pneumophilia*[15] and *B pertussis*[16] should improve the ability to diagnose these pathogens. Real-time PCR technology to diagnose tuberculosis is relatively new, but may prove useful for achieving a rapid diagnosis for this slow-growing organism.[17] Acid fast bacillus culture will still need to be performed because of the growing problem of drug resistance in *M tuberculosis*. Also exciting is the development of new multiplex assays that evaluate for multiple respiratory pathogens rapidly and simultaneously from a single sample.[18] These multiplex platforms are designed for use in local clinical microbiology laboratories such that results can be available in hours, as discussed later. **Table 2** lists the individual pathogens that are typically assayed by these multiplex platforms, but there is variation regarding how many and which organisms are tested depending on the particular platform.

As illustrated in **Table 2**, individual real-time PCR assays currently exist for each of the bacterial, viral, and fungal pathogens. In the case of influenza and RSV, the rapid antigen assays can be verified with real-time PCR. Given that influenza A/B and RSV may cause illness that is clinically indistinguishable, a real-time PCR panel test that includes both influenza A/B and RSV (Mayo Diagnostic Test: PROD) should be considered. As already mentioned, innovative PCR-based multiplex molecular diagnostic tests are currently under development that can screen multiple respiratory pathogens at once. For example, the eSensor instrument (GenMark Dx, Carlsbad, CA) can identify the following pathogens in its respiratory viral panel: Influenza A (generic), Influenza A (H1 Seasonal Subtype), Influenza An H1 Mexico strain, Influenza A (H3 Seasonal Subtype) Influenza B, Respiratory Syncytial Virus subtypes A and B, Parainfluenza viruses 1, 2, 3, and 4, Human Metapneumovirus, Rhinovirus, Adenoviruses B, C, and E, and Coronaviruses NL63, 229E, OC43, and HKU1. Currently being considered for FDA approval, this technology has the ability to allow clinical laboratories to rapidly identify the causative agent in a matter of hours. The recent development of PCR assays for *Pneumocystis*[19] and *Aspergillus*[20] in immune-compromised hosts will likely improve detection over current technologies.

CARDIAC (MYOCARDITIS AND PERICARDITIS)
Clinical Perspective and Molecular Diagnosis

This section focuses on diagnostic tests for the evaluation of infectious origins of myocarditis and pericarditis (**Table 3**). Although these are relatively rare events

Table 3
Molecular diagnostics for cardiac infections: myocarditis and pericarditis

Normal Host	Microorganism	Methods	Specimens	Diagnostic Test
	Enterovirus	PCR	Blood	MAYO: LENT
	Adenovirus	PCR	Blood	MAYO: LADV
	Parvovirus	PCR	Blood	MAYO: PARVP
	HIV	qPCR	Blood	MAYO: HIVQU
	Mycobacterium tuberculosis	PCR	Pericardial fluid, blood	MAYO: MTBRP
Compromised	*Toxoplasma gondii*	PCR	Blood, other	MAYO: PTOX
	Cryptococcus neoformans	Antigen	Blood, other	MAYO: SCRYR/ SCRYP
	Aspergillus spp	Antigen, PCR	Blood, other	MAYO: ASPBA QUEST: 87798 (×3)

Abbreviations: HIV, human immunodeficiency virus; MAYO, Mayo Medical laboratories test identifier; QUEST, Quest Diagnostics test identifier.

clinically, they frequently are life-threatening emergencies for both normal and immune-compromised hosts. Enteroviruses and adenoviruses are the most common infectious causes of myocarditis[21] and real-time PCR is the best technology to evaluate for viremia caused by these organisms. These organisms are also the major ones implicated in cardiac transplant rejection.[22] In addition, *Toxoplasma* infections are associated with heart transplantation[23] as well as myocarditis in immune-compromised hosts.[24] Real-time PCR methodology is currently available for the various pathogens associated with cardiac infections except for *C neoformans* which, as mentioned earlier, currently relies on antigen-based tests such as latex agglutination or enzyme immunosorbent assays (see **Table 3**).

GASTROINTESTINAL (ENTERITIS, COLITIS, HEPATITIS, PANCREATITIS)
Clinical Perspective and Molecular Diagnosis

The diagnostic tests in this section focus on infectious causes of enteritis, colitis, hepatitis, and pancreatitis (**Table 4**). Real-time PCR for diagnosis of *Clostridium difficile* infection[25] is replacing the standard *C difficile* toxin assay in many centers. Real-time PCR assays are now available for bacterial enteric pathogens typically diagnosed for by standard stool culture.[26] These real-time PCR assays for bacterial enteric pathogens can be ordered as a panel (eg, Mayo Diagnostic Test: EPRP). Antibiotic resistance can occur for *Salmonella* species in particular, such that stool culture is necessary for testing antibiotic susceptibilities. Real-time PCR for shiga-toxin producing *E coli* can be used to identify O157/H7 strains that can cause hemolytic uremic syndrome.[27] Standard stool-culture techniques will not recover enteroinvasive *E coli*, which can now be assayed for by real-time PCR. Antigen detection for *Giardia* and *Cryptosporidium* is significantly more sensitive than assaying for these organisms by standard ova-and-parasite examination of stool.[28,29] Adenovirus serotypes associated with enteritis (ie, 40 and 41) do not grow in standard viral culture and must be

Table 4
Molecular diagnostics for gastrointestinal infections: enteritis and hepatitis

Normal Host	Microorganism	Methods	Specimens	Diagnostic Test
	Clostridium difficile	PCR	Stool	FOCUS: 87493, 87798
	Salmonella spp	PCR	Stool	MAYO: EPRP
	Shigella spp	PCR	Stool	MAYO: EPRP
	Campylobacter jejuni/coli	PCR	Stool	MAYO: EPRP
	Yersinia spp	PCR	Stool	MAYO: EPRP
	Escherichia coli, enteroinvasive	PCR	Stool	MAYO: EPRP
	Escherichia coli, shiga-toxin prod.	PCR	Stool	MAYO: EPRP
	Giardia lamblia	Antigen	Stool	MAYO: GIAR
	Cryptosporidium spp	Antigen	Stool	MAYO: CRYPS
	Adenovirus, enteric	Antigen, PCR	Stool, other	FOCUS: 87798 MAYO: LADV
	Hepatitis B virus	qPCR	Blood	MAYO: HBVQU
	Hepatitis C virus	qPCR	Blood	MAYO: HCVQU
Compromised	CMV	qPCR	Blood, other	MAYO: QCMV
	HSV	PCR	Blood, other	MAYO: VDER

Abbreviations: CMV, cytomegalovirus; HSV, herpes simplex virus; MAYO, Mayo Medical laboratories test identifier; QUEST, Quest Diagnostics test identifier.

assayed by antigen detection or real-time PCR.[30,31] Adenovirus can be grown in viral culture of stool, but these are not enteritis-causing serotypes. Real-time PCR for hepatitis B and hepatitis C are quantitative, and used in diagnosis and monitoring of patients with chronic infection with these pathogens both on and off of antiviral therapy.[32] Testing for hepatitis virus is routinely used for patients presenting with or developing acute liver disease.

BLOODSTREAM AND SYSTEMIC INFECTIONS
Clinical Perspective and Molecular Diagnosis

This section focuses on molecular diagnostics that can be used in settings of likely bloodstream infection, sepsis, or systemic infection (**Table 5**). In the setting of a sepsis-like illness or severe systemic illness likely to be due to an infectious etiology, bacteremia remains the most common and important cause.[33] Thus, blood cultures remain the gold standard in the evaluation of these patients. In addition to blood culture, molecular diagnostics can be useful in the evaluation of these patients depending on the clinical scenario.[34] HIV is included in this section because acute HIV infection (ie, acute retroviral syndrome) can present as an acute febrile illness with multiple manifestations.[35] There is real-time PCR testing available for multiple tick-borne illnesses, with Rocky Mountain spotted fever (*Rickettsia rickettsii*) being potentially fatal.[36] EBV, CMV, HSV, varicella zoster virus (VZV), adenovirus, and parvovirus are included in the immune-compromised section because these infections are typically self-limited in the normal host, but potentially fatal in the immune-compromised host.

As shown in **Table 5**, specific real-time PCR assays are available for many bloodstream pathogens unlikely to be detected via standard blood cultures. In the case of HIV, the real-time PCR reaction involves an initial reverse transcription step because HIV is a retrovirus containing a bipolar, plus-sense RNA genome. Because of the well-studied relationship of HIV RNA copy number to the stage of HIV disease and efficacy of HIV therapy, many truly quantitative real-time RT-PCR assays exist for HIV, with analytical sensitivity commonly as low as 20 copies/mL.[37]

In the United States ticks are a significant vector of infectious diseases, and rank second only to mosquitoes in disease transmission across the world.[38] Given the many different agents associated with tick-borne disease (eg, *R rickettsia*, *Borrelia burgdorferi*, *Ehrlichia* spp, and *Babesia microti*), commercial real-time PCR tick-borne panels are currently available to differentially identify the causative agent. In

Table 5
Molecular diagnostics for bloodstream and systemic infections

Normal Host	Microorganism	Methods	Specimens	Diagnostic Test
	HIV	qPCR	Blood	MAYO: HIVQU
	Rickettsia rickettsii	PCR	Blood, skin	MAYO: PTICK EHRL
	Borrelia burgdorferi	PCR	Blood, other	MAYO: PTICK EHRL
	Ehrlichia spp	PCR	Blood	MAYO: PTICK EHRL
	Babesia microti	PCR	Blood	MAYO: PTICK EHRL
Compromised	EBV	qPCR	Blood	MAYO: QEBV
	CMV	qPCR	Blood, other	MAYO: QCMV
	HSV	PCR	Blood, swab, other	MAYO: VDER
	VZV	PCR	Blood, swab, other	MAYO: VDER
	Adenovirus	PCR	Blood, other	MAYO: LADV
	Parvovirus	PCR	Blood, marrow	MAYO: PARVP

Abbreviations: CMV, cytomegalovirus; EBV, Epstein-Barr virus; HIV, human immunodeficiency virus; HSV, herpes simplex virus; MAYO, Mayo Medical laboratories test identifier; VZV, varicella zoster virus.

most cases this is a qualitative assay, and results are reported as either negative or positive for the targeted organisms. In the case of Rocky Mountain spotted fever, real-time PCR in a skin biopsy can be more useful for detecting the etiologic agent than an acute blood sample, owing to the low numbers of rickettsiae circulating in the blood in the absence of advanced disease or fulminant infection.[39]

In the immune-compromised category, the herpesviruses EBV and CMV are of significant concern in transplantation recipients.[40–42] Quantitative real-time PCR assays exist for both these pathogens, which can reliably detect between 2000 and 200 million copies per milliliter. It is important to recognize that there may be variation between results obtained from one laboratory and another laboratory. Clinically this can cause difficulty in interpreting whether a significant change in viral replication has occurred. A common example is when an EBV or CMV copy number is reported from one institution, after which the patient is transferred to another institution and a second quantitative PCR is performed. As these tests become more standardized over time, this should be less problematic. Qualitative real-time PCR assays are also available for herpesviruses HSV and VZV as well as adenovirus and parvovirus.[43,44]

SUMMARY

In the setting of infectious disease emergencies, rapid and accurate identification of the causative agent is critical to optimizing antimicrobial therapy in a timely manner. It is clearly evident that the age of molecular diagnostics is now upon us, with real-time PCR becoming the standard of diagnosis for many infectious disease emergencies in either monoplex or multiplex format. Other molecular techniques such as whole or partial genome sequencing, microarrays, broad-range PCR, restriction fragment length polymorphisms, and molecular typing are also being used. However, for most small clinical laboratories, implementation of these advanced molecular techniques is not feasible owing to the high cost of instrumentation and reagents. If these tests are not available in-house, samples can be sent to national reference laboratories (eg, Mayo Medical Laboratories and Quest Diagnostics) for real-time PCR assays that can be completed in 1 day. It is anticipated that over time commercial real-time PCR tests and instrumentation will become more standardized and affordable, allowing individual laboratories to conduct tests locally, thus further reducing turnaround time. Although real-time PCR has been proved to expand our diagnostic capability, it must be stressed that such molecular methodology constitutes only an additional tool in the diagnosis of infectious diseases in emergency situations. Phenotypic methodologies (staining, cultures, biochemical tests, and serology) still play a critical role in identifying, confirming, and providing antibiotic susceptibility testing for many microbial pathogens. As multiplex assays become increasingly available, there will be even greater temptation for taking a "shotgun" approach to diagnostic testing. These new technologies will not substitute for a proper history and physical examination leading to a thoughtful differential diagnosis. None the less, these new molecular tests increase the capability of the diagnostician to rapidly identify the microbiological etiology of an infection. An added advantage of rapid diagnostic tests often not emphasized is the capability to rule out certain diagnoses for which unnecessary antimicrobial therapy may otherwise be instituted and/or continued.

REFERENCES

1. Sibley CD, Peirano G, Chruch DL. Molecular methods for pathogen and microbial community detection and characterization: current and potential application in diagnostic microbiology. Infect Genet Evol 2012;12:505–21.

2. Procop GW. Molecular diagnostics for the detection and characterization of microbial pathogens. Clin Infect Dis 2007;45:S99–111.

3. Thompson MA, Aberg JA, Cahn P, et al. Antiretroviral treatment of adult HIV infection: 2010 recommendations of the International AIDS Society-USA panel. JAMA 2010;304:321–33.

4. Sankar S, Ramamurthy M, Nandagopal B, et al. Molecular and nanotechnologic approaches to etiologic diagnosis of infectious syndromes. Mol Diagn Ther 2011; 15:145–58.

5. Parikh V, Tucci V, Galwankar S. Infections of the nervous system. Int J Crit Illn Inj Sci 2012;2:82–97.

6. Gaeta A, Verzaro S, Cristina LM, et al. Diagnosis of neurological herpesvirus infections: real time PCR in cerebral spinal fluid analysis. New Microbiol 2009; 32:333–40.

7. de Crom SC, Obihara CC, van Loon AM, et al. Detection of enterovirus RNA in cerebrospinal fluid: comparison of two molecular assays. J Virol Methods 2012; 179:104–7.

8. Perkins MD, Mirrett S, Reller LB. Rapid bacterial antigen detection is not clinically useful. J Clin Microbiol 1995;33:1486–91.

9. Lu H, Zhou Y, Yin Y, et al. Cryptococcal antigen test revisited: significance for cryptococcal meningitis therapy monitoring in a tertiary Chinese hospital. J Clin Microbiol 2005;43:2989–90.

10. Warren NG, Hazen KC. *Candida*, *Cryptococcus*, and other yeasts of medical importance. In: Murray PR, editor. Manual of clinical microbiology. 7th edition. Washington, DC: ASM Press; 1999. p. 1184–99.

11. Landry ML. Diagnostic tests for influenza infection. Curr Opin Pediatr 2011;23: 91–7.

12. Jacobus CH, Raja AS. How accurate are rapid influenza diagnostic tests? Ann Emerg Med 2012. [Epub ahead of print].

13. Kumar S, Henrickson KJ. Update on influenza diagnostics: lessons from the novel H1N1 influenza A pandemic. Clin Microbiol Rev 2012;25:344–61.

14. Swenson PD, Kaplan MH. Rapid detection of respiratory syncytial virus in nasopharyngeal aspirates by a commercial enzyme immunoassay. J Clin Microbiol 1986;23:485–8.

15. Diederen BM, Kluytmans JA, Vandenbroucke-Grauls CM, et al. Utility of real-time PCR for diagnosis of Legionnaires' disease in routine clinical practice. J Clin Microbiol 2008;46:671–7.

16. Guthrie JL, Robertson AV, Tang P, et al. Novel duplex real-time PCR assay detects *Bordetella holmesii* in specimens from patients with pertussis-like symptoms in Ontario, Canada. J Clin Microbiol 2010;48:1435–7.

17. Sankar S, Ramamurthy M, Nandagopal B. An appraisal of PCR-based technology in the detection of *Mycobacterium tuberculosis*. Mol Diagn Ther 2011; 15:1–11.

18. Mahony JB, Petrich A, Smieja M. Molecular diagnosis of respiratory virus infections. Crit Rev Clin Lab Sci 2011;48:217–49.

19. Khot PD, Fredricks DN. PCR-based diagnosis of human fungal infections. Expert Rev Anti Infect Ther 2009;7:1201–21.

20. Chen SC, Kontoyiannis DP. New molecular and surrogate biomarker-based tests in the diagnosis of bacterial and fungal infection in febrile neutropenic patients. Curr Opin Infect Dis 2010;23:567–77.

21. Andréoletti L, Lévêque N, Boulagnon C, et al. Viral causes of human myocarditis. Arch Cardiovasc Dis 2009;102:559–68.

22. Cainelli F, Vento S. Infections and solid organ transplant rejection: a cause-and-effect relationship? Lancet Infect Dis 2002;2:539–49.
23. Derouin F, Pelloux H, ESCMID Study Group on Clinical Parasitology. Prevention of toxoplasmosis in transplant patients. Clin Microbiol Infect 2008;14: 1089–101.
24. Ferreira MS, Borges AS. Some aspects of protozoan infections in immunocompromised patients— review. Mem Inst Oswaldo Cruz 2002;97:443–57.
25. Crobach MJ, Dekkers OM, Wilcox MH, et al. European Society of Clinical Microbiology and Infectious Diseases (ESCMID): data review and recommendations for diagnosing *Clostridium difficile*-infection (CDI). Clin Microbiol Infect 2009; 15:1053–66.
26. Cunningham SA, Sloan LM, Nyre LM, et al. Three-hour molecular detection of *Campylobacter*, *Salmonella*, *Yersinia*, and *Shigella* species in feces with accuracy as high as that of culture. J Clin Microbiol 2010;48:2929–33.
27. Couturier MR, Lee B, Zelyas N, et al. Shiga-toxigenic *Escherichia coli* detection in stool samples screened for viral gastroenteritis in Alberta, Canada. J Clin Microbiol 2011;49:574–8.
28. Janoff EN, Craft JC, Pickering LK, et al. Diagnosis of *Giardia lamblia* infections by detection of parasite-specific antigens. J Clin Microbiol 1989;27:431–5.
29. Soave R, Johnson WD Jr. Cryptosporidium and *Isospora belli*. J Infect Dis 1988; 157:225–9.
30. Ebner K, Suda M, Watzinger F, et al. Molecular detection and quantitative analysis of the entire spectrum of human adenoviruses by a two-reaction real-time PCR assay. J Clin Microbiol 2005;43:3049–53.
31. Jothikumar N, Cromeans TL, Hill VR, et al. Quantitative real-time PCR assays for the detection of human adenoviruses and identification of serotypes 40 and 41. Appl Environ Microbiol 2005;71:3131–6.
32. Chevaliez S, Rodriguez C, Pawlotsky JM. New virologic tools for management of chronic hepatitis B and C. Gastroenterology 2012;142:1303–13.
33. Coburn B, Morris AM, Tomlinson G, et al. Does this adult patient with suspected bacteremia require blood cultures? JAMA 2012;308:502–11.
34. Riedel S, Carroll KC. Blood cultures: key elements for best practices and future directions. J Infect Chemother 2010;16:301–16.
35. Perrin L. Primary HIV infection. Antivir Ther 1999;4:13–8.
36. Graham J, Stockley K, Goldman RD. Tick-borne illnesses: a CME update. Pediatr Emerg Care 2011;27:141–7.
37. Panel on Antiretroviral Guidelines for Adults and Adolescents. Guidelines for the use of antiretroviral agents in HIV-1-infected adults and adolescents. Department of Health and Human Services; 2011. p. 1–166. Available at: http://www.aidsinfo.nih.gov/ContentFiles/AdultandAdolescentGL.pdf. Accessed August 15, 2012.
38. Mathieu ME, Wilson BB. Ticks (including tick paralysis). In: Mandell GL, Bennett JE, Dolin R, editors. Mandell, Douglas, and Bennett's principles and practice of infectious diseases, vol. 1, 5th edition. Philadelphia: Churchill Livingston; 2000. p. 2980–3.
39. Center for Disease Control and Prevention (CDC). Diagnosis and management of tickborne rickettsial diseases: Rocky mountain spotted fever, ehrlichioses, and anaplasmosis—United States. MMWR Morb Mortal Wkly Rep 2006;55:1–27.
40. Xuan L, Huang F, Fan Z, et al. Effects of intensified conditioning on Epstein-Barr virus and cytomegalovirus infections in allogeneic hematopoietic stem cell transplantation for hematological malignancies. J Hematol Oncol 2012;5:46 [Epub ahead of print].

41. Green M, Cacciarelli TV, Mazariegos GV, et al. Serial measurement of Epstein-Barr viral load in peripheral blood in pediatric liver transplant recipients during treatment for posttransplant lymphoproliferative disease. Transplantation 1998; 66:1641–4.

42. Kotton CN, Kumar D, Caliendo A, et al. International consensus guidelines on the management of cytomegalovirus in solid organ transplantation. Transplantation 2010;89:779–95.

43. Espy MJ, Ross TK, Teo R. Evaluation of LightCycler PCR for implementation of laboratory diagnosis of herpes simplex virus infections. J Clin Microbiol 2000; 38:3116–8.

44. Burrel S, Fovet C, Brunet C. Routine use of duplex real-time PCR assays including a commercial internal control for molecular diagnosis of opportunistic DNA virus infections. J Virol Methods 2012;185:136–41.

Choosing Optimal Antimicrobial Therapies

Thomas J. Lynch, PharmD

KEYWORDS

- Antimicrobial therapy • Multidrug resistance • *Streptococcus pneumoniae*
- Methicillin-resistant *Staphylococcus aureus* • *Enterococcus*
- *Pseudomonas aeruginosa* • Group A β-hemolytic *Streptococcus*

KEY POINTS

- Life-threatening infections require immediate and aggressive empiric use of parenteral bactericidal antibiotics.
- The recommended antibiotics are usually broad spectrum, are effective for the presumptive bacterial cause, readily achieve bactericidal concentrations at the site of infection, and are relatively safe to use in high doses.
- Vancomycin is most often used for gram-positive coverage, a carbapenem or piperacillin-tazobactam for gram-negative coverage, and metronidazole or clindamycin for anaerobic coverage.

Selecting appropriate antimicrobial agents for treating infections has always been a difficult task. Unlike selecting drugs to treat other disease processes, there are more variables to address. Not only does one have to consider the pharmacodynamic and pharmacokinetic properties of a drug as it relates to the patient to ensure tolerance and safety, one must also select an agent that the presumed microbe(s) will be susceptible to and that will reach the presumed site of infection with a high enough concentration to at least inhibit further microbial growth.

For treating life-threatening infectious disease emergencies, several properties of the appropriate antimicrobial agent are necessary. More often than not it will have to be given parenterally (intravenously or intramuscularly) to ensure 100% absorption and distribution and have an immediate onset of effect. It should also be bactericidal at achievable plasma and tissue concentrations to destroy and reduce the microbial load, rather than bacteriostatic, which only results in inhibition of further growth, relying on a competent immune system to slow the infectious process.

For the infectious disease emergencies discussed in this article, antimicrobial agents are recommended based on the presumed causative microorganisms and

Disclosures: No funding sources or conflict of interest to report.
Department of Family and Community Medicine, Eastern Virginia Medical School, PO Box 1980, Norfolk, VA 23501, USA
E-mail address: lyncht@evms.edu

Med Clin N Am 96 (2012) 1079–1094
http://dx.doi.org/10.1016/j.mcna.2012.08.006
0025-7125/12/$ – see front matter © 2012 Elsevier Inc. All rights reserved.

medical.theclinics.com

site of infection. Once the microorganism has been cultured and sensitivities reported, antimicrobial selection can be streamlined to target the pathogen or pathogens.

HEAD AND NECK INFECTIONS
Meningitis

Infections of the central nervous system (CNS) require the maximum doses of suggested antimicrobial agents in order for the agent to penetrate the blood-brain barrier. Agents such as β-lactam antibiotics and vancomycin penetrate poorly whereas others such as metronidazole have better bioavailability.[1] If meninges are inflamed, there is usually better penetration into the brain, but this is reduced once the meningitis starts to resolve. Vancomycin doses must be adjusted to obtain high serum trough levels of 15 to 20 mg/L.[2]

Empiric antimicrobial therapy for meningitis depends on the age of the patient. About 80% of cases in children and adults are due to *Streptococcus pneumoniae* or *Neisseria meningitidis*. The third-generation cephalosporins, ceftriaxone or cefotaxime, are drugs of choice for meningitis and vancomycin is added in case *S pneumoniae* is highly resistant to the cephalosporins (**Table 1**). Additional agents must be given for neonates and patients over 50 years old because of possible infection by *Listeria monocytogenes* or group B streptococci.[3]

Brain Abscess

Polymicrobial infections are common in patients with brain abscesses. Aerobic and anaerobic streptococci such as *Streptococcus anginosus* along with other anaerobic bacteria such as *Bacteroides fragilis* are common causes. Metronidazole as an antianaerobic agent is usually added to ceftriaxone or cefotaxime because of its excellent penetration into brain abscesses. If the potential source is penetrating trauma or postneurosurgical procedure, then *Staphylococcus aureus* (including methicillin-resistant *S aureus* [MRSA]) and *Pseudomonas aeruginosa* need to be considered as pathogens (see **Table 1**). Vancomycin would be added and the antipseudomonal cephalosporins, ceftazidime or cefepime, would be chosen as the cephalosporins.[4]

Encephalitis

By far the most common cause of encephalitis is infection by herpes simplex virus (HSV). More than 90% of herpes infections are due to HSV-1 and the rest by HSV-2. Intravenous acyclovir is the drug of choice (see **Table 1**). Other more rare viral causes of encephalitis include West Nile virus and Eastern equine encephalitis virus, which are arthropod-borne or arboviruses. At present, no antiviral therapy is available against these viruses.[5]

Jugular Septic Thrombophlebitis

Also known as Lemierre syndrome, jugular septic thrombophlebitis can be a rare complication of oropharyngeal or odontogenic infections. The most likely organisms involved are anaerobic streptococci, *Bacteroides* species, and *Fusobacterium necrophorum*. Three to 6 weeks of an antipseudomonal carbapenem plus metronidazole or ampicillin-sulbactam alone are the therapies of choice (see **Table 1**).[6]

Upper Airway Obstruction

Sudden obstruction of the upper airway usually is caused by acute epiglottitis, especially in children. The most common organism associated with epiglottitis is *Haemophilus influenzae*, although *S aureus*, including MRSA, can also cause it. Because *H influenzae* may be ampicillin resistant, ampicillin-sulbactam, ceftriaxone, or cefotaxime are recommended along with vancomycin to provide activity against MRSA

Table 1
Empiric treatment of life-threatening head and neck infections

Infection	Likely Organism(s)	First-Line Agent(s)	Alternative Agent(s) if Severe Allergy to First Line
Bacterial meningitis Age 1 mo to 50 y	Streptococcus pneumoniae, Neisseria meningitidis	Vancomycin + ceftriaxone or cefotaxime	Vancomycin + aztreonam
Bacterial meningitis Neonate or age >50 y	S pneumoniae, N meningitidis, Listeria monocytogenes	Vancomycin + ceftriaxone or cefotaxime + ampicillin	Aztreonam in place of cephalosporins and TMP-SMX in place of ampicillin
Brain abscess Community-acquired	Streptococcus anginosus Bacillus fragilis	Ceftriaxone or cefotaxime + metronidazole	Vancomycin + aztreonam + metronidazole
Brain abscess Nosocomial-acquired	S anginosus B fragilis Staphylococcus aureus Pseudomonas aeruginosa	Vancomycin + antipseudomonal cephalosporin + metronidazole	Vancomycin + aztreonam + metronidazole or vancomycin + antipseudomonal carbapenem
Encephalitis	Herpes simplex virus	Acyclovir	
Upper airway obstruction	Haemophilus influenzae S aureus	Vancomycin + third-generation cephalosporin	Trimethoprim-sulfamethoxazole (TMP-SMX)
Jugular septic thrombophlebitis	Streptococcus spp Peptostreptococcus spp Bacteroides spp Fusobacterium necrophorum	Antipseudomonal carbapenem + metronidazole or Ampicillin-sulbactam	Clindamycin

(see **Table 1**). For the severe penicillin-allergic patient, either trimethoprim-sulfamethoxazole or a fluoroquinolone (in adults) may be substituted for the ampicillin-sulbactam or cephalosporin.[7]

PULMONARY INFECTIONS
Pneumonia

When selecting antimicrobial agents for life-threatening pneumonia, it is important to first differentiate between community-acquired (CAP) and hospital-acquired (HAP) or heath care–associated pneumonia (HCAP). The most common bacterial causes of severe CAP are *S pneumoniae*, including drug-resistant strains, and atypical pathogens such as *Chlamydophila pneumoniae*, *Mycoplasma pneumoniae*, and *Legionella pneumophila*. For this reason the intravenous antibiotic combination of choice is a third-generation cephalosporin plus the macrolide, azithromycin, for the atypical pathogens. Respiratory fluoroquinolones (moxifloxacin or levofloxacin) also are usually effective against these pathogens.[8] For severe HAP and HCAP the presumption is that the pathogen(s) may include gram-negative bacilli, multiply drug-resistant (MDR) bacteria, or MRSA. A patient is considered to have HAP if pneumonia occurs at least 48 hours after admission. HCAP should be considered if the patient has a history of recent hospitalization within 90 days, is a resident of a long-term care facility, has received intravenous antibiotics, chemotherapy, or wound care within 30 days, or has attended a hemodialysis clinic. The most prevalent gram-negative organism to consider is *P aeruginosa*. For severe pseudomonal infections it is recommended that 2 agents be used, such as an antipseudomonal carbapenem and fluoroquinolone or the synergistic combination of an antipseudomonal β-lactam (meropenem, doripenem, cefepime, ceftazidime, piperacillin-tazobactam) with and aminoglycoside antibiotic. MDR pathogens may include extended-spectrum β-lactamase (ESBL)-producing bacteria such as *Klebsiella pneumoniae* or *Acinetobacter* species, which are resistant to cephalosporin antibiotics. Therefore for severe HAP or HCAP it is recommended that an antipseudomonal cephalosporin or carbapenem (meropenem or doripenem) be used with an additional antipseudomonal fluoroquinolone (ciprofloxacin or levofloxacin). If MRSA is suspected, vancomycin or linezolid should be added (**Table 2**). Although bacteriostatic, linezolid may be preferred because of its better lung-tissue penetration than vancomycin.[9]

Empyema

Empyema is an infection of the pleural space with pus and is usually a result of pneumonia. Pathogens associated with empyema include the same aerobic bacteria that cause pneumonia along with anaerobic bacteria such as *B fragilis*, *Prevetella* species, and *Fusobacterium nucleatum*. In previously healthy individuals the most common aerobic bacteria include *S pneumoniae*, *Streptococcus pyogenes*, and *S aureus*, including MRSA. Also to be considered is *S anginosus*, which is present in the oral cavity and gastrointestinal tract. Once drainage of the pleural space is performed, many antibiotics are available that readily penetrate the pleural space and are bactericidal for the most likely pathogens that cause empyema. Single agents would include piperacillin-tazobactam or a carbapenem. Double therapy would include a ceftriaxone or cefotaxime plus either metronidazole or clindamycin (see **Table 2**). Vancomycin or linezolid could be added if MRSA is a possible cause.[10]

Lung Abscess

Lung abscesses can occur as a complication of aspiration pneumonia and are due to the same bacteria that cause this particular pneumonia, usually anaerobic bacteria

Table 2
Empiric treatment of life-threatening pulmonary infections

Infection	Likely Organism(s)	First-Line Agent(s)	Alternative Agent(s) if Severe Allergy to First Line
Pneumonia community-acquired (CAP)	Streptococcus pneumoniae, Legionella pneumophila, Mycoplasma pneumoniae, Chlamydophila pneumoniae	Ceftriaxone or cefotaxime + azithromycin	Moxifloxacin or levofloxacin (also considered first-line agents)
Pneumonia HAP or HCAP	S pneumoniae, Klebsiella pneumoniae, Pseudomonas aeruginosa, Acinetobacter spp, MRSA	Cefepime or ceftazidime + ciprofloxacin +/- vancomycin	Meropenem or doripenem + gentamicin +/- linezolid
Empyema	S pneumoniae Streptococcus pyogenes, Streptococcus anginosus, Staphylococcus aureus, anaerobes	Piperacillin-tazobactam or carbapenem or ceftriaxone/cefotaxime + metronidazole	Fluoroquinolone + clindamycin
Lung abscess	Mouth flora anaerobes including Fusobacterium spp, Prevatella spp, and Peptostreptococcus spp	Ceftriaxone or cefotaxime + clindamycin or ampicillin-sulbactam alone	Moxifloxacin
Adult respiratory distress syndrome	See sepsis guidelines		

from the oral cavity. Initially a lung abscess is presumed to be polymicrobial and is treated with the combination of ceftriaxone or cefotaxime plus clindamycin (see **Table 2**). Metronidazole, although generally a very effective antianaerobic agent, is specifically inferior for gram-positive anaerobic mouth flora. A parenteral β-lactam plus a β-lactamase inhibitor such as ampicillin-sulbactam or piperacillin-tazobactam can also be used.[11] Alternatives for this polymicrobial infection could include a carbapenem or respiratory fluoroquinolone with anaerobic activity such as moxifloxacin.[12]

Adult Respiratory Distress Syndrome

Among other conditions, adult respiratory distress syndrome may be precipitated by a sepsis syndrome, either as a result of severe pneumonia or infection from an extrapulmonary source. Antimicrobial treatment guidelines for sepsis should be followed.

CARDIAC INFECTIONS
Endocarditis

Infective endocarditis is defined as infected vegetations on the heart valve composed of layers of fibrin, platelets, and bacteria. This resulting tough fibrin mesh lacks vasculature and impairs host response as leukocytes and complement are unable to reach the encased bacteria. Therefore, bacteria can continue to multiply with inoculum counts reaching as high as 10^9 to 10^{10} cfu/mL. Just as leukocytes cannot readily penetrate this fibrin mesh, antibiotics also find it a formidable barrier.[13] Treatment of infective endocarditis requires high doses of intravenous bactericidal antibiotics for an extended period of time, many times in synergistic combination, for a more rapid and reliable killing effect. Presumptive therapy is necessary for initial treatment in life-threatening situations, but the ultimate selection of antibiotics depends on blood culture results and subsequent antimicrobial susceptibility tests. Quantitative minimum inhibitory concentration (MIC) and minimum bactericidal concentration (MBC) determinations may be needed if the infection is due potentially to antibiotic-resistant isolates. Most cases of native valve infective endocarditis are due to either streptococci or staphylococci. S aureus is the leading single bacterial cause of acute infective endocarditis. Choice of therapy depends on whether the infecting organism is a penicillin-sensitive streptococcus (MIC ≤0.125 mg/L) such as viridans group streptococci or *Streptococcus bovis*, a penicillin-tolerant streptococcus (MIC >0.125 to ≤0.5 mg/L), or a penicillin-resistant enterococcus or staphylococcus, including MRSA (**Table 3**). Viridans streptococci are usually mouth flora and include *Streptococcus mitis, Streptococcus mutans, Streptococcus salivarius, Streptococcus sanguis*, and the *Streptococcus intermedius* group (*S intermedius, S anginosus*, and *Streptococcus constellatus*). Enterococcus must always be treated with 2 antibiotics, as no single agent is bactericidal for this organism. Duration of treatment should always be counted from the time of the first negative blood culture. The initial therapy for prosthetic valve endocarditis is similar to native valve endocarditis. The most reliable initial antibiotic combination, pending blood culture results, is vancomycin plus gentamicin. Piperacillin-tazobactam, ceftazidime, cefepime, or ciprofloxacin should be added for gram-negative coverage, including *P aeruginosa*, in patients with early prosthetic valve endocarditis.[14]

Pericarditis and Myocarditis

Pericarditis and myocarditis refer to inflammatory processes of the pericardium and myocardium, respectively, which can ultimately lead to heart failure. Viruses seem to be the most likely cause of these inflammatory disorders, but there are few antiviral

Table 3
Infective native valve endocarditis

Documented Infecting Organism	First Line Agent(s)	Treatment Duration	Alternative Agent(s) if Severe Allergy to First Line
Viridans streptococci/ *Streptococcus bovis* with penicillin MIC ≤0.12 mg/L	Penicillin G or ceftriaxone	4 wk	Vancomycin
Viridans streptococci/*S bovis* with penicillin MIC >0.12 mg/L and ≤0.5 mg/L	Penicillin G or ceftriaxone + high-dose gentamicin	4 wk 2 wk	Vancomycin
Viridans streptococci/*S bovis* with penicillin MIC >0.5 mg/L	See ampicillin-resistant enterococcal endocarditis	—	—
Methicillin-sensitive *Staphylococcus* spp	Nafcillin +/− low-dose gentamicin	6 wk/3–5 d	Vancomycin +/− low-dose gentamicin
Methicillin-resistant *Staphylococcus* spp	Vancomycin	6 wk	Daptomycin
Enterococcus spp susceptible to ampicillin	Ampicillin + low-dose gentamicin	4–6 wk	Vancomycin + low-dose gentamicin
Enterococcus spp resistant to ampicillin	Vancomycin + low-dose gentamicin	6 wk	Daptomycin

therapies available. In rare cases where the specific etiologic agent has been identified, such as tuberculosis or human immunodeficiency virus, targeted antimicrobial therapy can be initiated. However, in most cases supportive care is the treatment of choice along with immunosuppressive therapy where appropriate. When a bacterial cause is likely or documented, antimicrobial therapy is similar to that of infective endocarditis.[15]

INTRA-ABDOMINAL AND PELVIC INFECTIONS
Acute Peritonitis and Intra-Abdominal Abscess

Peritonitis can develop secondary to perforation of the gastrointestinal tract and spillage of bacterial contents into the peritoneum. The resulting infection is usually polymicrobial and the probable infecting organisms are determined by the site of the perforation along the gastrointestinal tract. The upper intestine usually contains relatively few oral gram-positive microorganisms such lactobacillus and streptococci. The ileum contains a much higher concentration of enteric gram-negative bacteria, such as *Escherichia coli*, gram-positive bacteria such as *Enterococcus*, and an equal number of obligate anaerobes such as *B fragilis*. The colon has, by far, the highest concentration of bacteria (10^{11} cfu/mL) leading to a high incidence of serious intra-abdominal infection if perforation occurs. Hundreds of bacterial species can be present, and anaerobes outnumber aerobic bacteria by a factor of 1000 to 1.[16] Treatment of acute secondary peritonitis therefore must be directed at gram-negative bacteria and anaerobes. Although *Enterococcus* species may be present, antibiotics without enterococcal activity, such as cephalosporins and fluoroquinolones, still appear to be effective. The selection of antibiotics is further determined by whether the infection is community-acquired or health care–acquired (usually as a result of surgical intervention and presumably due to more resistant organisms) (**Table 4**). Intraabdominal abscess may occur as a complication of peritonitis; however, the bacteriology is the same. Because antibiotics may not penetrate abscesses very well and there are very high concentrations of bacteria, drainage of the abscess is necessary for antibiotics to be effective.[17]

Cholecystitis and Cholangitis

Cholecystitis and cholangitis usually result from obstruction in the gallbladder or common bile duct, respectively. The most common pathogens associated with cholecystitis are E coli, Klebsiella species, and Enterococcus species. Cholangitis may, in addition, be caused by Enterobacter species and anaerobes. For severe biliary tract infections, empiric antibiotic therapy should cover enteric gram-negative organisms and anaerobic bacteria (see **Table 4**). If health care–associated, coverage should be expanded to include Enterococcus species.[17]

Pyelonephritis and Perinephric Abscess

Acute pyelonephritis with potentially life-threatening bacteremia requires empiric broad-spectrum intravenous antibiotic therapy. If community-acquired, a fluoroquinolone, piperacillin-tazobactam, or a third-generation cephalosporin may be used. If a Gram stain shows gram-positive cocci, vancomycin should be added for potential MRSA (see **Table 4**). Moxifloxacin should not be used because it is not renally eliminated. Also, if the patient is pregnant, fluoroquinolones are contraindicated. If it is a health care facility–acquired infection, alternative broad-spectrum agents may be needed based on the prevalence of antibiotic-resistant organisms.[18,19]

A perinephric abscess can be a rare complication of a urinary tract infection, and up to 25% of cases may be due to multiple bacterial species. Percutaneous aspiration and drainage will help determine the causative organisms and thus guide antibiotic therapy. Trimethoprim-sulfamethoxazole (TMP-SMX) and fluoroquinolones may be able to better penetrate the abscess site than other antibiotics.[19]

Infectious Colitis

There are several bacterial causes of severe, life-threatening colitis and diarrhea, each of which requires a different antimicrobial approach for treatment (see **Table 4**). Infection due to Clostridium difficile, a spore-forming bacteria, is associated with exposure to health care environments, previous antibiotic use, or both. For severe infection oral vancomycin, which is nonabsorbable, is the treatment of choice. Intravenous metronidazole may also be added, although supporting data are lacking. Intravenous vancomycin is ineffective and oral metronidazole is the treatment of choice for milder disease. Several new antibiotics, such as rifaximin, fidaxomicin, and tigecycline, are now available for treating recurrent infection unresponsive to the agents of choice.[20]

Complicated nontyphoidal Salmonella infections can usually be treated with a fluoroquinolone or TMP-SMX. However, if life threatening, a third-generation cephalosporin should be added to intravenous fluoroquinolone until susceptibilities are known.[21]

Shigellosis (bacillary dysentery) can be treated with a fluoroquinolone, such as ciprofloxacin, or azithromycin. TMP-SMX should not be used any longer because of the development of widespread resistance.[21]

Campylobacter jejuni gastroenteritis secondary to ingesting undercooked food is usually self-limiting. However, in high-risk individuals, antibiotics are recommended.

Table 4
Empiric treatment of serious intra-abdominal and pelvic infections

Infection	Likely Organism(s)	First-Line Agents	Alternative Agent(s) if Severe Allergy to First Line
Secondary peritonitis and intra-abdominal abscess (community-acquired)	Enteric gram-negative bacteria (*Escherichia coli, Klebsiella* spp, *Proteus* spp) Anaerobic bacteria (*Bacteroides* spp)	Piperacillin-tazobactam or antipseudomonal carbapenem	Levofloxacin or aztreonam + metronidazole
Secondary peritonitis and intra-abdominal abscess (health care–associated)	Above organisms + *Pseudomonas aeruginosa* and/or *Staphylococcus aureus*	Above agents + aminoglycoside and vancomycin	Above agents + aminoglycoside and vancomycin
Cholecystitis and cholangitis	Enteric gram-negative bacteria, *Enterococcus* spp, anaerobic bacteria	Piperacillin-tazobactam or carbapenem	Levofloxacin or aztreonam + metronidazole
Pyelonephritis	Enteric gram-negative bacteria	Levofloxacin or ciprofloxacin, piperacillin-tazobactam, or ceftriaxone	Aminoglycoside
Perinephric abscess	Enteric gram-negative bacteria	Levofloxacin or ciprofloxacin	TMP-SMX
Infectious colitis	*Clostridium difficile*	Oral vancomycin +/− intravenous metronidazole	Rifaximin or fidaxomicin
	Salmonella (nontyphoid)	Fluoroquinolone + ceftriaxone	TMP-SMX
	Shigella	Fluoroquinolone	Azithromycin
	Campylobacter jejuni	Azithromycin	Fluoroquinolone
	Yersinia enterocolitica	Fluoroquinolone	Azithromycin

The macrolide azithromycin is the agent of choice. Erythromycin and clarithromycin can also be used, but this increases the risk of metabolic interactions with drugs that inhibit or are metabolized by the cytochrome P450 3A4 enzyme. Fluoroquinolones are now considered alternative agents because there is a high level of *C jejuni* resistance to this class of drugs, attributed to its widespread use in the food animal industry.[21]

Yersinia enterocolitica is a zoonotic infection of rodents, birds, and other wild animals. The organism is transmitted to humans by fleas, and in the resulting infection symptoms of fever, diarrhea, and abdominal pain resemble acute appendicitis. Antibiotics of choice include fluoroquinolones and azithromycin.[21]

E coli serotype O157:H7 is an enterohemorrhagic *E coli* strain (EHEC) that produces a Shiga toxin associated with several severe complications including hemorrhagic colitis, hemolytic uremia syndrome, and thrombotic thrombocytopenic purpura. This EHEC strain is usually consumed in undercooked beef products. The role of antibiotic treatment of *E coli* O157:H7 remains controversial, and currently no particular antibiotic is recommended. In fact antibiotic treatment may lead to complications such as hemolytic uremic syndrome.[22]

NECROTIZING SOFT-TISSUE INFECTIONS
Necrotizing Fasciitis

Necrotizing fasciitis is a rapidly developing inflammation and infection of both superficial and deep fascia, which can quickly progress to septic shock. A wide variety of bacteria can potentially release toxins that cause necrosis, requiring empiric broad-spectrum antibiotic coverage until Gram stain and culture can help narrow the microbiological etiology. Along with immediate surgical debridement, initial empiric therapy with vancomycin plus a carbapenem is indicated to cover for gram-positive organisms, gram-negative Enterobacteriaciae, and *B fragilis*.[23] Virulent strains of Group A B-hemolytic *Streptococcus* are associated with a so-called flesh-eating necrotizing infection. High-dose penicillin G plus clindamycin is indicated for this particularly gruesome disease (**Table 5**). The clindamycin is added for its ability to reduce the production of bacterial toxins.

Clostridial Myonecrosis

Necrotizing infections involving the muscle are termed myonecrosis. Myonecrosis caused by *Clostridium perfringens*, a gram-positive bacillus, is also known as gas gangrene and is a very painful infection secondary to gas in the wound. Penicillin G

Table 5 Life-threatening necrotizing soft tissue infections			
Infection	**Likely Organism(s)**	**First-Line Agents**	**Alternative Agent(s) if Severe Allergy to First Line**
Necrotizing fasciitis	Unknown	Carbapenem or piperacillin-tazobactam + vancomycin + clindamycin	Fluoroquinolone + vancomycin + clindamycin
	Group A β-hemolytic *Streptococcus*	Penicillin G + clindamycin	
Clostridial myonecrosis	*Clostridium perfringens*	Penicillin G + clindamycin	Clindamycin or metronidazole

is the antibiotic of choice, after the diagnosis is confirmed, given along with parenteral clindamycin.[24] Those with a severe penicillin allergy history may be treated with clindamycin or metronidazole alone (see **Table 5**).

SEPSIS SYNDROME
Bloodstream Infections

Sepsis syndrome is a life-threatening condition secondary to infection and consequent end-organ dysfunction, hypotension, and hypoperfusion. In addition to supportive measures, immediate administration of appropriate antimicrobial agents is vital to prevent progression to septic shock and death. It is estimated that for every hour of delay in giving parenteral antibiotics, survival decreases by 8%. The choice of antibiotics for sepsis syndrome depends on the presumed source of the infection, causative organism, and the immune status of the patient. After blood cultures are obtained, a broad-spectrum bactericidal parenteral agent such as piperacillin-tazobactam or a carbapenem, plus vancomycin for gram-positive coverage, should be started.[25,26] Therapy can then be guided by culture results and susceptibility testing (**Table 6**). If sepsis occurs in a neutropenic patient or if *P aeruginosa* is a suspected cause, an aminoglycoside should be added for synergistic effect. If sepsis occurs after broad-spectrum antimicrobial therapy, a fungal organism, such as *Candida*, may be the cause and a parenteral antifungal agent should be considered.

Device-Related Infections

Device-related sepsis syndrome can be secondary to peripheral and central intravenous catheters, tunneled catheters, implanted ports, and arterial lines. *S aureus* and coagulase-negative staphylococcal organisms account for 70% to 90% of these infections. Gram-negative bacteria and fungal organisms are also implicated. Therefore, until culture results are available a broad-spectrum bactericidal agent for gram-negative coverage should be started along with vancomycin (see **Table 6**).[25]

TRAVEL-RELATED INFECTIONS
Malaria

For both chloroquine-sensitive and resistant *Plasmodium* species, quinidine gluconate is the only parenteral agent for severe malaria that is approved by the US Food and Drug Administration. Intravenous quinine is available outside the United States. If quinidine gluconate is not available, parenteral artemisinin derivatives are available from the Centers for Disease Control and Prevention (CDC) (**Table 7**).[27] Oral antibiotics such as doxycycline or clindamycin should be added when tolerated.

Table 6
Sepsis syndrome

Source	First-Line Agents	Alternative Agent(s) if Severe Allergy to First Line
Unknown	Piperacillin-tazobactam or carbapenem + vancomycin	Fluoroquinolone + vancomycin
Neutropenic	Piperacillin-tazobactam or carbapenem + aminoglycoside + vancomycin	Fluoroquinolone + aminoglycoside + vancomycin
Device-related	Piperacillin-tazobactam or carbapenem + vancomycin	Fluoroquinolone + vancomycin

Table 7			
Travel-related severe infections			
Infection	**Likely Organism(s)**	**First-Line Agent(s)**	**Alternative Agent(s) if Severe Allergy to First Line**
Malaria	*Plasmodium* spp	Intravenous quinidine gluconate	Artemisinin derivatives (from CDC)
Dengue fever	*Flavivirus*	Symptomatic treatment only	

Dengue Hemorrhagic Fever

Dengue and dengue hemorrhagic fever are viral illnesses caused by several *Flavivirus* serotypes and transmitted by the mosquito, *Aedes aegypti*. There is currently no known antiviral therapy, and treatment is symptomatic.

POTENTIAL MULTIDRUG-RESISTANT ORGANISMS AND ANTIMICROBIAL AGENTS OF CHOICE
Streptococcus pneumoniae

S pneumoniae (pneumococcus) is a common bacterial cause of CNS and respiratory infections. Resistance in pneumococcus is defined by its susceptibility to penicillin. In 2008, the Clinical Laboratory and Standards Institute revised susceptibility breakpoints to penicillin for meningitis and nonmeningeal infections. For meningitis, penicillin breakpoints are 0.06 mg/L and 0.12 mg/L for sensitive and resistant strains, respectively. For nonmeningeal infections, breakpoints are 2 mg/L, 4 mg/L, and 8 mg/L for sensitive, intermediate, and resistance strains, respectively.[28] Using these new breakpoints it has been estimated that, for non-CNS infections in the United States, 65% of pneumococci are sensitive to oral penicillin and 93% are sensitive to parenteral penicillin or oral amoxicillin. For meningitis, 65% of pneumococci are susceptible to parenteral penicillin. However, these rates may vary considerably depending on locality. As pneumococcus acquires resistance to penicillin, it also becomes resistant to other common non–β-lactam antibiotics such as macrolides, doxycycline, clindamycin, and TMP-SMX. Most isolates remain sensitive to the respiratory fluoroquinolones, and all are susceptible to vancomycin.[29]

Staphylococcus aureus

S aureus is a common bacterial cause of skin and soft-tissue infections and sepsis. It is now estimated that 50% to 60% of *S aureus* infections are due to methicillin-resistant strains. By definition, all MRSA infections are resistant to β-lactam and carbapenem antibiotics. Antimicrobial susceptibility of MRSA depends on whether it is community-acquired (CA) or health care–acquired (HA), 2 phenotypically and genotypically distinct strains. It is essential that culture and sensitivity testing be done for all suspected MRSA infections. Most CA-MRSA strains carry the Panton-Valentine leukocidin gene, which encodes for a cytotoxin that is associated with purulent skin and soft-tissue infections and severe necrotizing pneumonia. Although resistant to β-lactams, CA-MRSA is usually susceptible to such common antibiotics as TMP-SMX, clindamycin, and doxycycline. Infections attributable to HA-MRSA, on the other hand, are resistant to most common antibiotics and the drug of first choice is parenteral vancomycin. Linezolid, a bacteriostatic agent that is available in both parenteral and oral dosage forms, is an alternative but expensive choice for both strains of MRSA. Other new alternative parenteral agents include daptomycin, tigecycline, and ceftaroline. These antibiotics may take on greater importance as vancomycin intermediate-resistant and fully-resistant strains become more prevalent.[30,31]

Enterococcus

Enterococcus is part of the normal gastrointestinal flora and occasionally may contribute to intra-abdominal, biliary tract, or urinary tract infections. For life-threatening enterococcal infections, such as endocarditis, it is necessary that 2 antibiotics be administered to achieve a bactericidal killing effect; this usually consists of a β-lactam or vancomycin combined with an aminoglycoside. Unlike with other bacterial species, there is no single antibiotic that is bactericidal against Enterococcus. Penicillin-susceptible strains can be treated with ampicillin or piperacillin, with vancomycin being used for patients with severe penicillin allergy. Cephalosporins have very weak or no activity. Some Enterococcus species, particularly Enterococcus faecium, are now resistant to penicillin, ampicillin, and vancomycin (vancomycin-resistant enterococcus or VRE). For these strains options include linezolid, daptomycin, or tigecycline.[32]

Pseudomonas aeruginosa

P aeruginosa is an opportunistic organism that easily colonizes moist surfaces and is usually associated with nosocomial bacterial infections. Several broad-spectrum β-lactam antibiotics have been developed over the last several decades specifically with activity against P aeruginosa. These agents include piperacillin-tazobactam, the cephalosporins ceftazidime and cefepime, and the carbapenems imipenem, meropenem, and doripenem. For infections such as bacteremia and pneumonia, the highest doses recommended should be used in order for serum and tissue levels of antibiotic to be above the MIC for more than 50% of the time. Initial treatment with an antipseudomonal β-lactam and fluoroquinolone or aminoglycoside improves the likelihood that one or the other antibiotic class will be effective until sensitivity results are available. There is still controversy regarding whether to continue high-dose aminoglycoside therapy for a synergistic bactericidal effect. Multiresistant strains are now emerging that will not respond to β-lactam, fluoroquinolone, or aminoglycoside therapy. In such cases old antibiotics such as colistin and polymyxin are being tried.[33]

MONITORING PARAMETERS FOR SELECTED ANTIMICROBIAL AGENTS

Bactericidal antibiotics can generally be divided into 2 categories based on how they best kill bacteria. Knowing the difference in these mechanisms helps in determining the best dosing strategies to ensure early success in treating a life-threatening infection. β-Lactam antibiotics such as the penicillins, cephalosporins, and carbapenems kill bacteria in a time-dependent manner. Vancomycin falls in this same category. Active growth inhibition only occurs as long as antibiotic concentration at the site of infection is above the MIC. For antibiotics to be bactericidal, concentrations usually have to be 4 to 5 times higher than the MIC. This level can be measured in vitro and is known as the minimum bactericidal concentration or MBC. With inappropriately low doses and/or prolonged dosing intervals, time-dependent antibiotics will not be effective for serious infections.[34] The second category of antibiotics kills bacteria in a concentration-dependent manner and includes the aminoglycosides, fluoroquinolones, and daptomycin. For this group of antibiotics, peak levels should be at least 8 to 10 times the MIC for a bactericidal effect. As serum concentration levels decline after a dose, bactericidal activity continues (postantibiotic effect). If a bacteria MIC is relatively high and/or the site of infection is difficult for antibiotics to penetrate, concentrations of single antibiotics will not achieve bactericidal levels, which is often the case for treating endocarditis or infections due to *Enterococcus* and *P aeruginosa*.[34] In these cases, the use of 2 agents with different mechanisms of action is necessary for either an additive or synergistic bactericidal effect. Although somewhat controversial, it may also be necessary to expose a positive bacterial culture to a patient's serum containing antibiotics to measure serum bactericidal titers (SBT) as a guide to therapy. For endocarditis, SBTs of 1:8 or greater are recommended.[35]

The recommended antibiotic regimens in this article are based on current national bacterial-resistant trends. To ensure optimal success, it is necessary to follow local and regional antibiotic resistance data. Local data are made available every 6 to 12 months by diagnostic laboratories at the local hospitals.

Several antibiotics require routine measurement of serum levels to guide treatment. The most important is vancomycin, which is frequently used in empiric regimens to cover for MRSA. Because the MIC for MRSA has been gradually rising over the last few years (MIC creep), new guidelines now recommend that vancomycin trough levels be 15 to 20 mg/L.[2] Peak levels are not measured. These new target levels require higher doses that can potentially cause nephrotoxicity. Therefore it is also necessary to routinely monitor renal function. Aminoglycoside antibiotics traditionally required frequent serum-level determinations when dosed as a time-dependent antibiotic because of their nephrotoxic potential. Once it was discovered that bactericidal activity is concentration dependent, once-daily high-dose therapy is now the norm. If more frequent low-dose therapy is required, peak and trough serum levels should be monitored on a regular basis.

SUMMARY

Life-threatening infectious disease emergencies require immediate, aggressive parenteral administration of antimicrobial agents to ensure high bactericidal concentrations of drug at the site of infection. Usually initial treatment is empiric until culture results and antimicrobial sensitivities are reported. This approach necessitates the use of broad-spectrum bactericidal agents that will eradicate the presumed infecting organism(s), which potentially could be multidrug resistant. For infections potentially attributable to gram-positive bacteria, vancomycin is commonly used because it will be effective for highly resistant strains such as MRSA and multidrug-resistant *S pneumoniae*. For gram-negative infections, broad-spectrum β-lactams, such as ceftriaxone, piperacillin-tazobactam, and the carbapenems, are commonly chosen. Excellent alternatives include the fluoroquinolone antibiotics. For nosocomial infections whereby *P aeruginosa* and other highly resistant organisms may be the cause, antipseudomonal β-lactams such as cefepime, ceftazidime, piperacillin-tazobactam, or doripenem may be used as well as the fluoroquinolone, ciprofloxacin. For anaerobic infections, it is usually necessary to add either metronidazole or clindamycin. Once an infection is under control and the culture and sensitivity results are reported, it is important to switch to the most narrow-spectrum agent possible. Taking this action will decrease the potential for adverse drug effects and the risk of development of antibiotic-induced resistance.

REFERENCES

1. Lutsar I, McCracken GH, Friedland IR. Antibiotic pharmacodynamics in cerebrospinal fluid. Clin Infect Dis 1998;27:1117–27.
2. Rybak M, Lomaestro B, Rotschafer JC, et al. Therapeutic monitoring of vancomycin in adult patients: a consensus review of the American Society of Health-System

Pharmacists, the Infectious Diseases Society of America, and the Society of Infectious Diseases Pharmacists. Am J Health Syst Pharm 2009;66:82–98.

3. Tunkel AR, Hartman BJ, Kaplan SL, et al. Practice guidelines for the management of bacterial meningitis. Clin Infect Dis 2004;39:1267–84.

4. Tunkel AR, Glaser CA, Bloch KC, et al. The management of encephalitis: Clinical practice guidelines by the Infectious Disease Society of America. Clin Infect Dis 2008;47:303–27.

5. Mathisen GE, Johnson JP. Brain abscess. Clin Infect Dis 1997;25:763–79.

6. Chow AW. Infections of the oral cavity, neck, and head. In: Mandell GL, Bennett JE, Dolin R, editors. Mandell, Douglas, and Bennett's principles and practice of infectious diseases. Philadelphia: Churchill Livingstone; 2010. p. 855–71.

7. Guildfred LA, Lyhne D, Becker BC. Acute epiglottitis: epidemiology, clinical presentation, management and outcome. J Laryngol Otol 2008;122:818–23.

8. Mandell LA, Wunderink RG, Anzueto A, et al. Infectious Disease Society of America/American Thoracic Society Consensus Guidelines on the management of community acquired pneumonia in adults. Clin Infect Dis 2007;44:S27–72.

9. American Thoracic Society, Infectious Diseases Society of America. Guidelines for the management of adults with hospital-acquired, ventilator-associated, and healthcare-associated pneumonia. Am J Respir Crit Care Med 2005;171: 388–416.

10. Septimus EJ. Pleural effusion and empyema. In: Mandell GL, Bennett JE, Dolin R, editors. Mandell, Douglas, and Bennett's principles and practice of infectious diseases. Philadelphia: Churchill Livingstone; 2010. p. 917–23.

11. Levison ME. Anaerobic pleuropulmonary infection. Curr Opin Infect Dis 2001;14: 187–91.

12. Ott SR, Allewelt M, Lorenz J, et al. Moxifloxacin vs ampicillin/sulbactam in aspiration pneumonia and primary lung abscess. Infection 2008;36:23–30.

13. McDonald JR. Acute infective endocarditis. Infect Dis Clin North Am 2009;23: 643–64.

14. Baddour LM, Wilson WR, Bayer AS, et al. Infective endocarditis: diagnosis, antimicrobial therapy, and management of complications. A statement for healthcare professionals from the Committee on Rheumatic Fever, Endocarditis, and Kawasaki Disease, Council of Cardiovascular Disease in the Young, and the Councils on Clinical Cardiology, Stroke, and Cardiovascular Surgery and Anesthesia, American Heart Association. Circulation 2005;111:e394–434.

15. Knowlton KU, Savoia MC, Oxman MN. Myocarditis and pericarditis. In: Mandell GL, Bennett JE, Dolin R, editors. Mandell, Douglas, and Bennett's principles and practice of infectious diseases. Philadelphia: Churchill Livingstone; 2010. p. 1153–71.

16. Levison ME, Bush LM. Peritonitis and intraperitoneal abscesses. In: Mandell GL, Bennett JE, Dolin R, editors. Mandell, Douglas, and Bennett's principles and practice of infectious diseases. Philadelphia: Churchill Livingstone; 2010. p. 1011–34.

17. Solomkin JS, Mazuski JE, Bradley JS, et al. Diagnosis and management of complicated intra-abdominal infections in adults and children: guidelines by the Surgical Infection Society and the Infectious Disease Society of America. Clin Infect Dis 2010;50:13–64.

18. Gupta K, Hooten TM, Naber KG, et al. International clinical practice guidelines for the treatment of acute uncomplicated cystitis and pyelonephritis in women: a 2010 update by the Infectious Diseases Society of America and the European Society for Microbiology and Infectious Diseases. Clin Infect Dis 2011;52: e103–20.

19. Sobel JD, Kaye D. Urinary tract infections. In: Mandell GL, Bennett JE, Dolin R, editors. Mandell, Douglas, and Bennett's principles and practice of infectious diseases. Philadelphia: Churchill Livingstone; 2010. p. 957–85.

20. Cohen SH, Gerding DN, Johnson S, et al. Clinical practice guidelines for *Clostridium difficile* infection in adults: 2010 update by the Society for Healthcare Epidemiology of America and the Infectious Disease Society of America. Infect Control Hosp Epidemiol 2010;31:431–55.

21. DuPont HL. Approach to the patient with infectious colitis. Curr Opin Gastroenterol 2012;28:39–46.

22. Pennington H. *Escherichia coli* 0157. Lancet 2010;376:1428–35.

23. Anaya D, Dellinger P. Necrotizing soft tissue infection: diagnosis and management. Clin Infect Dis 2007;44:705–10.

24. Pasternack MS, Swartz MN. Myositis and myonecrosis. In: Mandell GL, Bennett JE, Dolin R, editors. Mandell, Douglas, and Bennett's principles and practice of infectious diseases. Philadelphia: Churchill Livingstone; 2010. p. 1313–22.

25. Munford RS, Suffredini AF. Sepsis, severe sepsis, and septic shock. In: Mandell GL, Bennett JE, Dolin R, editors. Mandell, Douglas, and Bennett's principles and practice of infectious diseases. Philadelphia: Churchill Livingstone; 2010. p. 987–1010.

26. Freifield AG, Ej Bow, Sepkowitz KA, et al. Clinical practice guideline for the use of antimicrobial agents in neutropenic patients with cancer: 2010 update by the Infectious Diseases Society of America. Clin Infect Dis 2011;52:e56–93.

27. Centers for Disease Control and Prevention (CDC). Availability and use of parenteral quinidine gluconate for severe or complicated malaria. MMWR Morb Mortal Wkly Rep 2000;49:1138–40.

28. Centers for Disease Control and Prevention (CDC). Effects of new penicillin susceptibility breakpoints for *Streptococcus pneumoniae*—United States, 2006-2007. MMWR Morb Mortal Wkly Rep 2008;57:1353–7.

29. Musher DM. *Streptococcus pneumoniae*. In: Mandell GL, Bennett JE, Dolin R, editors. Mandell, Douglas, and Bennett's principles and practice of infectious diseases. Philadelphia: Churchill Livingstone; 2010. p. 2623–42.

30. Yok-Ai Q, Moreillon P. *Staphylococcus aureus* (including staphylococcal toxic shock). In: Mandell GL, Bennett JE, Dolin R, editors. Mandell, Douglas, and Bennett's principles and practice of infectious diseases. Philadelphia: Churchill Livingstone; 2010. p. 2543–78.

31. Liu C, Bayer A, Cosgrove SE, et al. Clinical practice guidelines by the Infectious Disease Society of America for the treatment of methicillin-resistant *Staphylococcus aureus* infections in adults and children. Clin Infect Dis 2011;52:1–38.

32. Arias CA, Murray BE. *Enterococcus* species, *Streptococcus bovis* group, and *Leuconostoc* species. In: Mandell GL, Bennett JE, Dolin R, editors. Mandell, Douglas, and Bennett's principles and practice of infectious diseases. Philadelphia: Churchill Livingstone; 2010. p. 2642–53.

33. Pier GB, Ramphal R. *Pseudomonas aeruginosa*. In: Mandell GL, Bennett JE, Dolin R, editors. Mandell, Douglas, and Bennett's principles and practice of infectious diseases. Philadelphia: Churchill Livingstone; 2010. p. 2835–60.

34. Bergman SJ, Speil C, Short M, et al. Pharmacokinetic and pharmacodynamic aspects of antibiotic use in high-risk populations. Infect Dis Clin North Am 2007;21:821–46.

35. Stratton CW. Serum bactericidal test. Clin Microbiol Rev 1988;1:19–26.

Endocrine and Metabolic Changes During Sepsis: An Update

Romesh Khardori, MD, PhD[a,b,*], Danielle Castillo, MD[a]

KEYWORDS

- Hyperglycemia • Adrenal insufficiency • Thyroid dysfunction • Glucocorticoids
- Insulin • Hypoglycemia

KEY POINTS

- Strict glycemic control need not be stringent.
- Mineralocorticoid use does not modify outcome.
- Thyroid dysfunction does not require treatment.
- Fluid and electrolyte abnormalities must be corrected.
- Aggressive management of sepsis with appropriate and judicious use of antibiotics remains a top priority.
- Use of glucocorticoids in persistently hypotensive and vasopressin-dependent patients appears to be beneficial.

INTRODUCTION

Stress of critical illness/sepsis brings about several and serious changes in hormonal concentrations and metabolism that become difficult to interpret and manage. Some of the changes are adaptive to accommodate stress and protect tissues from catabolic breakdown. Others are the consequence of the impact of factors such as toxins and cytokines released during stress related to infection/sepsis. Alternatively, changes may be the consequence of treatments such as antifungal therapy, particularly in immunocompromised patients.

Sepsis is one of the most stressful situations encountered by humans and animals alike. Sepsis-related stress is not only acute in onset but also is sustained until the incriminating source has been eliminated. Stress-related endocrine/metabolic changes reflect this temporal profile. Ordinarily responses may be choreographed based on degree of stress, and if the stress remains unabated a metabolic chaos

[a] Division of Endocrinology and Metabolism, Department of Internal Medicine, Strelitz Diabetes Institute for Endocrine and Metabolic Disorders, Eastern Virginia Medical School, 855 West Brambleton Avenue, Norfolk, VA 23510, USA; [b] Endocrinology Fellowship Training Program, Division of Endocrinology and Metabolism, Department of Internal Medicine, Strelitz Diabetes Center for Endocrine and Metabolic Disorders, Eastern Virginia Medical School, 855 West Brambleton Avenue, Norfolk, VA 23510, USA
* Corresponding author.
E-mail address: khardoRK@evms.edu

Med Clin N Am 96 (2012) 1095–1105
http://dx.doi.org/10.1016/j.mcna.2012.09.005
0025-7125/12/$ – see front matter © 2012 Elsevier Inc. All rights reserved.

may set in, placing a patient in harm's way. Stress comprises a set of complex biological perturbations imposed by aggression on the body's defense systems. Two systems, the endocrine and autonomic nervous systems, provide mechanisms to provide rapid adaptation thus maintaining homeostasis. This concept has been further expanded by the introduction of the term allostasis by Sterling and Eyer[1] in 1988. In attempting to explain how the cardiovascular system adjusts to the changing state of body, this paradigm can be easily applied to other concurrent systems undergoing resetting such as the hypothalamo-pituitary-adrenal (HPA) axis and the hypothalamo-pituitary-thyroid (HPT) axis. Humans try to cope with stress through modulation of the autonomic nervous system, neuroendocrine axis, and the metabolic and immune systems. When stress abates rapidly, these systems come into quick equilibration with the prestress state. However, unrelenting stress leads to decompensation and breakdown of these systems, with development of a pathologic illness. When there is repeated stress, a certain degree of wear and tear is to be expected. This phenomenon is now referred to as allostatic load, resulting from repeated cycles of allostasis.

In situations such as sepsis, the rapidity with which an organism must respond depends on genetic, developmental, and experiential factors. This aspect would explain some of the differences often reported in cohorts of people for whom such factors may not have been considered. However, in general most patients exhibit a predictable response during acute stress of sepsis. It must be noted that activation of neuroendocrine and autonomic nervous system responses is an energy-consuming process, and the robustness of a response is determined by energy stores and availability of energy (nutrients) to tissues facing the brunt of stress. Thus in patients in a dysglycemic state, such as diabetes mellitus, tissues may still be starving in the face of concurrent insulinopenia or insulin resistance even though there might be surfeit of energy (glucose) in circulation.

Specific Neuroendocrine and Metabolic Perturbations
1. Activation and depression of HPA axis
2. Biphasic vasopressin secretory response
3. Hyperglycemia/dysglycemia
4. Depression of pituitary-thyroid
5. Depression of gonadotropins and hypogonadism
6. Disorders of Na/K balance, hypophosphatemia, hypocalcaemia, and hypomagnesaemia.

PITUITARY-ADRENAL AXIS IN SEPSIS

During infection several factors collude together; for example, viral and bacterial products such as bacterial lipopolysaccharides (LPS) cause release of cytokines from immune cells that then travel to the brain. In addition, LPS may induce cytokines such as interleukin (IL)-1 within the neurons in the brain. Cytokines can freely diffuse into pituitary because of the absence of the blood-brain barrier. Several cytokines are produced by glial cells as well as IL-1, IL-2, and IL-6.[2] There is evidence for expression of anti-inflammatory mediators such as IL-1 receptor antagonist, IL-10, and IL-13 in pituitary and pineal glands. These cytokines possibly antagonize the effects of proinflammatory mediators on neurohormones.[3] IL-2, by stimulation of cholinergic neurons, leads to activation of nitric oxide (NO) synthase and release of NO. NO diffuses into corticotropin-releasing hormone (CRH)-secreting neurons, and releases CRH.[4] Cytokines are capable of directly acting on the pituitary to stimulate synthesis and release of corticotropin (formerly adrenocorticotropic hormone).[5] The neural axis independently also participates in the activation of CRH release via interaction with cholinergic interneurons in the parvocellular nucleus.[6] In general, the magnitude of HPA-axis activation is proportional to the severity of stress. Rising cortisol levels have a significant impact on immunomodulation and preservation of vascular reactivity to circulating catecholamines. Cortisol is important in maintaining vascular reactivity to norepinephrine, and is important in preserving perfusion to vital organs. As the stress of sepsis progresses there is blunting of HPA activation, leading to transient or permanent adrenal insufficiency in critically ill subjects.[7]

During critical illnesses such as sepsis, adrenal hypofunction can result from overwhelming destruction of adrenal glands themselves (bleeding/ischemic necrosis or Waterhouse-Friderichsen syndrome). Often the presenting signs are hemodynamic instability and persistent hypotension, and a petechial/purpuric rash. This syndrome is complicated by hypoglycemia, hyponatremia, and hyperkalemia. It is a medical emergency and needs to be treated urgently with antibiotics and hydrocortisone.

In less severe forms of HPA-axis infection pattern, activation followed by hypocortisolemia may be seen. In all patients with sepsis-persistent hypotension, hypoglycemia, hyponatremia, and hyperkalemia should be treated as adrenal insufficiency unless proved otherwise.

Much controversy surrounds what constitutes biochemical hypoadrenalism. This debate has also brought attention to the so-called relative or functional hypoadrenalism of critical illness, usually unaccompanied by any structural insult to the HPA axis. Theoretically it is possible that circulating cytokines and other inflammatory products may lead to suppression of corticotropin production/release and consequent hypocortisolemia. Alternatively, some mediators may lead to a state of peripheral glucocorticoid resistance.[7]

Ordinarily, stress imposed by sepsis itself should serve the function of a dynamic test to assess adrenal response. However, objections have been raised based on total cortisol measurement being less reliable than measurement of free cortisol.[8] In a later study it was found that even though free cortisol could be used to diagnose adrenal insufficiency in sepsis, free cortisol was not superior to total cortisol levels despite theoretical advantages.[9] The argument put forth to use free plasma cortisol is based on observed reductions in plasma albumin and cortisol-binding globulin (CBG) during critical illness (these normally bind 20% and 70% of cortisol, respectively). Another difficulty with diagnosing adrenal insufficiency arises from the lack of uniform diagnostic cutoffs for plasma cortisol levels.

Interest in using glucocorticoids in infections in not new, actually dating back to 1940 when Perla and Marmorston[10] demonstrated beneficial effects of such therapy in infections such as malaria and pneumonia. The use of steroids has seen ups and downs. In a review of glucocorticoid use at supraphysiologic doses in unselected patients with sepsis, no favorable effect on morbidity and mortality was seen.[11] More recently, however, using the cosyntropin stimulation test (CST) in patients with septic shock, relative adrenal insufficiency has been better defined as lack of incremental increase in plasma cortisol of less than 9 μg/dL following standard high-dose CST.[12] In a study of 300 patients with septic shock, use of hydrocortisone (50 mg intravenously every 6 hours) plus fludrocortisones (50 μg by mouth daily) for 7 days, a significant reduction in mortality and duration of vasopressin therapy was demonstrated.[13] The best evidence from which to draw definitive conclusions is still elusive. In a more recent randomized trial in adult patients with septic shock, addition of fludrocortisone did not result in statistically significant improvement in in-hospital mortality. Furthermore, use of hydrocortisone at a dose of 50 mg every 6 hours was associated with higher basal blood glucose levels.[14] It can, however, be inferred that corticosteroid therapy will most likely benefit patients in severe septic shock (blood pressure <90 mm Hg, no response to fluid resuscitation, and vasopressin administration). It should preferably be started within 8 hours of the onset of shock. Impact of drugs often used in seriously ill patients (etomidate, ketoconazole and phenytoin) must lead one to interpret dynamic testing with caution because of the impact of such drugs on glucocorticoid synthesis. Commonly used laboratory tests may be unreliable because of cross-reactivity with other steroids.

Finally, adrenal dysfunction in septic shock may represent a sick euadrenal state rather than true adrenocortical insufficiency, and should be treated as such.[15] It is quite possible that end-organ sensitivity to corticotropin and glucocorticoids itself may be altered to protect against tissue wasting under catabolic states. This position is supported by the evidence of the glucocorticoid receptor being a target for toxins related to bacterial infection.[16]

IMPACT OF INFECTION/SEPSIS ON OTHER PITUITARY HORMONES

- The key impact of sepsis is on blocking release of luteinizing hormone–releasing hormone, thereby affecting release of luteinizing hormone; this may in part be accomplished by stimulation of γ-aminobutyric acid neurons and β-endorphins.[17–19]
- Growth hormone levels are initially elevated, with concurrent peripheral resistance leading to low levels of insulin-like growth factor 1. However, this state transitions then to a state of low growth hormone, depending on the duration of critical illness.[20,21]
- Initially the prolactin levels are increased, and these drop off as stress enters the chronic phase.[22]
- Vasopressin levels are almost always increased at the initial stage of septic shock, and decline thereafter.[23]

Implications of these findings for possible targets for therapy need to be carefully considered. When growth hormone therapy was instituted in critically ill adult patients to decrease catabolism, increased mortality was seen.[24] Despite observed low levels of vasopressin, no cases of sepsis-related diabetes insipidus are reported in adults. Rarely cases of diabetes insipidus (central) have been reported in neonates with sepsis.[25]

SEPSIS AND GLUCOSE METABOLISM

During infection and critical illness hyperglycemia is a common occurrence, and it has generated much heated debate. Hyperglycemia is seen even in those not previously diagnosed to have diabetes. Hyperglycemia is indeed one of the most striking metabolic derangements seen with sepsis, and has been independently associated with increased mortality in patients with undiagnosed diabetes.[26] Critically ill patients with known diabetes fare better than those who present with hyperglycemia without known diabetes. This phenomenon, referred to as the diabetes paradox, remains of heightened interest.[27] Given the understanding that sepsis is associated with activation of overwhelming production of both proinflammatory and anti-inflammatory mediators, a serious impact on glucose stability is not unexpected.[28] Hyperglycemia is largely a consequence of lipolysis and muscle glycolysis associated temporally with hepatic glycogenolysis and neoglucogenesis. In the state of shock this is further augmented by muscle lactate released into circulation being used by the liver to produce glucose (the Cori cycle).[29] Furthermore, all of this is happening in the setting of insulin resistance mediated through actions of counterregulatory hormones (catecholamines, cortisol, growth hormone, and so forth), and numerous cytokines affecting actions of insulin through mechanisms involving insulin receptor and postreceptor signaling. Hyperglycemia is a marker of severity of illness and is a predictor of poor outcome.[30] Hyperglycemia impairs the host's ability to combat infection through an adverse impact on innate immunity, leading to reduced chemotaxis and phagocytosis, formation of reactive oxygen species, increased concentration of proinflammatory cytokines IL-1, IL-6, and tumor necrosis factor (TNF)-α, and impairment in the generation of endothelial NO.[31,32] Severe sepsis remains a major cause of mortality in critically sick patients.[33] The Surviving Sepsis Campaign Guidelines recommend a glycemic target of below150 mg/dL.[34] Undoubtedly, attention needs to be paid simultaneously to managing infections/sepsis through emergent, judicious, effective use of antibiotics (and drainage of abscesses/debridement of necrotic tissue where possible), and effective glucose control.

The rigor and extent of glycemic control has been a matter of great interest and study. In a ground-breaking article published in 2001 by Van den Bergh and colleagues[35] in the setting of the surgical intensive care unit (ICU), marked improvements in survival, length of hospital stay, bloodstream infections, acute renal failure requiring dialysis or hemofiltration, number of red blood cell transfusions, and critical illness neuropathy were reported when intensive insulin therapy was used to maintain blood glucose at or below 110 mg/dL. In another study by the same authors in the medical ICU setting, mortality with intensive insulin therapy was increased if the patient spent less than 3 days in the ICU.[36] In those who stayed for more than 3 days, improvements in morbidity were noted. While Van den Bergh and associates continued to promote the advantages of tight glycemic control (glucose level <110 mg/dL), several other subsequent studies have concluded that tight glycemic control as defined by Van den Bergh's group does not reduce the hospital mortality significantly, and is associated with a significant risk of hypoglycemia. The German Multicenter Efficacy of Volume Substitutions and Insulin Therapy in Severe Sepsis (VISEP) Study of Intensive Insulin Therapy (IIT) for septic patients in multidisciplinary ICUs was stopped prematurely because of a higher risk of hypoglycemia (17.0% vs 4.1% in intensified treatment group).[37] A much larger and long awaited study, the NICE-SUGAR (Normoglycemia in Intensive Care Evaluation—Survival Using Glucose Algorithm Regulation) trial, showed that intensive glucose control increased mortality in adults in the ICU.[38] This study further concluded that a blood glucose target of 180 mg/dL or less resulted in lower mortality than seen with a target of 81 to 108 mg/dL. The mean difference of blood glucose levels for 2 treatment groups was 29 mg/dL. Furthermore, severe hypoglycemia was noted more frequently in the intensified insulin-treated groups. No difference was seen between groups in terms of corticosteroid therapy, length of stay in the ICU, length of stay in hospital, need for renal replacement therapy, or duration of mechanical ventilation.

The meta-analysis by Wiener and colleagues[39] concluded that tight glycemic control does not lead to reduced hospital mortality, but rather results in a significantly increased risk of hypoglycemia. A subsequent meta-analysis of 29 randomized trials came to similar conclusions.[40] These developments lead to revised recommendations in 2009 by the Surviving Sepsis Campaign Guidelines Committee Subgroup for glucose control. It was recommended that teams seeking to implement glucose control should consider initiating insulin therapy when blood glucose levels exceed 180 mg/dL with a goal blood glucose approximating 150 mg/dL, as was observed in the beneficial arm of NICE-SUGAR trial (posted on the Surviving Sepsis Campaign Web site and list server 6/12/2009).

Patients who are critically ill remain at high risk for hypoglycemia, and these patients also remain at greater risk of death.[41] Hypoglycemia remains a strong limitation in intensified insulin treatment strategies. A carbohydrate-restrictive strategy with the aim of maintaining blood glucose levels less than 180 mg/dL, ideally less than 150 mg/dL, receiving regular insulin subcutaneously 4 times daily, when compared with intensified insulin treatment with insulin infusion targeting glucose between 80 and 120 mg/dL, revealed a 5-fold reduction in the incidence of hypoglycemia. No difference in mortality and morbidity was reported.[42] However, this finding remains to be verified in larger trials. For now, intensified insulin therapy implies a formidable risk for hypoglycemia. Sepsis further enhances the risk for hypoglycemia and glycemic variability.[43] Krinsley and Grover[44] indicated that even a single episode of hypoglycemia increased the risk of mortality. Several factors predisposing to hypoglycemia have been reported.[44,45]

1. Sepsis
2. Insulin use
3. Continuous renal replacement therapy with bicarbonate based substitution fluid
4. Diabetes
5. Nutritional decrease without adjustment for insulin use
6. Inotropic support

At present, evidence supports a glycemic target between 140 and 180 mg/dL for most of the patients admitted to ICUs without a prior history of diabetes mellitus.[46] To avoid hypoglycemia and also to achieve the recommended target, frequent bedside glucose monitoring becomes essential. Several factors may confound results in a critically sick patient, and these must be taken into account:

1. Source of sample (capillary, venous blood, whole blood)
2. State of peripheral perfusion (vasoconstriction/vasospasticity)
3. Speed of sample processing
4. Amount of blood sample (when using strips)
5. Substances interfering with glucose measurement (L-dopa, aspirin, mannitol, acetaminophen, maltose, icodextrin, ascorbic acid); the effects vary with the methodology used in bedside glucose monitoring[47,48]

Mechanisms of beneficial effects of glycemic control in sepsis remain of considerable interest, and include the direct anti-inflammatory role of insulin, the inhibitory effect of insulin on glycogen synthase kinase 3β, and reductions in inflammatory response mediated through advanced glycation end-product and receptor for advanced glycation end-product.[49] Interesting new directions are being pursued to facilitate glucose control in sepsis, including use of a cytokine-absorbing hemofilter (made from polymethylmethacrylate [PMMA]) for continuous hemodiafiltration (CHDF). In patients with hypercytokinemia (IL-6 blood level >10,000 pg/mL), blood glucose management became easier once the level of cytokines was lowered with PMMA-CHDF.[50] Modulation of glucose use and gluconeogenesis in sepsis with adrenergic β-receptor blockade has been proposed.[51]

HYPOTHALAMO-PITUITARY-THYROID AXIS IN SEPSIS/STRESS

Critical illness such as sepsis is often associated with alterations in thyroid hormone concentrations. A vast body of literature has evolved, but its clinical significance remains elusive. This state of abnormalities in thyroid function tests is often referred to as low T3 syndrome, euthyroid sick syndrome, or nonthyroidal illness syndrome

(NTIS). It has been debated whether changes in the HPT axis reflect an adaptive response or a pathologic state that requires hormone replacement.

The initial and most commonly observed abnormality is a decrease in total triiodothyronine (total T3) concentration secondary to a block in the action of type 1 deiodinase (5'-monodeiodinase) that catalyzes conversion of thyroxin (T4) in the periphery to T3 (type 1 deiodinase is located in the kidney, liver, and muscle). Several factors have been proposed as possible candidates involved in reducing 5'-deiodinase activity (hypocaloric state, endogenous or exogenous glucocorticoids, high-dose propranolol, free fatty acids, iodinated contrasts, amiodarone, and cytokines such as TNF, IL-6, interferon-α, and nuclear factor κB).[52,53] While total T3 levels are reduced, thyroxin conversion to reverse T3 (rT3) still occurs. However, because 5'-deiodinase is a downstream enzyme for degradation of rT3, reduction in its activity leads to a significant accumulation of rT3.

The typical progression of abnormalities is an initial low total T3 followed by a drop in total T4 (caused by a decrease in thyroxin-binding globulin [TBG]) as well as a reduction in its binding affinity; or inhibition of binding caused by other mediators such as circulating cytokines, or drugs such as salicylates, phenytoin furosemide, and carbamazepine. Some drugs accelerate clearance of T4, thereby effectively reducing its circulating levels (antiseizure medications, rifampin). Despite reductions in total T3 and T4 levels, free hormone levels remain normal initially. These levels should be interpreted with caution, because of the impact of binding protein abnormalities that may result in both overestimation and underestimation of free hormone levels, owing to changes in binding protein concentrations.[54] Even though free T4 measurement by equilibrium dialysis is the most touted and trusted, this technique is also prone to spurious results. An interesting in vitro phenomenon, the heparin effect, may lead to spurious increases in free T4. Heparin induces lipase activity in the blood, leading to the generation of free fatty acids that then displace T4 from binding sites on the TBG.[55]

Parallel with decreases in serum T4 concentrations, there is a decline in pituitary secretion of thyrotropin. Again, this can be multifactorial (magnitude of illness, suppression from glucocorticoids, caloric deprivation [importantly carbohydrates], use of medications such as dopamine, cytokines, and compromise of the biological activity of the TSH molecule due to glycosylation).[56–60]

Recently, the mechanisms behind hormonal changes seen in the NTIS have become somewhat clearer. Defects can be traced to effects of malnutrition and reduced leptin, leading to decreased thyrotropin-releasing hormone (TRH) and enhanced D2 deiodinase (tancyte) activity because of sepsis/inflammation causing local generation of more T3, leading to reductions in TRH secretions at the level of the hypothalamus. Cytokines elaborated during sepsis also directly suppresses TSH release. Defects in thyroid hormone binding proteins occur due to changes in quantity, affinity, and binding inhibition, as discussed earlier. Defects in tissue transport activity and changes in intracellular deiodination exist as well. Furthermore, alterations (depression) in nuclear thyroid hormone receptors and coactivators have been suggested. A recent review discusses these mechanisms in detail.[61]

Unless there is strong suspicion of primary thyroid disease (preexisting conditions and strong clinical evidence such as hypothermia, bradycardia, dry skin, and effusion in serosal spaces), treatment is not warranted.[62]

HYPOGONADISM OF SYSTEMIC ILLNESS

Hypogonadism has been associated with systemic acute and chronic illness. Acute systemic stress as seen in sepsis is indeed associated with marked and sharp reductions.[63] Acute central hypogonadism occurs with acute illness in both genders, and is evident within 24 to 48 hours.[64]

Suppression of the hypothalamo-pituitary gonadal axis is proportional to the severity of illness in critically ill patients. There is no established role for the treatment of critically ill patients with sex steroids.[65] Gonadotropin suppression is consequent to reduction in pulsatility of the gonadotropin-releasing hormone (GnRH) pulse generator. This process may be due to an increase in glucocorticoids/administration of glucocorticoids, hyperprolactinemia (stress or drug related), use of opioids, or possible inflammation-related reduction in kisspeptin and decreased responsiveness to it.[66] Exact implication of acute hypogonadism is far from clear. Restoration of the axis can be seen following administration of GnRH, verifying the hypothalamus as the dominant site for the downregulated axis.

ELECTROLYTE DISTURBANCES IN CRITICALLY ILL PATIENTS

Fluid and electrolyte disturbances in acutely ill patients with sepsis are common. Volume resuscitation in a volume-depleted septic patient is of paramount importance. Changes seen in electrolytes may be a consequence of sepsis/disease itself or result from use of medication such as antibiotics, antifungal agents, vasopressors, or a host of other medications used in septic sick patients. Practically any abnormality may be seen:

1. Hyponatremia/hypernatremia
2. Hypocalcemia/hypercalcemia
3. Hyperkalemia/hypokalemia
4. Hypophosphatemia/hyperphosphatemia
5. Hypomagnesaemia/hypomagnesaemia (less common).[67–69]

SUMMARY

The authors have reviewed the most recent and relevant literature from which reasonable conclusions may be drawn. This article highlights important endocrine and metabolic changes, and provides possible explanations for observed perturbations. Obviously infectious disease specialists are not charged with the primary responsibility of addressing these issues, which have largely remained the domain of endocrinologists and intensivists. However, infectious disease specialists use a variety of drugs that can contribute to these abnormalities. Therefore, a constant dialogue between specialists would enhance the quality of care and also contribute immensely to favorable outcomes.

REFERENCES

1. Sterling D, Eyer J. Allostasis: a new paradigm to explain arousal pathology. In: Fisher S, Reason J, editors. Handbook of life stress-cognition and health, vol. 34. New York: John Wiley & Sons; 1988. p. 629–49.
2. Koenig JI. Presence of cytokines in the hypothalamic-pituitary axis. Prog Neuro-endocrinoimmunol 1991;4:143–53.
3. Wong ML, Bongiorno PB, Rettori V, et al. Interleukin (IL) 1b, IL-1 receptor antagonist, IL-10, and IL113 gene expression in the central nervous system and anterior pituitary during systemic inflammation: Pathophysiological implications. Proc Natl Acad Sci U S A 1997;93:23–232.
4. McCann SM, Kimura M, Karanth S, et al. Ann NY Acad. Sci 2000;917:4–18.

5. Rettori V, Dels WL, Hiney JK, et al. An interleukin-1 alpha like neuronal system in the pre-optic-hypothalamic region and its induction by bacterial liposaccharide in concentration which alter pituitary hormone release. Neuroimmunomodulation 1997;1:251–8.

6. Karanth S, Lyson K, McCann SM. Role of nitric oxide in interleukin 2 induced corticotrophin-releasing factor release on incubated hypothalami. Proc Natl Acad Sci U S A 1993;90:3383–7.

7. Cooper MS, Stewart PM. Corticosteroid insufficiency in acutely ill patients. N Engl J Med 2003;348:727–34.

8. Hamrahian AH, Oseri TS, Arafah BM. Measurement of serum free cortisol in critically ill patients. N Engl J Med 2004;350:1629–38.

9. Annane D, Maxime V, Ibrahim F, et al. Diagnosis of adrenal insufficiency in severe sepsis and septic shock. Am J Respir Crit Care Med 2006;174:1319–26.

10. Perla D, Marmorston J. Suprarenal cortical hormone and salt in treatment of pneumonia and other severe infection. Endocrinology 1940;27:367–74.

11. Cronin L, Cook DJ, Carlet J, et al. Corticosteroid treatment for sepsis: a critical appraisal and meta-analysis of literature. Crit Care Med 1995;23:1430–9.

12. Annane D, Sebille V, Troche G, et al. A 3-level prognostic classification in septic shock based on cortisol levels and cortisol response to corticotrophin. JAMA 2000;283:1038–45.

13. Annane D, Sebille V, Charpentier C, et al. Effect of treatment with low dose hydrocortisone and fludrocortisones on mortality in patients with septic shock. JAMA 2002;288:862–71.

14. The COIITSS Study Investigators. Corticosteroid treatment and intensive insulin therapy for septic shock in adults—a randomized controlled trial. JAMA 2010;303(4):341–8.

15. Venkatesh B, Cohen J. Adrenocortical (dys)function in septic shock—a sick euadrenal state. Best Pract Res Clin Endocrinol Metab 2011;25:719–33.

16. Weber Marketon JI, Sternberg EM. The glucocorticoid receptor: a revisited target for toxins. Toxins (Basel) 2010;2:1359–80.

17. Seilicovich A, Duvilanski BH, Pisera D, et al. Nitric oxide inhibits hypothalamic luteinizing hormone releasing hormone release by releasing γ-aminobutyric acid. Proc Natl Acad Sci U S A 1995;92:3421–4.

18. Faleti AG, Mastonardi CA, Lominczi A. Beta-endorphin blocks luteinizing hormone-releasing hormone release by inhibiting the nitricoxidergic pathway controlling its release. Proc Natl Acad Sci U S A 1999;96:1722–6.

19. Kimura M, Yu WH, Rettori U, et al. Granulocyte-macrophage colony stimulating factor suppresses LHRH release by inhibition of nitric oxide synthase and stimulation of γ-aminobutyric acid release. Neuroimmunomodulation 1997;4:237–43.

20. Van den Bergh GH. The neuroendocrine stress response and modern intensive care: the concept revisited. Burns 1999;25:7–16.

21. Van den Bergh GH, Wouters P, Weekers F, et al. Reactivation of pituitary hormone release and metabolic improvement by infusion of growth hormone releasing peptides and thyrotropin-releasing hormone in patients with protracted illness. J Clin Endocrinol Metab 1999;84:788–91.

22. Van den Bergh G, de Zegher F, Veldhuis JD, et al. Thyrotropin and prolactin release in prolonged critical illness: dynamics of spontaneous secretion and effect of growth hormone secretagogues. Clin Endocrinol (Oxf) 1997;47:599–612.

23. Sharshar T, Blanchard A, Paillard M, et al. Circulating vasopressin in septic shock. Crit Care Med 2003;31(6):1752–8.

24. Takala J, Roukonen E, Webster NR, et al. Increased mortality associated with growth hormone treatment in critically ill adults. N Engl J Med 1999;341:785–92.

25. Jenkins HR, Hughes IA, Gray OP. Cranial diabetes insipidus in early infancy. Arch Dis Child 1988;63:434–5.

26. Umipierrez GE, Isaacs SD, Bazargan N, et al. Hyperglycemia: an independent marker of in-hospital mortality in patients with undiagnosed diabetes. J Clin Endocrinol Metab 2002;87:978–82.

27. Krinsley JS, Fisher M. The diabetes paradox: diabetes is not independently associated with mortality in critically ill patients. Hosp Pract (Minneap) 2012;40(2): 31–5.

28. Cinel I, Opal SM. Molecular biology of inflammation and sepsis: a primer. Crit Care Med 2009;37:291–304.

29. Levy B. Lactate and shock state: the metabolic view. Curr Opin Crit Care 2006;12: 315–21.

30. Taylor JH, Beilman GJ. Hyperglycemia in the intensive care unit: no longer just a marker of illness severity. Surg Infect (Larchmt) 2005;6:233–45.

31. Turina M, Fry DE, Polk HC Jr. Acute hyperglycemia and innate immune systems: clinical, cellular and molecular aspects. Crit Care Med 2005;33:1624–33.

32. Mizock BA. Alterations in fuel metabolism in critical illness hyperglycemia. Best Pract Res Clin Endocrinol Metab 2001;15:533–51.

33. Russell JA. Management of sepsis. N Engl J Med 2006;355:1699–713.

34. Dellinger RP, Levy MM, Carlet JM, et al. Surviving sepsis campaign: international guidelines for management of sepsis and septic shock: 2008. Crit Care Med 2008;36:296–327.

35. Van den Bergh G, Wouters P, Weekers F, et al. Intensive insulin therapy in critically ill patients. N Engl J Med 2001;345(19):1359–67.

36. Van den Bergh G, Wilmer A, Hermans G, et al. Intensive insulin therapy in the medical ICU. N Engl J Med 2006;354(5):449–61.

37. Brunkhorst FM, Engel C, Bloos F, et al. Intensive insulin therapy and pentastarch resuscitation in severe sepsis. N Engl J Med 2008;358:125–39.

38. Finfer S, Chittock DR, Su SY, et al. NICE-SUGAR study investigators. Intensive versus conventional glucose control in critically ill patients. N Engl J Med 2009; 360:1283–97.

39. Wiener RS, Wiener DC, Larson RJ. Benefits and risks of tight glucose control in critically ill adults: a meta-analysis. JAMA 2008;300:933–44.

40. Griesdale DE, de Souza RJ, Van Dam RM, et al. Intensive insulin therapy and mortality among critically ill patients: a meta-analysis including NICE-SUGAR study data. CMAJ 2009;180(8):821–7.

41. Egi M, Belloma R, Stachowski E, et al. Hypoglycemia and outcomes in critically ill patients. Mayo Clin Proc 2010;85(3):217–24.

42. de Azevedo JR, de Araujo LO, da Silva WS. A carbohydrate-restrictive strategy is safer and as efficient as intensive insulin therapy in critically ill patients. J Crit Care 2010;25:84–9.

43. Walschle RM, Morer O, Hilgers R, et al. The impact of the severity of sepsis on the risk of hypoglycemia and glycaemic variability. Crit Care 2008;12:R129.

44. Krinsley JS, Grover A. Severe hypoglycemia in critically ill patients: risk factors and outcomes. Crit Care Med 2007;35:2262–7.

45. Vriesendrop TM, Van Santen S, Devries JH, et al. Predisposing factors for hypoglycemia in intensive care unit. Crit Care Med 2006;34:96–101.

46. Farrokhi F, Smiley D, Umpierrez G. Glycemic control in non-diabetic critically ill patients. Best Pract Res Clin Endocrinol Metab 2011;25:813–24.

47. Dungan K, Chapman J, Braithwaite SS, et al. Glucose measurement confounding issues in setting target for in patient management. Diabetes Care 2007;30(2):403–9.

48. Fahy BG, Coursin DB. Critical glucose control: the devil is in the details. Mayo Clin Proc 2008;83:394–7.

49. Hirasawa H, Oda S, Nakamura M. Blood glucose control in patients with severe sepsis and septic shock. World J Gastroenterol 2009;15(33):4132–6.

50. Nakad T, Oda S, Matsuda K, et al. Continuous hemodiafiltration with PMMA hemofilters in the treatment of patients with septic shock. Mol Med 2008;14:257–63.

51. Novotny NM, Lahm T, Markel TA, et al. Beta blockers in sepsis: reexamining the evidence. Shock 2009;31:113–9.

52. Sakharova OV, Inzucchi S. Endocrine assessment in critical illness. Crit Care Clin 2007;23:467–90.

53. Economidou F, Douka E, Taznela M, et al. Thyroid function during critical illness. Hormones 2011;10(2):117–24.

54. Elkins R. Analytical measurements of free thyroxin. Clin Lab Med 1993;13:599–630.

55. Mendel CM, Kunitake ST, Cavalieri RR. Mechanism of heparin induced increase in the concentration of free thyroxin in plasma. J Clin Endocrinol Metab 1987;65: 1259–64.

56. Wehmann RE, Gregerman RI, Burns WH, et al. Suppression of thyrotropin in low thyroxin state of severe non-thyroidal illness. N Engl J Med 1985;312:546–52.

57. Faglia G, Ferrari C, Beck-Pecooz P. Reduced plasma thyrotropin response to thyrotropin releasing hormone after dexamethasone administration in normal subjects. Horm Metab Res 1973;5:289–92.

58. Van den Bergh G, de Zegher F, Lauwers P. Dopamine and sick euthyroid syndrome in critical illness. Clin Endocrinol (Oxf) 1994;41:731–7.

59. Papanicolaou DA. Euthyroid sick syndrome and role of cytokines. Rev Endocr Metab Disord 2000;1:43–8.

60. Lee HY, Suhl J, Pekary AE, et al. Secretion of thyrotropin with reduced concanavalin A-binding activity in patient with severe non-thyroid illness. J Clin Endocrinol Metab 1999;65:942–5.

61. Warner MH, Beckett GF. Mechanism behind non-thyroidal illness syndrome—an update. J Endocrinol 2010;205:1–13.

62. Adler SH, Wartofsky L. The non-thyroidal illness syndrome. Endocrinol Metab Clin North Am 2007;36(2):657–72.

63. Luppa P. Serum androgens in intensive care patients: correlations with clinical findings. Clin Endocrinol (Oxf) 1991;34(4):305–10.

64. Woolf PD. Transient hypo-gonadotropic hypogonadism caused by critical illness. J Clin Endocrinol Metab 1985;60(3):444–50.

65. Kalyani RR, Gavini S, Dobs AS. Male hypogonadism in systemic disease. Endocrinol Metab Clin North Am 2007;36:333–48.

66. Castellano JM, Bensten AH, Romero M, et al. Acute inflammation reduces kisspeptin immunoreactivity at the arcuate nucleus and decreases responsiveness to kisspeptin independently of it anorectic effects. Am J Physiol Endocrinol Metab 2010;229:E54–61.

67. Buckley MS, LeBlanc JM, Cawley MJ. Electrolyte disturbances associated with commonly prescribed medications in the intensive care unit. Crit Care Med 2010;38(Suppl 6):S253–64.

68. Lee JW. Fluid and electrolyte disturbances in critically ill patients. Electrolyte Blood Press 2010;8:72–81.

69. Limaye CS, Londhey VA, Nadkar MY, et al. Hypomagnesemia in critically ill medical patients. J Assoc Physicians India 2011;59:19–22.

Head and Neck Emergencies
Bacterial Meningitis, Encephalitis, Brain Abscess, Upper Airway Obstruction, and Jugular Septic Thrombophlebitis

Catherine J. Derber, MD*, Stephanie B. Troy, MD

KEYWORDS

- Meningitis • Encephalitis • Brain abscess • Epiglottitis • Ludwig angina
- Lemierre syndrome

KEY POINTS

- Head and neck infectious disease emergencies can be rapidly fatal without prompt recognition and treatment.
- Empiric intravenous (IV) antibiotics, tailored to the patient's age and predisposing factors, should be initiated immediately in any patient with suspected bacterial meningitis.
- IV acyclovir should be started immediately in any patient with suspected encephalitis.
- Surgical intervention in addition to prompt initiation of antibiotics is often necessary for brain abscesses, epiglottitis, and Ludwig angina.
- A high index of suspicion is needed to diagnose epiglottitis, Ludwig's angina, and Lemierre's syndrome.

BACTERIAL MENINGITIS

Bacterial meningitis carries a high morbidity and mortality, requiring emergent intervention and treatment. The classic triad associated with community-acquired bacterial meningitis (fever, neck stiffness, and altered mental status) is uncommon, appearing in less than half of patients in 1 study, although 95% of patients had at least 2 of the following 4 symptoms: headaches, fever, neck stiffness, or altered mental status.[1] Headache is the most common presentation in several reviews.[1–3] Additional symptoms seen in patients with community-acquired meningitis include nausea and vomiting, photophobia, and rash (most commonly in the setting of meningococcal meningitis).[2,4] Physical examination findings associated with meningitis, such as Kernig's sign and Brudzinski's sign, are typically not helpful in the diagnosis of meningitis.[2] Given the lack of consistency of clinical features, a high index of suspicion is the cornerstone of diagnosis.

Department of Internal Medicine, Division of Infectious Diseases, Eastern Virginia Medical School, Suite 572, 825 Fairfax Avenue, Norfolk, VA, USA
* Corresponding author.
E-mail address: derbercj@evms.edu

Med Clin N Am 96 (2012) 1107–1126
http://dx.doi.org/10.1016/j.mcna.2012.08.002
0025-7125/12/$ – see front matter © 2012 Elsevier Inc. All rights reserved.

medical.theclinics.com

Causes

In a review of 1670 cases of bacterial meningitis in the United States from 2003 to 2007, the most common pathogen was *Streptococcus pneumoniae* (58.0%), followed by group B streptococcus (18.1%), *Neisseria meningitidis* (13.9%), *Haemophilus influenzae* (6.7%), and *Listeria monocytogenes* (3.4%).[5] Bacterial meningitis secondary to *S pneumoniae* tends to be associated with a more severe clinical presentation and worse outcome.[1] Since the introduction of pneumococcal and *Haemophilus influenzae* type B (Hib) vaccinations, the rate of bacterial meningitis has decreased and the affected population has shifted toward adults.[5]

Nosocomial bacterial meningitis, defined as meningitis occurring within 2 to 6 days of admission, can be divided into 2 categories.[6] The first category includes patients with prior neurosurgical intervention or head trauma, and is most often associated with a cerebrospinal fluid (CSF) leak. In 1 review, the most common pathogen found in this category was *Staphylococcus aureus*.[6] The second category includes immunocompromised patients and individuals with a secondary bacterial meningitis from a distant infectious focus.

Recurrent meningitis is seen most commonly with prior neurosurgical trauma or surgery, especially in the setting of CSF leak.[4] Pathogens associated with certain predisposing factors are identified in **Table 1**.

Diagnostic Tests

The following diagnostic tests are important for the evaluation of bacterial meningitis:

- Lumbar puncture with opening pressure. CSF should be sent for:
  - Gram stain and culture
  - Cell count

Table 1
Specific pathogens more frequently seen associated with certain predisposing factors

Predisposing Factors	Bacterial Pathogens
Immunocompetent adult <50 y old	*Streptococcus pneumoniae, Neisseria meningitidis*
Immunocompetent adult >50 y old	*Streptococcus pneumoniae, Neisseria meningitidis, Listeria monocytogenes*, aerobic gram-negative bacilli
Immunocompromised adults	*Streptococcus pneumoniae, Neisseria meningitidis, Listeria monocytogenes*, aerobic gram-negative bacilli (including *Pseudomonas aeruginosa*)
Basilar skull fracture	*Streptococcus pneumoniae, Haemophilus influenzae*, group A streptococci
Penetrating head trauma or postneurosurgery	*Staphylococcus aureus*, coagulase-negative staphylococci, aerobic gram-negative bacilli (including *Pseudomonas aeruginosa*)
CSF shunt	Coagulase-negative staphylococci, *Staphylococcus aureus*, aerobic gram-negative rods (including *Pseudomonas aeruginosa*), *Propionibacterium acnes*

Adapted from Tunkel AR, Hartman BJ, Kaplan SL, et al. Practice guidelines for the management of bacterial meningitis. Clin Infect Dis 2004;39(9):1267–84; and Tunkel AR, van de Beek D, Scheld WM. Acute Meningitis. In: Mandell GL, Bennett JE, Dolin R, editors. Mandell, Douglas, and Bennett's principles and practice of infectious diseases, vol. 1(7). Philadelphia: Churchill Livingstone Elsevier; 2009:1190–93.

- o Glucose
- o Protein
- Two sets of blood cultures collected before initiation of antibiotics

Because of the risk of brain herniation during lumbar puncture in patients with intracranial masses, a computed tomography (CT) scan of the head should be obtained before lumbar puncture in any immunocompromised patient or any patient with papilledema, focal neurologic deficits, CSF shunts, history of hydrocephalus, or trauma.[7] Additional factors associated with an abnormal head CT include age 60 years or older and a seizure within 1 week of presentation.[3] If CT of the head is deemed necessary before a lumbar puncture, it is important to start antibiotics before imaging to avoid delays in treatment.[3,7]

A blood lactic acid level is useful in patients with suspected meningitis after a recent neurosurgical procedure. A level of 4.0 mmol/L or greater is more consistent with bacterial meningitis rather than aseptic postsurgical meningeal inflammation.[7]

Typical CSF findings associated with bacterial meningitis as well as fungal/tuberculous and viral meningitis are listed in **Table 2**.

Latex agglutination to detect capsular polysaccharides of bacterial pathogens may be useful in patients with a negative CSF Gram stain caused by prior antibiotic use, but in general, is not recommended because it does not seem to change treatment decision and false-positive results can occur.[7] Broad-range polymerase chain reaction (PCR) may allow rapid diagnosis of bacterial meningitis in patients with a negative CSF Gram stain and culture caused by prior antibiotics with a sensitivity of 100% and a specificity of 98.2%[9]; however, it is not readily available and the cost may be prohibitive.

Additional studies should be ordered if initial CSF findings suggest a nonbacterial meningitis or encephalitis, including CSF venereal disease research laboratory (VDRL) test, CSF PCR test for enteroviruses and herpes viruses, and CSF fungal stain/culture and stain/culture for mycobacteria. These tests are not included in this section given the focus on acute bacterial meningitis, but most of them are included in the section on diagnostic tests for encephalitis.

Treatment

The definitive treatment of bacterial meningitis depends on the isolated pathogen and antimicrobial sensitivities. In patients with negative CSF Gram stains and cultures, but

Table 2
Typical CSF findings associated with bacterial, fungal/tuberculous, and viral meningitis

Study	Bacterial Meningitis[8]	Fungal/Tuberculous Meningitis	Viral Meningitis/ Encephalitis
Opening Pressure	Increased (200–500 mm H_2O)	Often increased	Rarely increased
White blood cell count (cells/mm³)	1000–5000	10–500	10–500
Predominant cells	Neutrophils (>80%)	Lymphocytes (can be neutrophils early on)	Lymphocytes (can be neutrophils early on)
Glucose	Usually low (≤40 mg/dL)	Often low	Rarely low
Protein	Usually increased (100–500 mg/dL)	Moderately increased	Normal to slightly increased

with a high clinical suspicion for bacterial meningitis, treatment must be chosen based on the host presentation. Suggested initial presumptive antimicrobial regimens for adults with normal renal function are outlined in **Table 3**.

Antimicrobial resistance patterns are especially important when narrowing coverage for pneumococcal meningitis.[7] When the penicillin minimum inhibitory concentration (MIC) is less than 0.1 μg/mL, penicillin G or ampicillin is adequate. For a penicillin MIC of 0.1 to 1.0 μg/mL, a third-generation cephalosporin (such as ceftriaxone), cefepime, or meropenem is necessary. In cases in which the penicillin MIC is 2.0 μg/mL or greater or the cefotaxime/ceftriaxone MIC is 1.0 μg/mL or greater, a combination of vancomycin plus a third-generation cephalosporin should be used. Addition of rifampin should be considered when the ceftriaxone MIC is greater than 2 μg/mL.

Dexamethasone should be given at a dose of 0.15 mg/kg every 6 hours for the first 2 to 4 days of suspected pneumococcal meningitis.[7] The dexamethasone should be given only before or during the first dose of antibiotics, and it may be stopped if the Gram stain and cultures do not show *S pneumoniae*.[7] Early studies suggested that adjunctive dexamethasone, given 15 to 20 minutes before administration of antibiotics and continued for 4 days, significantly reduced the risk for adverse outcomes in patients with pneumococcal meningitis.[10] Use of dexamethasone may be most effective in adults older than 55 years, with increased central nervous system (CNS) inflammation (as suggested by an increased CSF protein level), and without prior receipt of antibiotics.[11]

Patients with suspected meningococcal meningitis should be placed on respiratory isolation for the first 24 hours of therapy, and close contacts should be treated prophylactically.[12]

A repeat lumbar puncture should be considered for patients who have not improved after 48 hours of appropriate antimicrobial therapy.[7] Neck stiffness seems to lag behind other signs of clinical improvement and may persist for more than 7 days.[4]

Table 3
Suggested initial presumptive antimicrobial regimens for adults with normal renal function

Predisposing Factors	Empiric Antibiotic Regimen
Immunocompetent adult <50 y old	Vancomycin 15 mg/kg IV every 8–every 12 h (for goal trough of 15–20) + ceftriaxone 2 g IV every 12 h
Adults older than 50 y	Above + ampicillin 2 g IV every 4 h (for coverage of *Listeria monocytogenes*)
Immunocompromised adults	Vancomycin + ampicillin + either ceftazidime 2 g IV every 8 h, cefepime 2 g IV every 8 h, or meropenem 2 g IV every 8 h (for coverage of aerobic gram-negative rods, including *Pseudomonas aeruginosa*)
Basilar skull fracture	Vancomycin + ceftriaxone
Penetrating head trauma or postneurosurgery	Vancomycin + either ceftazidime, cefepime, or meropenem
CSF shunt	Above + consider addition of intraventricular antibiotics

Adapted from Tunkel AR, Hartman BJ, Kaplan SL, et al. Practice guidelines for the management of bacterial meningitis. Clin Infect Dis 2004;39(9):1267–84; and Tunkel AR, van de Beek D, Scheld WM. Acute Meningitis. In: Mandell GL, Bennett JE, Dolin R, editors. Mandell, Douglas, and Bennett's principles and practice of infectious diseases, vol. 1(7). Philadelphia: Churchill Livingstone Elsevier; 2009:1211–14.

The duration of antibiotics depends on the organism isolated and should be extended if necessary based on the patient's clinical response.[7] Current guidelines suggest a minimum of 7 days for *N meningitidis* or *H influenzae*, 10 to 14 days for *S pneumoniae,* 14 to 21 days for *Streptococcus agalactiae,* and 21 days for aerobic gram-negative bacilli or *L monocytogenes.*

Prognosis

The mortality associated with bacterial meningitis is high. In an analysis of adults with acute bacterial meningitis treated at Massachusetts General Hospital from 1962 to 1988,[4] the mortality for a single episode of community-acquired bacterial meningitis was 25%; factors associated with a significantly increased mortality were age greater than 60 years, obtunded mental status on admission, and onset of seizures within 24 hours of admission. In another review of adult meningitis cases in the Netherlands from 1998 to 2002,[1] the overall mortality was 21%, but increased to 30% in cases of pneumococcal meningitis. One recent study of bacterial meningitis cases in the United States from 1998 to 2007,[5] showed an overall case fatality rate of 16.4% in adults with bacterial meningitis, with mortality increasing linearly with age.

Survivors can also have significant morbidity. In 1 review, cognitive impairment was greatest in the first few years after meningitis, particularly with pneumococcal meningitis, but then improved slowly over the following decade.[13] In a meta-analysis of bacterial meningitis articles published from 1980 to 2008, the most common complications were hearing loss, followed by seizures, cognitive impairment, hydrocephalus, and visual deficits.[14] Multiple impairments were cited in almost 20% of cases.[14]

ENCEPHALITIS

Encephalitis is defined as an inflammation of the brain associated with clinical signs of neurologic dysfunction. Similar to meningitis, with which there is often overlap, classic presenting symptoms include the triad of fever, headache, and altered level of consciousness. Some patients with encephalitis also display acute cognitive dysfunction, behavioral changes, focal neurologic deficits, or seizures.[15]

Causes

An underlying cause for encephalitis is identified in only about one-third of cases. When the cause is determined, viruses are most often the culprit (accounting for two-thirds of cases with known cause). Less commonly, encephalitis can be caused by bacteria, prions, parasites, fungi, or noninfectious causes (such as acute disseminated encephalomyelitis [ADEM], which is an autoimmune process that can occur after an infection or vaccination).[15]

The possible causes of encephalitis vary based on season of the year, location, travel history, vaccination history, immune function of the host, and exposure to different animals, animal products, and insects. The most common cause of nonepidemic acute encephalitis in the United States is herpes simplex virus (HSV), which is also one of the only causes for which there is effective treatment.[16] Japanese encephalitis virus is the most common cause of acute encephalitis worldwide, causing 30,000 to 50,000 cases and 10,000 to 15,000 deaths annually, but it is limited to Asia and parts of Australia.[17] West Nile virus, which first spread to North America in 1999, caused the largest outbreak of arboviral encephalitis in US history in 2002 to 2003, with approximately 3000 cases per year.[18]

Diagnostic Tests

Any patient with suspected encephalitis should be evaluated promptly with neuroimaging and a lumbar puncture. Brain magnetic resonance imaging (MRI) is preferred over CT because it is more sensitive and specific.[15] Neuroimaging is necessary to rule out mass lesions such as brain abscess, which may present with similar symptoms and require surgical intervention. In addition, characteristic patterns on neuroimaging can suggest a specific cause; bilateral temporal lobe involvement is often seen with HSV encephalitis, and multifocal enhancing signal abnormalities in the subcortical white matter $\pm$ gray matter suggest ADEM.[15] The basic CSF tests (protein, glucose, and cell count) can rule out bacterial meningitis and the need for antibiotics. Furthermore, the pattern can suggest whether the cause is viral, fungal, or mycobacterial, and at times can point to a specific diagnosis (eg, HSV encephalitis can increase the number of red blood cells in the CSF).[19]

Given the numerous possible causes for encephalitis, the diagnostic workup can be extensive, and should be tailored by epidemiologic and host risk factors.[15] In the workup of North American patients with suspected encephalitis, diagnostic tests should be selected from the following:

- Neuroimaging (MRI preferred over CT)
- Chest radiograph (to evaluate for tuberculosis)
- Blood tests
  - Complete blood count
  - Comprehensive metabolic panel
  - Coagulation studies
  - Two sets of blood cultures
  - Cryptococcal antigen (cryptococcal infections are more common in immunocompromised hosts, but can occur in patients without obvious immunodeficiency)
  - Serologic testing for
    - Human immunodeficiency virus (HIV)
    - *Treponema pallidum*
    - *Borrelia burgdorferi* (enzyme-linked immunosorbent assay and Western blot)
    - *Mycoplasma pneumoniae* (acute and convalescent)
    - Epstein-Barr virus (EBV)
  - In patients with epidemiologic risk factors, serologic testing for:
    - *Coccidioides* species (primarily southwestern United States, Mexico)
    - *Taenia solium* (past travel to endemic areas such as Mexico or South America; usually has compatible lesions on neuroimaging)
    - *Toxoplasma gondii* (immunocompromised host)
  - In patients with risk factors, serologic testing (acute and convalescent) for:
    - West Nile virus (summer/fall)
    - *Rickettsia rickettsi* (tick bite, primarily southeastern United States)
    - *Ehrlichia chaffeensis* (tick bite, primarily southeastern United States)
    - *Anaplasma phagocytophilum* (tick bite, primarily southeastern United States)
- CSF tests
  - Gram stain and culture
  - Stain and culture for mycobacteria
  - Fungal stain and culture
  - VDRL (for syphilis)
  - PCR for HSV-1 and HSV-2

- ○ Cryptococcal antigen
- ○ PCR for *Mycobacterium tuberculosis*
- ○ PCR and IgM for varicella zoster virus
- ○ PCR for enteroviruses
- ○ PCR for EBV
- ○ *Borrelia burgdorferi* serology
- ○ In patients with epidemiologic risk factors:
  - ■ Histoplasma antigen (primarily Midwestern United States and Central America)
  - ■ *Coccidioides* complement fixation antibodies
  - ■ West Nile virus IgM
  - ■ Cytomegalovirus PCR (immunocompromised)
  - ■ JC virus PCR (immunocompromised)
  - ■ Human herpesvirus 6 (HHV-6) PCR (immunocompromised)
- • Urine tests (in patients with epidemiologic risk factors, urine histoplasma antigen).

Electroencephalograms are generally nonspecific, but they can be helpful in suggesting HSV encephalitis, in which focal abnormalities involving the temporal lobes are often seen, or in diagnosing nonconvulsive seizures.[15] Brain biopsies are infrequently used except when the cause is unknown despite an extensive workup and when there is rapid neurologic deterioration on acyclovir.

Treatment

Any patient with suspected encephalitis should be promptly started on acyclovir (10 mg/kg every 8 hours intravenously [IV] in adults with good renal function) until HSV encephalitis is ruled out. HSV is the most common nonepidemic cause of encephalitis in the United States, and one of the only types of encephalitis that responds well to antiviral therapy. Mortality from HSV encephalitis without treatment is more than 70% (with most survivors developing neurologic sequelae), but decreases to 30% with use of acylovir[20] and to 8% when acyclovir is initiated within 4 days of onset of clinical symptoms.[15] If HSV encephalitis is diagnosed or cannot be ruled out, acyclovir should be continued for 14 to 21 days. If patients have not had an appropriate clinical response by the end of treatment, a repeat CSF sample should be sent for HSV PCR test, and therapy extended if the result is positive. Although rare, HSV can be resistant to acyclovir because of a mutation in the viral thymidine kinase; in these cases, foscarnet can be used as alternate therapeutic agents.[21]

Any patient with suspected encephalitis and epidemiologic risk factors (tick bite, residence in the southeastern United States) and clinical signs (rash, myalgias, transaminitis) suggestive of rickettsial or ehrlichial infection should also be treated with doxycycline 100 mg twice a day,[15] because definitive diagnosis for these infections is often delayed. Furthermore, if there is any suspicion of bacterial meningitis, appropriate antibacterials should be promptly initiated and continued until bacterial meningitis is ruled out.

Specific antiviral therapies are mainly limited to the herpesviruses (including HSV, varicella zoster virus, CMV, and HHV-6), with only supportive care available for most other types of viral encephalitis. Effective therapy is available for most nonviral infectious causes of encephalitis; please refer to the 2008 guidelines for the management of encephalitis produced by the Infectious Diseases Society of America (http://www.idsociety.org/uploadedFiles/IDSA/Guidelines-Patient_Care/PDF_Library/Encephalitis.pdf) for an exhaustive list.[15]

Prognosis

Prognosis varies based on the cause but is in general poor, with a large proportion of survivors developing neurologic sequelae. Mortality for HSV encephalitis ranges from more than 70% to close to 0% depending on if and how soon the patients receive acyclovir. Among patients with HSV encephalitis who are treated promptly with acyclovir and survive, two-thirds have moderate to severe neurologic sequelae.[16] Rabies encephalitis, which can be prevented even after exposure with immunization, has a mortality close to 100%. Japanese encephalitis has a mortality of 30%, and 50% of survivors have serious neurologic sequelae. Although less than 1% of people infected with West Nile virus develop encephalitis, West Nile encephalitis has a mortality of 4% to 16%, with ~50% of survivors developing neurologic sequelae.[18]

BRAIN ABSCESS

Brain abscess is a focal purulent collection in the brain parenchyma usually caused by a bacterial or fungal infection. A brain abscess can develop because of spread of infection from a contiguous focus (such as the sinuses, middle ear, or dental infection) in 25% to 50% of cases, from hematogenous spread from a distant focus of infection (such as endocarditis) in 15% to 30% of cases, or from direct inoculation (such as head trauma or neurosurgery) in 8% to 19% of cases.[22] Presentation varies based on the origin of infection and location of the abscess, but frequently patients present with symptoms of increased intracranial pressure (headache, nausea/vomiting, and altered mental status), focal neurologic deficits, and fever (although fever can be absent in 30% to 76% of cases).[23,24]

Causes

The microbial cause depends on how the brain abscess develops and whether the patient is immunocompromised. Streptococci (both aerobic and anaerobic) are the most common pathogens, comprising about 70% of isolates cultured from bacterial brain abscesses.[25] However, other anaerobes (particularly in polymicrobial infections), enteric gram-negative bacilli, *Staphylococcus aureus* (particularly in abscesses originating from cranial trauma or endocarditis), and fungi (immunocompromised patients) are also frequently identified. The most common pathogens found in brain abscesses are listed in **Table 4**.[25]

Our understanding of the microbial spectrum of brain abscesses has recently expanded because of 16S ribosomal DNA amplification. In a recent study, this technology could identify pathogens in 9 of 21 (43%) culture-negative brain abscesses. Polymicrobial infections were identified at a significantly higher rate than by culture, and 44 distinct bacterial species not previously described in brain abscesses were identified.[22] However, it is unclear if all the bacteria identified by 16S ribosomal DNA amplification in brain abscess are clinically significant. For example, *Mycobacteria faucium* was identified in 4 polymicrobial brain abscesses, but all 4 patients recovered without receiving any specific therapy.[22,26]

Diagnostic Tests

Brain abscess is diagnosed by neuroimaging, with brain MRI favored over contrast head CT because of its higher sensitivity.[25] Neuroimaging can also frequently identify an otogenic, mastoid, sinus, or dental source if the brain abscess developed from contiguous spread. When surgical drainage is performed, the material should always be sent for Gram stain, aerobic and anaerobic culture, stain and culture for mycobacteria, and fungal stain and culture, as well as for histopathology. Other diagnostic tests

Table 4
Most common pathogens found in brain abscesses

Risk Factor	Usual Microbial Causes
Otitis media or mastoiditis	Streptococci (particularly *Streptococcus pneumoniae*)[22] Anaerobes (*Bacteroides* and *Prevotella* spp) Aerobic gram-negative bacilli (eg, *Proteus*, *Escherichia coli*, *Klebsiella*, *Pseudomonas*, and *Enterobacter* spp)
Sinusitis	Streptococci Anaerobes (*Bacteroides* spp) Aerobic gram-negative bacilli *Staphylococcus aureus* *Haemophilus* spp ***Often polymicrobial***[22]
Dental infection	Anaerobes, usually polymicrobial (*Fusobacterium*, *Actinomyces*, *Bacteroides*, and *Prevotella* spp) Streptococci *** Often polymicrobial***[22]
Penetrating trauma or postneurosurgical	*Staphylococcus aureus* Streptococci Aerobic gram-negative bacilli (including *Pseudomonas aeruginosa*) *Clostridium* spp
Endocarditis	*Staphylococcus aureus* Streptococci
Lung abscess, empyema, or bronchiectasis	Anaerobes (*Fusobacterium*, *Actinomyces*, *Bacteroides*, and *Prevotella* spp) Streptococci *Nocardia* spp
Immunocompromised: neutropenic	Aerobic gram-negative bacilli Fungi (*Aspergillus*, *Mucorales*, *Candida*, and *Scedosporium* spp)
Immunocompromised: transplant patients	Fungi (*Aspergillus*, *Candida*, *Mucorales*, and *Scedosporium* spp) Aerobic gram-negative bacilli *Nocardia* spp *Toxoplasma gondii*
Immunocompromised: AIDS	*Toxoplasma gondii* *Nocardia* spp *Mycobacterium* spp *Listeria monocytogenes* *Cryptococcus neoformans*

Adapted from Tunkel A. Brain abscess. In: Mandell GL, Bennett JE, Dolin R, editors. Mandell, Douglas, and Bennett's principles and practice of infectious diseases. Vol. 1(7). edition. Philadelphia: Churchill Livingston Elsevier; 2009. p. 1265–6.

that can be useful, particularly in patients who do not go promptly for surgical drainage, are the following:

- Two sets of blood cultures
- CSF Gram stain, aerobic and anaerobic cultures, stain and culture for mycobacteria, and fungal stain and culture (unless lumbar puncture is contraindicated because of increased intracranial pressure)
- Gram stain, aerobic and anaerobic cultures, acid fast bacilli stain and culture, and fungal stain and culture of material aspirated from the suspected source of infection (eg the sinuses, middle ear, or lung abscess material)

- HIV antibody and CD4 count (to evaluate for undiagnosed HIV infection and immunosuppression)
- Chest radiograph or chest CT (particularly when the source is unknown, the patient has respiratory symptoms, or the patient is immunocompromised)
- Echocardiogram (particularly when the source is unknown or *Staphylococcus aureus* grows from blood or abscess cultures)
- In immunocompromised patients, the following tests are also helpful:
  - Serum *Toxoplasma* IgG antibody
  - CSF EBV PCR (often increased in patients with AIDS with CNS lymphoma, which is the main differential diagnosis in patients with AIDS with suspected CNS toxoplasmosis)
  - Serum aspergillus galactomannan
  - Serum and CSF cryptococcal antigen
  - Urine and CSF histoplasma antigen
  - Serum and CSF *Coccidioides* serology
  - Biopsy/cultures of skin lesions in patients with suspected disseminated fungal infection

Treatment

Treatment often involves a combined medical and surgical approach. Surgical drainage of the brain abscess, either by craniotomy or by CT-guided aspiration, is often necessary to relieve increased intracranial pressure. Drainage also allows for sampling of the material so that a definitive microbiological diagnosis can be made.

In cases in which the intracranial pressure is not dangerously increased, medical treatment alone can be considered for brain abscesses on a case-by-case basis (this is in contrast to a subdural empyema, which is always a surgical emergency[19]). In general, medical treatment alone has the best odds of success if the abscess is small (<2.5 cm), if there are multiple abscesses, if the microbial cause is already known (from a blood or CSF culture), and if the patient is in good clinical condition (with a Glasgow Coma Scale >12).[23] In the case of patients with AIDS with a positive anti-*Toxoplasma* IgG and lesions consistent with cerebral toxoplasmosis, standard of care is to treat presumptively for toxoplasmosis and limit surgical intervention to patients who worsen or do not respond (radiographically or clinically) after 10 to 14 days of treatment.[25]

The optimal type of surgical intervention (surgical excision by craniotomy vs CT-guided aspiration) was evaluated in a recent review.[24] The investigators found that in studies after 1990, the mean mortality associated with CT-guided aspiration (6.6%) was less than the mean mortality associated with surgical excision by craniotomy (12.7%). However, they did not evaluate the baseline characteristics of the patients in each group; one would presume that patients in whom neurosurgeons chose to perform a surgical excision by craniotomy may have been sicker and have higher intracranial pressure than those who received a CT-guided aspiration. Consequently, we believe the choice of surgical approach should still be determined on a case-by-case basis.

Empiric antibiotic therapy should be broad, started promptly, and narrowed only when a specific microbial cause is known. For abscesses that are not surgically drained, regimens containing metronidazole are preferred given the excellent penetration of metronidazole into brain abscess cavities.[25] Empiric therapy is based on the usual microbial causes associated with the patient's risk factors for brain abscess, with possible options listed in **Table 5**.

Empiric therapy is not so clearly defined in the immunocompromised patient, and varies greatly based on the appearance of the lesion and the results of

Table 5
Empiric antibiotic therapy based on patient's risk factors

Risk Factor	Empiric Antibiotic Therapy
Otitis media, mastoiditis, or sinusitis	Vancomycin (15 mg/kg IV every 8–12 h, goal trough 15–20) and cefepime (2 g IV every 8 h) and metronidazole (7.5 mg/kg IV every 6 h)[25]
Dental infection	Ceftriaxone (2 g IV every 12 h) and metronidazole
Penetrating trauma or postneurosurgical	Vancomycin and cefepime and metronidazole or vancomycin and meropenem (2 g IV every 8 h)
Endocarditis	Vancomycin and gentamicin (5 mg/kg IV every 8 h)[25]
Lung abscess, empyema, or bronchiectasis	Meropenem and trimethoprim-sulfamethoxazole (15 mg/kg/d of trimethoprim and 75 mg/kg/d of sulfamethoxazole IV divided in 2–4 doses)
Unknown	Vancomycin and meropenem or vancomycin and cefepime and metronidazole

diagnostic tests. In general, we treat empirically with vancomycin, meropenem, and trimethoprim-sulfamethoxazole (which covers broadly for bacteria, including *Pseudomonas aeruginosa* and *Nocardia*, and also covers *Toxoplasma gondii*). In addition, if a fungal cause is suspected, we also add voriconazole, plus liposomal amphotericin B if *Mucorales* is suspected (such as in a patient with fungal sinusitis).

Coverage should be narrowed when the microbial cause is definitively determined, although anaerobic coverage should be continued regardless of culture results for abscesses that originate from contiguous spread. For bacterial abscesses, IV antibiotics are generally recommended for 4 to 6 weeks when the abscess was surgically drained or 6 to 12 weeks when there was no surgical intervention.[23,25] However, treatment duration may vary based on clinical course and follow-up imaging. For fungal abscesses, or those caused by *Nocardia* or *Toxoplasma gondii*, treatment duration is longer.

Prognosis

Although historically high, with the recent development of more effective antibiotics and better imaging modalities, mortality from brain abscess now ranges from about 8% to 25%.[25] However, mortality increases to 27% to 85% when the abscess ruptures into the ventricle. Neurologic sequelae develop in 20% to 70% of survivors. Poor prognostic factors include rapid progression of the disease before hospitalization, altered mental status on admission, sepsis, and an underlying immunodeficiency.

UPPER AIRWAY OBSTRUCTION

Infections associated with upper airway obstructions include epiglottitis, Ludwig's angina, retropharyngeal abscesses, and diphtheria. Of these 4 diseases, only epiglottitis and Ludwig's angina are commonly described in North American adults. Diphtheria is a vaccine-preventable disease characterized by pseudomembrane formation over the upper respiratory tract after exposure to toxigenic strains of *Corynebacterium diptheriae*.[27] Although endemic in some countries where vaccines against diphtheria are not consistently used, no cases of diphtheria have been reported in the United States since 2003.[27] Retropharyngeal abscesses often result from lymphatic spread of upper respiratory infections.[28] Because lymph nodes tend to get smaller with age, these infections are predominantly seen in children.[28] Because diphtheria and retropharyngeal abscess are rarely seen in North American adults, the rest of this section focuses on epiglottitis and Ludwig's angina.

Epiglottitis is often termed supraglottitis in adults because of the involvement of additional anatomic structures above the epiglottis, including the base of the tongue and the pharynx.[29] As a result, adults tend to have a generalized, erythematous swelling of the supraglottic structures rather than the classic cherry red epiglottitis.[30] Epiglottitis in adults also differs from childhood infections by having a slower progression of symptoms, less likelihood of being caused by Hib, and different clinical presentation.[30] Since the implementation of childhood Hib vaccination, multiple analyses have shown an increased percentage of epiglottitis cases in adult populations worldwide.[31–38]

Ludwig's angina is a common cause of deep space neck infections, and may be more common in populations of lower socioeconomic status having less access to routine dental care.[39] Ludwig's angina results in airway obstruction by swelling and upward displacement of the tongue.[28] The traditional definition provided by Grodinsky in 1939 includes: (1) origin in the floor of the mouth, usually from infected teeth; (2) invasion of the submandibular space; and (3) development of complications, such as tongue edema and mediastinitis, secondary to direct spread across fascial planes rather than through the lymphatic system or blood stream.[40] This situation accounts for the characteristic bilateral woody cellulitis, rather than discrete abscess formation.[40,41]

Causes

The cause of acute epiglottitis has changed since the widespread use of Hib vaccine. Hib is an uncommon cause of epiglottitis in adults.[29,34] In a review of cases of acute epiglottitis in Iceland, no Hib has been isolated from blood or pharyngeal cultures since 1991.[31] Since that time, several different organisms have been isolated, most commonly *Streptococcus* species.[31] Patients with epiglottitis secondary to Hib may have a more virulent form, with a shorter duration of symptoms and a higher rate of respiratory complications.[34]

Most cases of Ludwig's angina are odontogenic in origin, accounting for almost 90% of cases in some studies.[42,43] Other potential causes include facial trauma and oral malignancies.[41] Cultures are often polymicrobial,[44] reflecting normal oral flora. The distribution may vary depending on the immune status of the host. Streptococcus viridans was the most commonly isolated pathogen in patients in 1 review of deep neck infections, including Ludwig's angina; however, when analyzing only patients with diabetes mellitus, *Klebsiella pneumoniae* was most common.[45]

Diagnosis and Diagnostic Tests

A high index of clinical suspicion is needed to diagnose epiglottitis and deep neck infections in adults. Most adults with acute epiglottitis present with a sore throat and odynophagia, findings that could be mistaken for a routine upper respiratory tract infection.[29,36,38,46,47] Fewer adults with acute epiglottitis present with the classic signs of airway compromise, such as drooling, a muffled voice, or respiratory distress.[29,36,47] Patients with Ludwig's angina tend to be more apparent and frequently present with fever, bilateral submandibular and neck swelling, and tongue elevation.[42] Pain with tongue movement is also described in patients who have Ludwig's angina.[44]

Blood cultures should be obtained in all patients, although many are negative.[29,33,37,38,47] Pharyngeal cultures may also be useful. One study of 31 children and adults with acute epiglottitis in Iceland revealed a match between throat and blood cultures in 58% of cases, although half of these matched sets were negative.[31] Some authorities also advocate serology and PCR testing to increase the yield of diagnosis, and in 1 study, isolation of a pathogen increased from 28% when only blood cultures were obtained to 57% when all 3 modalities were used.[48]

Imaging or direct visualization by endoscopy are useful adjuncts to diagnosis of acute epiglottitis. Abnormal findings on a routine oropharyngeal examination are present in less than half of patients.[29,46] A lateral plain film may show a thumb sign, consistent with a swollen epiglottitis; however, direct visualization by flexible fiber-optic nasopharyngoscopy is more reliable.[30,38,49] In 1 analysis of adults diagnosed with acute epiglottitis, 81.4% had abnormal plain films, whereas 100% had abnormal findings on flexible laryngoscopy.[38] CT imaging may be used to diagnose adult epiglottitis when flexible laryngoscopy is not an option; findings include swelling of the supraglottis, loss of the surrounding fat, and thickening of the platysma muscles and prevertebral fascia.[50] CT or MRI of the neck may also be useful to evaluate for complications of epiglottitis, such as abscess formation.[30]

The diagnostic workup of suspected epiglottitis or deep neck infection should include the following:

- Two sets of blood cultures
- Pharyngeal cultures
- CT scan of the neck
- Ear, nose and throat consult for a flexible fiber-optic nasopharyngoscopy
- In suspected Ludwig's angina, a chest CT to evaluate for mediastinal spread of infection

Additional workup for underlying immunodeficiencies and concurrent illnesses should be considered. Comorbid medical conditions have been found in almost a quarter of patients with epiglottitis,[38] and in up to a third of patients with deep neck infections.[45,51] Using data from the Nationwide Inpatient Sample, researchers[35] found that 39% of patients with epiglottitis admitted to US hospitals had concurrent cardiac diseases, 23% had underlying respiratory diseases, and 13% had diabetes mellitus. In another review of patients with Ludwig's angina,[43] diabetes mellitus was the most common associated illness, many of whom were newly diagnosed. Depending on the clinical scenario, an investigation for underlying cardiopulmonary, renal, or gastrointestinal diseases, malignancies, long-term steroid use, and HIV may be appropriate.[29,35,36,38,39,45,51]

Treatment

The initial focus of managing acute epiglottitis should be protecting the airway. Conservative management without intubation may be considered for adults without respiratory distress and with at least a 50% laryngeal lumen on flexible laryngoscopy.[49] The following factors have been associated with increased need for airway intervention in acute epiglottitis: drooling, diabetes mellitus, shorter onset of symptoms, and development of epiglottic abscess.[36] Katori and Tsukuda[52] reported that severe swelling of the epiglottis (less than 50% of posterior vocal cord visible) and extension of swelling to the arytenoids were also associated with an increased need for airway intervention. In 1 review, authorities who opted to provide only conservative medical management for cases with mild airway obstruction were able to avoid airway intervention in approximately two-thirds of patients.[30]

Broad-spectrum antibiotics should be initiated immediately for both epiglottitis and deep neck infections. For acute epiglottitis, antibiotics should include activity against β-lactamase–producing Hib.[29,30,32] If no improvement is seen by flexible laryngoscopy after 36 to 48 hours of appropriate medical therapy, evaluation for complications, such as abscess formation, should be pursued.[30,37] Antibiotics directed toward deep neck infections should also target β-lactamase–producing pathogens as well as anaerobes.[51,53] Additional coverage should be considered for methicillin-resistant *Staphylococcus aureus* until cultures are available.[51] Antibiotics should be continued for 7 to 10 days in cases of acute epiglottitis without complications [49]; however, the duration of antibiotics for deep neck infections has not been clearly defined and depends on the clinical course and follow-up imaging.

Presumptive antibiotic choices (before culture results are back) in adults with normal renal function are shown in **Table 6**.

The role of steroids in the treatment of acute epiglottitis to reduce airway edema is unclear. Several studies have not shown improved outcomes in patients treated with steroids,[34,38] but most of these data were collected retrospectively and may be a reflection of more severe cases.[47] Steroid use in patients with Ludwig's angina to reduce airway edema is reported but is controversial.[39,54] One authority recommends dexamethasone (10 mg IV, followed by 4 mg IV every 6 hours) for the first 48 hours in addition to antibiotics and surgical intervention in cases of Ludwig's angina.[55]

Abscesses arising from deep neck infections, including Ludwig's angina, may require surgical intervention. Some authorities advocate urgent surgical intervention if there are any signs or symptoms of sepsis or airway compromise, descending infection, anterior visceral space involvement, abscess involving 2 or more deep neck spaces, and abscesses larger than 3.0 cm.[51] In patients who did not meet the criteria for immediate debridement, repeat contrast-enhanced CT was obtained at 48 hours, and surgery was performed if no improvement in abscess size was seen.[51]

Prognosis

Mortality has been reported as close to 7% in cases of adult supraepiglottitis,[49] although other reviews have cited lower percentages. In a review of US cases from 1998 to 2006, the mean weighted mortality was 0.89%, which remained relatively constant throughout the study period.[35] Several reports from Hong Kong have reported no mortalities.[38,56] In addition to airway obstruction, other potential complications of acute epiglottitis include epiglottitis abscess formation and pneumonia.[32,34,36,38,46]

Most deaths in cases of Ludwig's angina result from an impaired airway.[54] Other potentially fatal complications include descending mediastinitis.[43] Concurrent systemic illnesses may contribute to adverse outcomes. The mortality in 1 series of patients with Ludwig's angina was 9%, but when analyzing patients with diabetes mellitus, the mortality increased to 19%.[43] Many of the diabetic patients who died were newly diagnosed, raising concerns for metabolic derangements as a contributing factor.[43]

JUGULAR SEPTIC THROMBOPHLEBITIS (LEMIERRE'S SYNDROME)

Jugular septic thrombophlebitis, or Lemierre's syndrome, was first described by Dr André Lemierre in 1936 in a series of primarily young adults with anaerobic

Table 6 Presumptive antibiotic choices in adults with normal renal function	
Epiglottitis	Ceftriaxone 2 gm IV daily and vancomycin 15 mg/kg IV every 12 h
Deep neck infections	Vancomycin 15 mg/kg IV every 12 h and ampicillin/sulbactam 3 g IV every 6 h or meropenem 1 g IV every 8 h

septicemia after an oropharyngeal infection, resulting in metastatic complications and frequently death. Lemierre's syndrome is also referred to as postanginal septicemia, reflecting the diffuse inflammatory response that occurs several days after the initial sore throat.[57] Although multiple anaerobes have been described, *Fusobacterium nec-rophorum* is most commonly isolated.[58–62] The following case definition of Lemierre's syndrome was recently proposed:

- "History of anginal illness (sore throat) in the preceding 4 weeks or compatible clinical findings
- Evidence of either metastatic lung lesions or another remote site, and
- Evidence of internal jugular vein thrombophlebitis or isolation of *F. necrophorum* or *Fusobacterium* sp. from blood cultures or a normally sterile site"[63]

Although uncommon, the number of reported cases of Lemierre's syndrome may be increasing. A prospective study in Denmark from 1998 to 2001 revealed an increased overall incidence of 3.6 cases per million per year, and 14.4 cases per million per year occurred among individuals aged 15 to 24 years.[64] Similar findings have been reported in other reviews.[65,66] Potential explanations for this increase in cases include the reduced tendency for clinicians in recent years to prescribe antibiotics for pharyngitis, much of which is believed to be viral in cause; changes in antibiotic sensitivity profiles; improved detection, and a decreased number of tonsillectomies in recent decades.[61,66–69]

Causes

Lemierre's syndrome most commonly affects young, immunocompetent individuals.[59,62] In 1 review, 73.6% of patients were aged 16 to 25 years, most of whom were described as healthy.[59] Most cases arise from the throat and peritonsillar tissues.[58,59,62] The spread through the lateral pharyngeal space eventually leads to internal jugular thrombophlebitis and metastatic complications, which characterize Lemierre's syndrome.[59]

Fusobacterium necrophorum is believed to be a part of the normal oropharyngeal flora,[70–72] although some authorities disagree.[63] In 1 literature review of 222 cases of Lemierre's syndrome since 1970, anaerobes were isolated in 90% of cases, *Fusobacterium* species in 86% of cases, and *F necrophorum* in 69% of cases.[63] In this same analysis, cultures were negative in 6% of cases, and blood cultures that grew *Fusobacterium* species were mixed in 12% of cases. In addition to anaerobes, multiple other pathogens have been described in Lemierre's syndrome, including methicillin-resistant *Staphylococcus aureus*.[73]

Diagnostic Tests

The clinician should have a high index of suspicion for Lemierre's syndrome in any patient presenting with sepsis and complaints of a sore throat in the preceding few weeks, especially if the patient was not prescribed antibiotics or received antibiotics without anaerobic coverage. The 2 most important diagnostic tests are blood cultures and a CT scan of the neck with contrast (to evaluate for a septic clot in the internal jugular vein). According to some authorities, "patients with blood cultures growing *F. necro-phorum* should be assumed to have Lemierre syndrome until proven otherwise."[74] Anaerobic blood cultures can grow slowly (5–8 days of incubation in 1 review).[71]

Although occasionally internal jugular vein thrombophlebitis can be suggested by characteristic clinical features in the absence of imaging (painful jaw and neck swelling, sepsis and evidence of pulmonary emboli),[62] 1 review found that almost half of cases had no significant neck findings.[59] A CT scan of the neck with contrast is preferred over ultrasonography because ultrasonography is unable to image beneath the clavicular and jaw bones and is less sensitive for recent clots.[59,63,74,75]

Involvement of the internal jugular vein allows the infection to invade the bloodstream and spread to distant organs, and an investigation for mestastatic sites should be pursued. Various organ systems may be affected, particularly the lungs followed by the large joints.[59,74,76] Additional laboratory findings associated with Lemierre's syndrome include leukocytosis, an increased C-reactive protein (CRP) level, hyperbilirubinemia, and mild disseminated intravascular coagulation with thrombocytopenia.[77]

A diagnostic workup for Lemierre's syndrome should include the following tests:

- Two sets of blood cultures (with both sets containing an anaerobic bottle)
- CT scan of the neck with contrast
- CT scan of the lungs (or chest radiograph) to look for pulmonary septic emboli
- If clinical evidence of a septic joint, joint aspiration with fluid sent for aerobic and anaerobic cultures
- Complete blood count, comprehensive metabolic panel, and CRP

Treatment

Antibiotics should be started promptly before culture results, because delays in appropriate therapy have been associated with higher mortality.[71] Because of the polymicrobial nature of most infections, regimens directed solely at anaerobes should be avoided.[74,76] In 1 analysis, 41.1% of Fusobacteria species were β-lactamase positive.[78] In another analysis, 15% of F necrophorum isolates were resistant to erythromycin.[67] F necophorum is intrinsically resistant to gentamicin.[76] On the other hand, moxifloxacin has good in vitro activity against most Fusobacteria.[79] Based on these sensitivities, appropriate regimens (for adults with normal renal function) include the following:

- Beta-lactam/beta-lactamase inhibitor (such as ampicillin/sulbactam 3 gm IV every 6 hours) OR a carbapenem (such as ertapenem 1 gm IV daily) OR moxifloxacin 400 mg IV daily plus
- Clindamycin 600 mg IV every 8 hours OR metronidazole 500 mg IV every 6 hours

Because Lemierre's syndrome is an endovascular syndrome, most authorities advocate higher-dose antibiotic therapy for an extended period.[62] A commonly cited duration of antibiotic therapy is 3 to 6 weeks,[59,74] although IV antibiotics may be changed to an oral regimen when the patient is afebrile and neck pain has resolved.[80]

Clinical improvement may be delayed despite adequate antibiotic treatment secondary to the decreased ability of antibiotics to penetrate clots and abscesses.[69,71,74] In 1 review,[76] fevers persisted for 8 to 12 days despite appropriate antibiotic regimens. Surgical drainage of infected fluid collections and debridement of abscesses are important adjuncts to medical therapy.[62] Surgical ligation of the internal jugular vein is probably unnecessary unless there is persistent septic embolization.[74,75,77] In our experience, respiratory decompensation requiring intubation is not unusual, and clinicians should have a low threshold for transferring patients with suspected Lemierre's syndrome to the intensive care unit (ICU).

Use of anticoagulation for the infected thrombus is controversial and is typically reserved for cases with retrograde cavernous sinus thrombosis.[75,77,80] If anticoagulation is warranted, a 3-month duration has been suggested.[77]

Prognosis

With the advent of appropriate antibiotic therapy, mortality in Lemierre's syndrome has decreased but remains high at approximately 17%.[77] Although most survivors recover completely, it is our experience that a prolonged hospitalization, including an ICU stay, is often required.

REFERENCES

1. van de Beek D, de Gans J, Spanjaard L, et al. Clinical features and prognostic factors in adults with bacterial meningitis. N Engl J Med 2004;351(18):1849–59.
2. Thomas KE, Hasbun R, Jekel J, et al. The diagnostic accuracy of Kernig's sign, Brudzinski's sign, and nuchal rigidity in adults with suspected meningitis. Clin Infect Dis 2002;35(1):46–52.
3. Hasbun R, Abrahams J, Jekel J, et al. Computed tomography of the head before lumbar puncture in adults with suspected meningitis. N Engl J Med 2001;345(24): 1727–33.
4. Durand ML, Calderwood SB, Weber DJ, et al. Acute bacterial meningitis in adults. A review of 493 episodes. N Engl J Med 1993;328(1):21–8.
5. Thigpen MC, Whitney CG, Messonnier NE, et al. Bacterial meningitis in the United States, 1998–2007. N Engl J Med 2011;364(21):2016–25.
6. Weisfelt M, van de Beek D, Spanjaard L, et al. Nosocomial bacterial meningitis in adults: a prospective series of 50 cases. J Hosp Infect 2007;66(1):71–8.
7. Tunkel AR, Hartman BJ, Kaplan SL, et al. Practice guidelines for the management of bacterial meningitis. Clin Infect Dis 2004;39(9):1267–84.
8. Tunkel AR, van de Beek D, Scheld WM. Acute meningitis. In: Mandell GL, Bennett JE, Dolin R, editors. Mandell, Douglas, and Bennett's principles and practice of infectious diseases, vol. 1(7). Philadelphia: Churchill Livingston Elsevier; 2009. p. 1189–229.
9. Saravolatz LD, Manzor O, VanderVelde N, et al. Broad-range bacterial polymerase chain reaction for early detection of bacterial meningitis. Clin Infect Dis 2003;36(1):40–5.
10. de Gans J, van de Beek D. Investigators EDiABMS. Dexamethasone in adults with bacterial meningitis. N Engl J Med 2002;347(20):1549–56.
11. Brouwer MC, Heckenberg SG, de Gans J, et al. Nationwide implementation of adjunctive dexamethasone therapy for pneumococcal meningitis. Neurology 2010;75(17):1533–9.
12. van de Beek D, de Gans J, Tunkel AR, et al. Community-acquired bacterial meningitis in adults. N Engl J Med 2006;354(1):44–53.
13. Schmand B, de Bruin E, de Gans J, et al. Cognitive functioning and quality of life nine years after bacterial meningitis. J Infect 2010;61(4):330–4.
14. Edmond K, Clark A, Korczak VS, et al. Global and regional risk of disabling sequelae from bacterial meningitis: a systematic review and meta-analysis. Lancet Infect Dis 2010;10(5):317–28.
15. Tunkel AR, Glaser CA, Bloch KC, et al. The management of encephalitis: clinical practice guidelines by the Infectious Diseases Society of America. Clin Infect Dis 2008;47(3):303–27.
16. Whitley RJ, Gnann JW. Viral encephalitis: familiar infections and emerging pathogens. Lancet 2002;359(9305):507–13.
17. Tyler KL. Emerging viral infections of the central nervous system: part 1. Arch Neurol 2009;66(8):939–48.
18. Solomon T. Flavivirus encephalitis. N Engl J Med 2004;351(4):370–8.

19. Smith TL, Nathan BR. Central nervous system infections in the immune-competent adult. Curr Treat Options Neurol 2002;4(4):323–32.

20. Whitley RJ, Lakeman F. Herpes simplex virus infections of the central nervous system: therapeutic and diagnostic considerations. Clin Infect Dis 1995;20(2): 414–20.

21. Schulte EC, Sauerbrei A, Hoffmann D, et al. Acyclovir resistance in herpes simplex encephalitis. Ann Neurol 2010;67(6):830–3.

22. Al Masalma M, Lonjon M, Richet H, et al. Metagenomic analysis of brain abscesses identifies specific bacterial associations. Clin Infect Dis 2012;54(2): 202–10.

23. Arlotti M, Grossi P, Pea F, et al. Consensus document on controversial issues for the treatment of infections of the central nervous system: bacterial brain abscesses. Int J Infect Dis 2010;14(Suppl 4):S79–92.

24. Ratnaike TE, Das S, Gregson BA, et al. A review of brain abscess surgical treatment–78 years: aspiration versus excision. World Neurosurg 2011;76(5):431–6.

25. Tunkel A. Brain abscess. In: Mandell GL, Bennett JE, Dolin R, editors. Mandell, Douglas, and Bennett's principles and practice of infectious diseases. vol. 1. 7th edition. Philadelphia: Churchill Livingstone Elsevier; 2009. p. 1265–78.

26. Al Masalma M, Armougom F, Scheld WM, et al. The expansion of the microbiological spectrum of brain abscesses with use of multiple 16S ribosomal DNA sequencing. Clin Infect Dis 2009;48(9):1169–78.

27. Tiwari T. Infectious diseases related to travel–diphtheria. The Yellow Book: CDC Health Information for International Travelers. Chapter 3. Atlanta (GA): CDC; 2012.

28. Vieira F, Allen SM, Stocks RM, et al. Deep neck infection. Otolaryngol Clin North Am 2008;41(3):459–83, vii.

29. Frantz TD, Rasgon BM, Quesenberry CP. Acute epiglottitis in adults. Analysis of 129 cases. JAMA 1994;272(17):1358–60.

30. Al-Qudah M, Shetty S, Alomari M, et al. Acute adult supraglottitis: current management and treatment. South Med J 2010;103(8):800–4.

31. Briem B, Thorvardsson O, Petersen H. Acute epiglottitis in Iceland 1983-2005. Auris Nasus Larynx 2009;36(1):46–52.

32. Torkkeli T, Ruoppi P, Nuutinen J, et al. Changed clinical course and current treatment of acute epiglottitis in adults a 12-year experience. Laryngoscope 1994; 104(12):1503–6.

33. Hafidh MA, Sheahan P, Keogh I, et al. Acute epiglottitis in adults: a recent experience with 10 cases. J Laryngol Otol 2006;120(4):310–3.

34. Mayo-Smith MF, Spinale JW, Donskey CJ, et al. Acute epiglottitis. An 18-year experience in Rhode Island. Chest 1995;108(6):1640–7.

35. Shah RK, Stocks C. Epiglottitis in the United States: national trends, variances, prognosis, and management. Laryngoscope 2010;120(6):1256–62.

36. Berger G, Landau T, Berger S, et al. The rising incidence of adult acute epiglottitis and epiglottic abscess. Am J Otolaryngol 2003;24(6):374–83.

37. Wong EY, Berkowitz RG. Acute epiglottitis in adults: the Royal Melbourne Hospital experience. ANZ J Surg 2001;71(12):740–3.

38. Cheung CS, Man SY, Graham CA, et al. Adult epiglottitis: 6 years experience in a university teaching hospital in Hong Kong. Eur J Emerg Med 2009;16(4):221–6.

39. Larawin V, Naipao J, Dubey SP. Head and neck space infections. Otolaryngol Head Neck Surg 2006;135(6):889–93.

40. Grodinsky M. Ludwig's angina: an anatomical and clinical study with review of the literature. Surgery 1939;5:678–96.

41. Honrado CP, Lam SM, Karen M. Bilateral submandibular gland infection presenting as Ludwig's angina: first report of a case. Ear Nose Throat J 2001;80(4): 217–8, 222–3.

42. Srirompotong S, Art-Smart T. Ludwig's angina: a clinical review. Eur Arch Otorhinolaryngol 2003;260(7):401–3.

43. Bross-Soriano D, Arrieta-Gómez JR, Prado-Calleros H, et al. Management of Ludwig's angina with small neck incisions: 18 years experience. Otolaryngol Head Neck Surg 2004;130(6):712–7.

44. Costain N, Marrie TJ. Ludwig's angina. Am J Med 2011;124(2):115–7.

45. Huang TT, Liu TC, Chen PR, et al. Deep neck infection: analysis of 185 cases. Head Neck 2004;26(10):854–60.

46. Wick F, Ballmer PE, Haller A. Acute epiglottis in adults. Swiss Med Wkly 2002; 132(37–38):541–7.

47. Guldfred LA, Lyhne D, Becker BC. Acute epiglottitis: epidemiology, clinical presentation, management and outcome. J Laryngol Otol 2008;122(8):818–23.

48. Trollfors B, Nylén O, Carenfelt C, et al. Aetiology of acute epiglottitis in adults. Scand J Infect Dis 1998;30(1):49–51.

49. Sobol SE, Zapata S. Epiglottitis and croup. Otolaryngol Clin North Am 2008;41(3): 551–66, ix.

50. Smith MM, Mukherji SK, Thompson JE, et al. CT in adult supraglottitis. AJNR Am J Neuroradiol 1996;17(7):1355–8.

51. Boscolo-Rizzo P, Da Mosto MC. Submandibular space infection: a potentially lethal infection. Int J Infect Dis 2009;13(3):327–33.

52. Katori H, Tsukuda M. Acute epiglottitis: analysis of factors associated with airway intervention. J Laryngol Otol 2005;119(12):967–72.

53. Kinzer S, Pfeiffer J, Becker S, et al. Severe deep neck space infections and mediastinitis of odontogenic origin: clinical relevance and implications for diagnosis and treatment. Acta Otolaryngol 2009;129(1):62–70.

54. Saifeldeen K, Evans R. Ludwig's angina. Emerg Med J 2004;21(2):242–3.

55. Busch RF, Shah D. Ludwig's angina: improved treatment. Otolaryngol Head Neck Surg 1997;117(6):S172–5.

56. Ng HL, Sin LM, Li MF, et al. Acute epiglottitis in adults: a retrospective review of 106 patients in Hong Kong. Emerg Med J 2008;25(5):253–5.

57. Lemierre A. On certain septicaemias due to anaerobic organisms. Lancet 1936;1: 701–3.

58. Alvarez A, Schreiber JR. Lemierre's syndrome in adolescent children–anaerobic sepsis with internal jugular vein thrombophlebitis following pharyngitis. Pediatrics 1995;96(2 Pt 1):354–9.

59. Chirinos JA, Lichtstein DM, Garcia J, et al. The evolution of Lemierre syndrome: report of 2 cases and review of the literature. Medicine (Baltimore) 2002;81(6): 458–65.

60. Goldhagen J, Alford BA, Prewitt LH, et al. Suppurative thrombophlebitis of the internal jugular vein: report of three cases and review of the pediatric literature. Pediatr Infect Dis J 1988;7(6):410–4.

61. Karkos PD, Asrani S, Karkos CD, et al. Lemierre's syndrome: a systematic review. Laryngoscope 2009;119(8):1552–9.

62. Sinave CP, Hardy GJ, Fardy PW. The Lemierre syndrome: suppurative thrombophlebitis of the internal jugular vein secondary to oropharyngeal infection. Medicine (Baltimore) 1989;68(2):85–94.

63. Riordan T. Human infection with *Fusobacterium necrophorum* (Necrobacillosis), with a focus on Lemierre's syndrome. Clin Microbiol Rev 2007;20(4):622–59.

64. Hagelskjaer Kristensen L, Prag J. Lemierre's syndrome and other disseminated *Fusobacterium necrophorum* infections in Denmark: a prospective epidemiological and clinical survey. Eur J Clin Microbiol Infect Dis 2008;27(9):779–89.

65. Hagelskjaer LH, Prag J, Malczynski J, et al. Incidence and clinical epidemiology of necrobacillosis, including Lemierre's syndrome, in Denmark 1990-1995. Eur J Clin Microbiol Infect Dis 1998;17(8):561–5.

66. Ramirez S, Hild TG, Rudolph CN, et al. Increased diagnosis of Lemierre syndrome and other *Fusobacterium necrophorum* infections at a Children's Hospital. Pediatrics 2003;112(5):e380.

67. Brazier JS, Hall V, Yusuf E, et al. *Fusobacterium necrophorum* infections in England and Wales 1990-2000. J Med Microbiol 2002;51(3):269–72.

68. Love WE, Zaccheo MV. Lemierre's syndrome: more judicious antibiotic prescribing habits may lead to the clinical reappearance of this often forgotten disease. Am J Med 2006;119(3):e7–9.

69. Kuppalli K, Livorsi D, Talati NJ, et al. Lemierre's syndrome due to *Fusobacterium necrophorum*. Lancet Infect Dis 2012. [Epub ahead of print].

70. Burden P. *Fusobacterium necrophorum* and Lemierre's syndrome. J Infect 1991; 23(3):227–31.

71. Leugers CM, Clover R. Lemierre syndrome: postanginal sepsis. J Am Board Fam Pract 1995;8(5):384–91.

72. Jensen A, Hagelskjaer Kristensen L, Prag J. Detection of *Fusobacterium necrophorum* subsp. *funduliforme* in tonsillitis in young adults by real-time PCR. Clin Microbiol Infect 2007;13(7):695–701.

73. Chanin JM, Marcos LA, Thompson BM, et al. Methicillin-resistant *Staphylococcus aureus* USA300 clone as a cause of Lemierre's syndrome. J Clin Microbiol 2011; 49(5):2063–6.

74. Syed MI, Baring D, Addidle M, et al. Lemierre syndrome: two cases and a review. Laryngoscope 2007;117(9):1605–10.

75. Lustig LR, Cusick BC, Cheung SW, et al. Lemierre's syndrome: two cases of postanginal sepsis. Otolaryngol Head Neck Surg 1995;112(6):767–72.

76. Riordan T, Wilson M. Lemierre's syndrome: more than a historical curiosa. Postgrad Med J 2004;80(944):328–34.

77. Hagelskjaer Kristensen L, Prag J. Human necrobacillosis, with emphasis on Lemierre's syndrome. Clin Infect Dis 2000;31(2):524–32.

78. Appelbaum PC, Spangler SK, Jacobs MR. Beta-lactamase production and susceptibilities to amoxicillin, amoxicillin-clavulanate, ticarcillin, ticarcillin-clavulanate, cefoxitin, imipenem, and metronidazole of 320 non-*Bacteroides fragilis* Bacteroides isolates and 129 fusobacteria from 28 U.S. centers. Antimicrob Agents Chemother 1990;34(8):1546–50.

79. Edmiston CE, Krepel CJ, Seabrook GR, et al. In vitro activities of moxifloxacin against 900 aerobic and anaerobic surgical isolates from patients with intraabdominal and diabetic foot infections. Antimicrob Agents Chemother 2004; 48(3):1012–6.

80. Bondy P, Grant T. Lemierre's syndrome: what are the roles for anticoagulation and long-term antibiotic therapy? Ann Otol Rhinol Laryngol 2008;117(9):679–83.

Pulmonary Emergencies

Pneumonia, Acute Respiratory Distress Syndrome, Lung Abscess, and Empyema

Himanshu Desai, MD[a],*, Aarti Agrawal, MD[b]

KEYWORDS

- Pneumonia • Acute respiratory distress syndrome • Lung abscess • Empyema
- Respiratory infections • Pulmonary emergencies

KEY POINTS

- Lower respiratory tract infections are a leading cause of death in the United States.
- Community-acquired and hospital-acquired pneumonia, acute respiratory distress syndrome, lung abscess, and empyema can present as life-threatening infections of the respiratory system.
- Early diagnostic and treatment strategies are required to effectively treat these infections and prevent complications.

INTRODUCTION

Infections of the respiratory tract constitute a major source of morbidity and mortality in the United States. Lower respiratory tract infections are the third leading cause of death in the United States after ischemic heart disease and cerebrovascular disease, accounting for 6.6% of all deaths. Development of new antibiotics and vaccines has not been fully successful in eliminating the morbidity and mortality associated with respiratory infections. Antibiotic resistance among common respiratory pathogens has emerged in the last 2 to 3 decades. Community-acquired and hospital-acquired pneumonia, acute respiratory distress syndrome (ARDS), lung abscess, and empyema can present as life-threatening infections of the respiratory system, which require early diagnosis and treatment to prevent complications and mortality. This review discusses diagnostic and treatment interventions for these pulmonary emergencies.

Disclosure: Authors have no conflicts of interest to disclose.
[a] Department of Internal Medicine, Division of Pulmonary and Critical Care Medicine, Eastern Virginia Medical School, 825 Fairfax Avenue, Suite 410, Norfolk, VA-23507, USA; [b] Infectious Disease Consultants of Hampton Roads, 6161 Kempsville Circle, # 220, Norfolk, VA 23502, USA
* Corresponding author.
E-mail address: desaihd@evms.edu

Med Clin N Am 96 (2012) 1127–1148
http://dx.doi.org/10.1016/j.mcna.2012.08.007
0025-7125/12/$ – see front matter © 2012 Elsevier Inc. All rights reserved.

medical.theclinics.com

PNEUMONIA

Severe community-acquired pneumonia (CAP), hospital-acquired/health care-associated pneumonia (HCAP), and ventilator-associated pneumonia (VAP) constitute a large percentage of respiratory tract infections requiring admission to an intensive care unit (ICU).

CAP

CAP is defined as an acute infection of the lung parenchyma acquired outside hospitals or extended-care facilities and accompanied by symptoms of acute illness.[1] CAP remains a major health problem in the United States, with more than 60,000 deaths annually.[2] In adults, CAP results in approximately 600,000 hospital admissions annually and ranks as the eighth leading cause of death. Mortality from CAP varies dramatically depending on the severity of the illness and associated comorbidities. Mortality is less than 1% to 5% in the outpatient setting and it approaches 23% in hospitalized patients.[2] In more seriously ill patients with bacteremia who require ICU admission, mortality can approach more than 40%.[3,4]

Pathophysiology

The common mechanisms for the development of pneumonia are inhalation of microorganisms into the lower airways and aspiration of oropharyngeal contents. Other mechanisms include direct spread from a contiguous site and distant hematogenous spread from an extrapulmonary focus. *Streptococcus pneumoniae* is the most common pathogen isolated from patients with CAP.[5,6] The common pathogens responsible for CAP are listed in **Table 1**.[7] In addition to *Streptococcus pneumoniae*, other typical pathogens that account for CAP include *Haemophilus influenzae, Staphylococcus aureus,* group A *Streptococci, Moraxella catarrhalis,* anaerobes, and aerobic gram-negative bacteria. The classically described atypical pneumonia refers to pneumonia caused by *Legionella* species, *Mycoplasma pneumoniae, Chlamydophila pneumoniae,* and *Chlamydophila psittaci.* However, the term atypical should no longer be used. In recent years, community-acquired methicillin-resistant *Staphylococcus aureus* (MRSA) has emerged as an important pathogen responsible for severe, fulminant necrotizing pneumonia in young, healthy individuals without typical risk factors.[8,9]

Table 1
Common pathogens in CAP by level of care

Outpatients	*Streptococcus pneumoniae, Mycoplasma pneumoniae, Haemophilus influenzae, Chlamydophila pneumoniae,* respiratory viruses (influenza A and B, adenovirus, respiratory syncytial virus, parainfluenza)
Inpatients (non-ICU)	*Streptococcus pneumoniae, Mycoplasma pneumoniae, , Chlamydophila pneumoniae, Haemophilus influenzae, Legionella* spp, respiratory viruses
Inpatients (ICU)	*Streptococcus pneumoniae, Legionella* spp, *Haemophilus influenzae,* gram-negative bacilli, *Staphylococcus aureus*

Data from Leroy O, Santre C, Beuscart C, et al. A five-year study of severe community-acquired pneumonia with emphasis on prognosis in patients admitted to an intensive care unit. Intensive Care Med 1995;21(1):24–31.

Clinical evaluation

Common clinical features of CAP include cough, fever, sputum production, and pleuritic chest pain. Patients may have gastrointestinal symptoms such as nausea, vomiting, or diarrhea. Other symptoms may include fatigue, headache, myalgia, and arthralgia. Risk stratification is an important component in the management of a patient with CAP and various risk stratification indices have been used to determine appropriate care setting (outpatient, inpatient non-ICU, ICU). Various prediction scores including the Pneumonia Severity Index (PSI), CURB 65 (confusion, urea >19 mg/dL; respiratory rate >30; low blood pressure: systolic <90 mm Hg or diastolic <60 mm Hg; and age >65 years), and CRB 65 (confusion, respiratory rate >30; low blood pressure: systolic <90 mm Hg or diastolic <60 mm Hg; and age >65 years) have been shown to reliably predict mortality in patients with CAP.[10–12] CRB 65 is simple to calculate and is based solely on physical examination findings and does not require laboratory data. The indications for ICU admission besides patients in need for mechanical ventilation and those in septic shock are listed in **Box 1**.[7]

Diagnosis

Although it is thought that pathogen-directed therapy is better than empiric therapy, a randomized trial failed to show such benefit.[13] Routine diagnostic tests are optional for outpatient treatment of CAP. Patients with severe CAP requiring ICU admission should have

- Blood cultures
- Urinary antigen tests for *Legionella pneumophila* and *Streptococcus pneumoniae*
- Expectorated sputum for Gram stain and culture

Box 1
Criteria for ICU admission in CAP

Major Criteria

- Requirement for mechanical ventilation
- Septic shock (SBP <90 mm Hg despite fluids)

Minor Criteria (3 or more)

- White blood cell count >30 × 10^9/L or <4 × 10^9/L
- Blood urea nitrogen >20 mg/dL
- Pao_2 (partial pressure of oxygen, arterial)/Fio_2 (fraction of inspired oxygen) <250
- Multilobe involvement
- Respiratory rate >30/min
- Platelet count <100,000 × 10^9/L
- Confusion/disorientation
- Hypothermia (temperature <36°C)
- Hypotension requiring fluid resuscitation

Modified from Mandell LA, Wunderink RG, Anzueto A, et al. Infectious Diseases Society of America/American Thoracic Society consensus guidelines on the management of community-acquired pneumonia in adults. Clin Infect Dis 2007;44(Suppl 2):S27–72.

- Intubated patients require endotracheal aspirate (ETA) (fresh) or m-BAL (blind bronchoalveolar lavage)
- Nasopharyngeal swab for influenza during seasonal influenza (rapid antigen test and viral polymerase chain reaction)

Even with extensive diagnostic evaluation, the cause is not identified in as many as 50% of patients.[5,6,14,15]

Treatment

Antimicrobial agents are the cornerstone of treatment in patients with CAP. Antibiotic therapy is typically begun on an empiric basis. Macrolides, quinolones, and second-generation/third-generation cephalosporins are considered the antimicrobial agents of choice for patients with CAP. However, resistance to antibiotics has been an increasingly recognized problem in the therapy for CAP. Risk factors for drug-resistant *Streptococcus pneumoniae* in adults include:

- Age >65 years
- β-lactam, macrolide, or fluoroquinolone therapy within the past 3 to 6 months
- Alcoholism
- Medical comorbidities
- Immunosuppressive illness or therapy
- Exposure to a child in a day care center

Two retrospective analyses of large Medicare databases identified that the time between presentation to the hospital and the time to the first antibiotic dose is a predictor of patient outcome when patients require hospital admission.[16,17] The antibiotic regimens advocated by a collaboration between the Infectious Disease Society of America and the American Thoracic Society (IDSA/ATS) in 2007 are summarized in **Figs. 1** and **2**.[7] The antibiotic therapy should be continued for a minimum of 5 days,

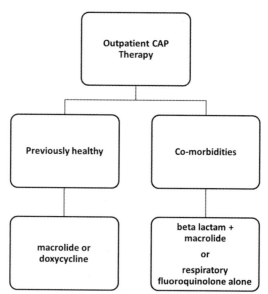

Fig. 1. ATS/IDSA guidelines for outpatient CAP treatment. (*Data from* Mandell LA, Wunderink RG, Anzueto A, et al. Infectious Diseases Society of America/American Thoracic Society consensus guidelines on the management of community-acquired pneumonia in adults. Clin Infect Dis 2007;44(Suppl 2):S29.)

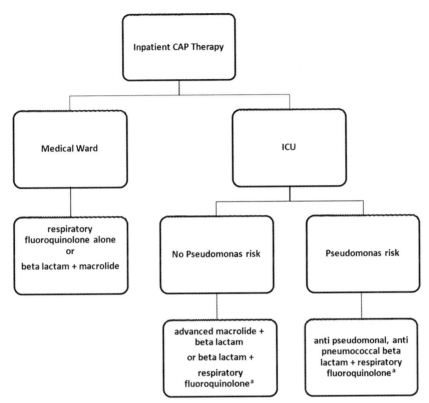

Fig. 2. ATS/IDSA guidelines for inpatient CAP treatment. [a] Add vancomycin or linezolid for suspected community-acquired MRSA infection. (*Data from* Mandell LA, Wunderink RG, Anzueto A, et al. Infectious Diseases Society of America/American Thoracic Society consensus guidelines on the management of community-acquired pneumonia in adults. Clin Infect Dis 2007;44(Suppl 2):S30.)

except for azithromycin, which has a long half-life and for which a shorter duration might be adequate. Longer duration of therapy may be needed in patients with necrotizing pneumonia, lung abscess, or empyema; those with associated extrapulmonary infections; pneumonia caused by *Pseudomonas aeruginosa* or *Legionella* species; and those with inappropriate initial empiric therapy.

HCAP

HCAP refers to patients with pneumonia who had recent hospitalization in the last 90 days, had residence in a nursing home or extended-care facility, were receiving chronic hemodialysis, were receiving home wound care, or had exposure to a family member with a drug-resistant pathogen infection.[18] HCAP is the second most common health care-related infection after urinary tract infection. HCAP accounts for 17% to 18% of pneumonia requiring hospitalization.[19,20]

Pathophysiology

The pathogenesis of HCAP includes a combination of immune impairment caused by underlying comorbidities, acquisition of a resistant strain, and exposure to large inocula of bacteria. Colonization of the upper respiratory tract followed by aspiration of bacteria-laden oropharyngeal secretions in to the lower respiratory tract is the most likely mechanism for development of HCAP. Common pathogens responsible for HCAP are listed in **Box 2**.[19–21]

Clinical evaluation

The clinical presentation of patients with HCAP is similar to patients with CAP. However, elderly patients and patients residing in long-term care (LTC) facilities might not have classic signs of infection. Compared to patients with CAP, these patients are less likely to have a productive cough, chills, myalgia, or arthralgia.[22] Patients from LTC facilities are more likely to present with altered mental status, tachypnea, and hypotension.[23] These atypical findings could be responsible for a delay in diagnosis and treatment, contributing to increased morbidity and mortality in this group of patients.

Diagnosis

There is no established gold standard for the diagnosis of HCAP. Fever, purulent cough, and new infiltrate on chest radiograph are considered to be the mainstay of diagnosis of pneumonia. In contrast to CAP, the value of sputum Gram stain in non-intubated patients with HCAP is questionable because of higher rates of oropharyngeal colonization in recently hospitalized patients or older patients residing in LTC facilities.[24,25] Transtracheal aspiration and bronchial washings are more accurate means of obtaining specimens for Gram stain and culture. Blood cultures and urinary antigen detection can be helpful in identifying the cause.

Treatment

Patients with HCAP are at higher risk of receiving inadequate antimicrobial therapy compared with CAP and are more likely to have a worse outcome.[19] Lack of adequate coverage for multidrug-resistant (MDR) pathogens is considered to be a contributing factor for this discrepancy between HCAP and CAP outcomes. Risk factors for isolation of MDR pathogens include severely ill patients requiring ICU admission, low functional status, and exposure to antibiotics for more than 3 days in previous 6 months.[26] The approach to initial empiric antimicrobial treatment of HCAP is summarized in **Fig. 3**.[27]

Box 2
Common pathogens for HCAP

Gram-Positive Bacteria

Staphylococcus aureus

Streptococcus pneumoniae

MRSA

Gram-Negative Bacteria:

Pseudomonas aeruginosa

Klebsiella pneumoniae

Escherichia coli

Haemophilus influenza

Data from Refs.[19–21]

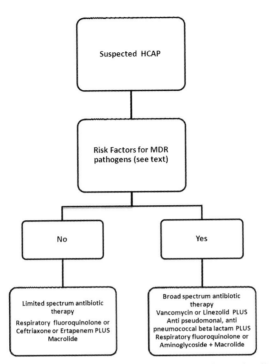

Fig. 3. Initial empiric antimicrobial therapy for HCAP. (*Data from* El-Solh AA. Health care-associated pneumonia. In: Sethi S, editor. Respiratory infections. 1st edition. New York: Informa Healthcare; 2010. p. 114–25.)

VAP

VAP is defined as a pneumonia that develops after 48 hours of mechanical ventilation. Pathogens causing late-onset VAP (≥5 days) are more likely to have MDR compared to those responsible for early-onset VAP (<5 days). VAP is the commonest nosocomial infection in the ICU, leading to increased morbidity, mortality, and health care costs.[18,28] VAP complicates the hospital course of about 20% of patients receiving mechanical ventilation. Rates of VAP increase with the duration of mechanical ventilation, with attack rates estimated to be approximately 3% per day.[18,28]

Pathophysiology

VAP pathogenesis begins with bacterial colonization that may progress to ventilator-associated tracheobronchitis and in some patients to VAP. In mechanically ventilated patients, colonization of the oropharynx with potentially pathogenic organisms occurs within 36 hours of intubation. Leakage of bacteria around the endotracheal tube cuff is a major route of access to the lower respiratory tract and a target for VAP prevention efforts. The common pathogens causing VAP are listed in **Table 2**. VAP caused by MDR organisms is associated with increased mortality. The risk factors for VAP caused by MDR organisms are listed in **Box 3**.

Clinical evaluation

The clinical criteria that have traditionally been used to diagnose VAP include a new or progressive pulmonary infiltrate, fever, leukocytosis, and increase in tracheobronchial

Table 2 Pathogens in VAP	
Common Pathogens	**Less Common Pathogens**
Pseudomonas aeruginosa	*Escherichia coli*
MRSA	*Enterobacter* spp
Klebsiella pneumoniae	*Citrobacter* spp
Acinetobacter spp	*Serratia* spp
Stenotrophomonas maltophilia	*Legionella* spp
Streptococcus pneumoniae (early VAP)	
Haemophilus influenzae (early VAP)	

secretions. However, these clinical criteria are nonspecific and of little clinical usefulness in the diagnosis of VAP.[29,30] The Clinical Pulmonary Infection Score (CPIS) was developed as a noninvasive method to diagnose VAP[31] and uses a combination of clinical features together with the culture of a tracheal aspirate to diagnose pneumonia. The CPIS assigns 0 to 12 points based on 6 clinical criteria:

- Fever
- Leukocyte count
- Oxygenation
- Quantity and purulence of secretions
- Type of radiographic abnormality
- Results of respiratory (tracheal aspirate) Gram stain and culture

Diagnosis
Because the clinical criteria of VAP lack specificity, several diagnostic techniques have been reported that attempt to distinguish patients with lung infection from those colonized with potentially pathogenic organisms or those with tracheobronchitis. ETA, BAL, and protective specimen brush (PSB) have been used to detect pathogenic bacteria in the lower respiratory tract. Studies have shown conflicting results in outcomes when noninvasive and invasive techniques to collect lower respiratory tract samples were compared.[32,33] Biological markers, such as procalcitonin, C-reactive protein, and soluble triggering receptor expressed on myeloid cells, may be helpful adjuncts for the diagnosis and management of VAP.[34]

Box 3
Risk factors for infection by MDR organisms

- Intubation for longer than 7 days
- Previous broad-spectrum antibiotics
- Hemodialysis
- Hospitalization for 2 days or more in the last 90 days
- Previous admission to the ICU
- Nursing home residence
- Immunosuppression
- Chronic wound care

Treatment

The most important factor determining the outcome of VAP is the early initiation of appropriate antibiotic therapy. Because of the spectrum of potential pathogens and the increasing prevalence of MDR organisms, a broad-spectrum, multidrug, empiric antibiotic protocol is required in most patients with suspected VAP (except those at low risk of infection with an MDR organism). BAL and quantitative culture allows for the de-escalation of antibiotics once a pathogen(s) is identified. Initial empiric antimicrobial therapies for early-onset and late-onset VAP are summarized in **Tables 3** and **4**.[18] Antibiotic therapy should be modified based on the identification and drug resistance of pathogens. Antimicrobial therapy is recommended for 7 to 8 days for uncomplicated VAP except when VAP is caused by *Pseudomonas aeruginosa* when antimicrobial therapy should be continued for longer duration (10–14 days).[18,35]

ARDS

ARDS is an important cause of ICU admission and is associated with high mortality.[36] ARDS is an acute, diffuse, inflammatory lung injury that is characterized by hypoxemia (Pao_2/Fio_2 <200), bilateral radiographic opacities, and no evidence of increased left atrial pressure. The common conditions associated with ARDS are listed in **Box 4**. Sepsis (both from pulmonary and extrapulmonary causes) is a leading cause of ARDS. Lung infection may account for 50% of cases of ARDS.[37,38] Superinfection with bacterial pathogen is also possible with ARDS from other causes because of impaired host defenses and prolonged mechanical ventilation.[39] Pneumonia can be a cause or complication of ARDS. The diagnosis of pulmonary infection in patients with ARDS is often difficult. The incidence of VAP during ARDS varied from 15% to 60% in different studies.[38,40–43]

Pathophysiology

CAP is a common cause for ARDS that develops outside the hospital.[44] Common pathogens include *Streptococcus pneumoniae*, *Legionella pneumophila*, *Pneumocystis jirovecii*, *Staphylococcus aureus*, enteric gram-negative organisms, and respiratory viruses.[6] Common pathogens responsible for pneumonia in patients with ARDS

Table 3 Initial empiric antimicrobial therapy for early-onset VAP	
HAP/VAP, Early-Onset (ie, No Risk Factors for MDR Pathogens), Any Disease Severity	
Potential Pathogen	**Recommended Antibiotic**
Streptococcus pneumoniae	Ceftriaxone
Haemophilus influenzae	or
Methicillin-sensitive *Staphylococcus*	ciprofloxacin, levofloxacin or moxifloxacin
aureus (MSSA)	or
Antibiotic-sensitive enteric gram-negative	ampicillin/sulbactam
bacilli:	or
• *Escherichia coli*	ertapenem
• *Klebsiella pneumoniae*	
• *Enterobacter* spp	
• *Proteus* spp	
• *Serratia marcescens*	

Data from American Thoracic Society, Infectious Diseases Society of America. Guidelines for the management of adults with hospital-acquired, ventilator-associated, and healthcare-associated pneumonia. Am J Respir Crit Care Med 2005;171(4):388–416.

Table 4
Initial empiric antimicrobial therapy for late-onset VAP

HAP/VAP/HCAP, Late-Onset (ie, Risk Factors for MDR pathogens), Any Disease Severity	
Potential Pathogen	Combination Antibiotic Therapy
Streptococcus pneumoniae	Antipseudomonal cephalosporin
Haemophilus influenzae	(cefepime, ceftazidime)
Staphylococcus aureus	or
Antibiotic-sensitive enteric	antipseudomonal carbepenem
gram-negative bacilli:	(imipenem or meropenem)
• *Escherichia coli*	or
• *Klebsiella pneumoniae*	β-lactam/β-lactamase inhibitor
• *Enterobacter* spp	(piperacillin-tazobactam)
• *Proteus* spp	plus
• *Serratia marcescens*	antipseudomonal fluoroquinolone
MDR Pathogens:	(ciprofloxacin or levofloxacin)
• *Pseudomonas aeruginosa*	or
• *Klebsiella pneumoniae* (ESBL+)	aminoglycoside (amikacin, gentamicin,
• *Acinetobacter* spp	or tobramycin)
• MRSA	plus
• *Legionella pneumophila*	linezolid or vancomycin

Data from American Thoracic Society, Infectious Diseases Society of America. Guidelines for the management of adults with hospital-acquired, ventilator-associated, and healthcare-associated pneumonia. Am J Respir Crit Care Med 2005;171(4):388–416.

include MRSA, *Pseudomonas aeruginosa*, *Acinetobacter baumannii*, *Stenotrophomonas maltophili*, and *Enterobacteriaceae*.[38,40] Effects of mechanical ventilation on bacterial growth, on lung inflammation, and on systemic inflammation have been believed to play a role in the pathogenesis of pneumonia during ARDS. Impaired

Box 4
Common conditions associated with ARDS

- Sepsis
- Aspiration
- Pneumonia
- Severe trauma
- Burns
- Multiple blood transfusions
- Pancreatitis
- Drug overdose
- Near drowning
- Smoke inhalation
- Cardiopulmonary bypass
- Pulmonary contusion
- Multiple fractures
- Venous air embolism
- Amniotic fluid embolism
- Neurogenic pulmonary edema

host defenses during ARDS and mechanical ventilation increase host susceptibility to infection with virulent or resistant organisms.

Clinical Evaluation

Initial clinical presentation is that of the underlying condition responsible for ARDS. Clinical symptoms of ARDS become apparent after 48 to 72 hours of inciting event. Dyspnea, tachypnea, hypoxia, and cough are generally present. Persistent or new fever, purulent respiratory secretions, oxygenation desaturation, tachycardia, hemo-dynamic instability or septic shock suggest VAP in mechanically ventilated patients with ARDS. The CPIS[31] can be helpful to diagnose new VAP in patients with ARDS.

Diagnosis

Diagnosis of new respiratory infection in patients with ARDS who are on mechanical ventilation is challenging. Physicians should have a low threshold for invasive proce-dures to diagnose new respiratory infections, because many of these patients have an abnormal chest radiograph with infiltrates, hypoxia, and fever at the time of initial presentation. Respiratory tract cultures can be obtained with ETA, BAL, PSB, or plugged telescopic catheter (PTC). Quantitative cultures of these samples help distin-guish colonization from true pulmonary infection (**Table 5**).[45] Efforts should be made to obtain bacteriologic samples before initiating or modifying antibiotic treatment.

Treatment

General goals of treatment of ARDS include treatment of underlying condition, lung protective mechanical ventilation, sedation, nutritional support, deep vein thrombosis and stress ulcer prophylaxis, and measures to avoid nosocomial infections. Principles of antimicrobial treatment of VAP during ARDS are similar to treatment of late-onset VAP, because infection with MDR pathogens is more likely in these patients. **Box 5** summarizes strategies for preventing VAP.

LUNG ABSCESS

Lung abscess is defined as necrosis of lung parenchyma as a result of microbial infec-tion. Lung abscesses were more common in the preantibiotic era as a result of the complication of bacterial pneumonia. The incidence and mortality of lung abscess have decreased significantly over the last few decades. In the postantibiotic era, most lung abscesses arise as a complication of aspiration pneumonia.[50] Lung abscesses can be classified as acute (<1 month of symptoms) or chronic (>1 month of symptoms), based on the causative organism (eg, pneumococcal lung abscess, anaerobic lung abscess) or on the underlying conditions. When an abscess develops

Table 5	
Microbiological culture thresholds for the diagnosis of VAP	
Sampling Technique	**Quantitative Culture Threshold (cfu/mL)**
ETA	10^6
BAL	10^4
PSB	10^3
PTC	10^3

Modified from Richard Jean-Damien DD, Roux D. Pneumonia in ARDS. In: Sethi S, editor. Respira-tory Infections. New York: Informa Healthcare; 2009. p. 153.

Box 5
Strategies for preventing VAP

- Semirecumbent position with head elevation up to 30° to 45°[46]
- Oral care with chlorhexidine[47]
- Implement weaning and wake-up protocols
- Limited use of proton pump inhibitors and sucralfate[38,48]
- Avoid gastric overdistention
- Early tracheotomy[49]
---

in individuals prone to aspiration or individuals in relatively good health, it is termed primary lung abscess. Secondary lung abscess implies underlying predisposing conditions like malignant neoplasm, complications of surgery, and immunosuppression. Approximately 80% of lung abscesses are primary.[51]

Pathophysiology

Anaerobic bacteria generally present in gingival crevices are responsible for aspiration pneumonia and lung abscess.[52] Primary lung abscess is rare in an edentulous person. Risk factors for aspiration pneumonia and lung abscess include reduced level of consciousness, periodontal disease, esophageal dysmotility, gastric reflux, dysphagia, vomiting, gastric overdistension, large-volume tube feedings, and recumbent position. After the initial inoculum of bacteria with large-volume aspiration, pneumonitis develops followed by tissue necrosis in 7 to 14 days depending on the host-pathogen interaction. This tissue necrosis results in lung abscess. Other mechanisms of development of lung abscess include septic embolization from right-sided infective endocarditis and hematogenous spread from suppurative thrombophlebitis. Lung abscesses from septic embolization are generally multiple, and involve noncontiguous areas of the lung. Both anaerobic and aerobic bacteria are known to cause lung abscess, with anaerobes being more common (**Box 6**). Anaerobic lung abscesses are typically polymicrobial. *Nocardia* is also known to cause lung abscesses in immunocompromised patients.

Box 6
Common pathogens for lung abscess

- *Peptostreptococcus*
- *Prevotella*
- *Bacteroides*
- *Fusobacterium*
- *Streptococcus milleri*
- *Streptococcus pyogenes*
- *Staphylococcus aureus*
- *Klebsiellae pneumoniae*
- *Escherichia coli*
- *Pseudomonas aeruginosa*

Certain parasites (*Entamoeba histolytica* and *Paragonimus westermani*) and fungi (*Aspergillus, Blastomyces,* and *Histoplasma*) can cause lung abscesses.

Clinical Evaluation

Primary lung abscess caused by anaerobic bacteria usually presents in a subacute fashion with symptoms for several weeks.[50,53] Cough, fever, and purulent sputum are common presenting symptoms of lung abscess. The sputum has a putrid smell in about 50% of cases. Patients may present with pleuritic chest pain, hemoptysis, weight loss, or night sweats. Physical examination findings include fever, poor dentition and gingival disease, and amphoric or cavernous breath sounds on auscultation. Clubbing of the fingers and absent gag reflex may also be present. Associated empyema is present in about one-third of cases and may be seen with or without bronchopleural fistula. Necrotizing pneumonia caused by *Staphylococcus aureus* or *Klebsiella pneumoniae* occasionally presents with a more rapid course, high-grade fever, marked leukocytosis, and early extension to pleural space.

Diagnosis

Lung abscess is usually diagnosed by chest radiograph showing a thick-walled cavity with air fluid level. However, computed tomography (CT) is more sensitive than chest radiography and is useful to detect small cavities, to identify associated malignancy, and to distinguish lung abscesses from empyema.[54] Multilobar involvement suggests secondary lung abscess and impaired host defenses.[55] It is difficult to isolate anaerobic bacteria in primary lung abscess because most respiratory tract specimens are contaminated by upper airway flora and are consequently inappropriate for anaerobic culture. As a result, treatment of anaerobic infection can be started without microbiological studies, with a classic presentation of subacute illness in a typical aspiration-prone patient with gingival disease and foul-smelling sputum with putrid odor.[51] Uncontaminated specimens can be obtained by transtracheal aspirates (TTA), transthoracic needle aspirates (TTNA), pleural fluid, or blood cultures.[56,57] The usefulness of BAL or PSB for diagnosis of lung abscess is not well established. Blood cultures are rarely positive in anaerobic lung abscess. TTA and TTNA are not routinely performed to confirm the diagnosis. Patients without the classic presentation and with secondary lung abscess should have expectorated sputum checked for aerobic bacteria, mycobacteria, fungi, and, in some instances, parasites. Bronchoscopy is indicated to detect underlying lesions in patients with atypical presentations and for those who fail standard therapy.

Treatment

Antibiotics

Patients with large abscesses and excessive coughing should be placed in a lateral decubitus position with the abscess side down to avoid sudden discharge of abscess contents causing asphyxiation or spread of infection to healthy lung segments. Standard treatment of primary lung abscess is clindamycin 600 mg intravenously every 8 hours initially, followed by 150 to 300 mg orally 4 times daily. Penicillin was considered to be the drug of choice for primary lung abscess for many years but recent studies have shown superiority of clindamycin over penicillin in time to defervescence, time to resolution of putrid sputum, and relapse rates.[58,59] Monotherapy with metronidazole is not very effective,[60] but combination of penicillin and metronidazole has yielded favorable results and is inexpensive. Other agents that could be used in the treatment of lung abscess include combinations of a penicillin with a β-lactamase inhibitor, carbapenems, and quinolones with good anaerobic activity (moxifloxacin and gatifloxacin).[61] Lung abscess caused by organisms other than anaerobes is best treated with antibiotics that are active against the infecting pathogen and penetrate the lung parenchyma. The preferred agents for MRSA are vancomycin and linezolid. The duration of antibiotic therapy is controversial. Patients are often treated for 6 to 8 weeks or more. One study using clindamycin to treat anaerobic lung abscess showed excellent efficacy with no advantage of 6 weeks over 3 weeks of therapy.[58] Some experts recommend continuing antibiotic treatment until the chest radiograph shows a small, stable residual lesion or is clear.

Bronchoscopic drainage

Studies in the preantibiotic era showed no advantage for bronchoscopic or postural drainage of abscesses compared with conservative management or surgery. Drainage of large abscesses may result in rapid unloading of the pus and necrotic material from the abscess into other lung segments and may produce acute asphyxiation or ARDS.[51] Bronchoscopy should be reserved for patients who fail standard therapy or patients with suspected endobronchial tumor.

Surgery

Lung abscesses, in contrast to other visceral abscesses, usually drain themselves, through communication with large airways. This drainage is indicated by the presence of air fluid levels. Almost all patients with lung abscess respond to appropriate antimicrobial therapy, and surgery (lobectomy or pneumonectomy) is reserved for the 10% to 15% of patients who do not improve with appropriate medical management. Causes of medical treatment failure include large cavities (>8 cm), abscesses caused by resistant organisms such as *Pseudomonas aeruginosa,* obstructing neoplasm, and massive hemoptysis. Percutaneous and endoscopic drainage can be tried in patients with poor surgical risk who fail medical treatment. Percutaneous procedures require special care to prevent contamination of the pleural space. Endoscopic drainage is performed by placing a pigtail catheter into the abscess cavity under bronchoscopic visualization, leaving the catheter in place until the cavity has drained.[62]

EMPYEMA

Empyema is characterized by aspiration of pus from pleural space or positive Gram stain on pleural fluid analysis. Infections of the pleural space most commonly follow pneumonia, accounting for 40% to 60% of all empyemas. Thoracotomy is the next most common precursor of empyema, accounting for 20%, and trauma accounts for 4% to 10%. Common causes of empyema are shown in **Table 6**.[63–66]

Pathophysiology

Pleural effusions develop because of increased hydrostatic pressure or decreased oncotic pressure caused by cardiac, renal, hepatic, or metabolic diseases or because of altered pleural permeability caused by noninfectious inflammatory disease, infection, toxic injury, malignancy, or trauma. Pleural effusions are nutritionally rich media in which phagocytic defenses are severely impaired. The formation of an empyema has been arbitrarily divided into an exudative phase, during which pus accumulates; a fibropurulent phase, during which fibrin deposition and loculation of pleural exudate occurs; and an organization phase, during which fibroblast proliferation and scar formation cause lung entrapment. However, if pneumonia associated with a parapneumonic effusion is treated promptly with an appropriate antimicrobial agent, the cellular and cytokine mediators of inflammation are aborted. Resolution of uncomplicated parapneumonic effusions leaves the pleura essentially normal without clinically significant

Table 6 Common causes of empyema	
Cause	Percentage
Pulmonary infection (pneumonia)	56
Surgery (thoracotomy)	22
Trauma	4
Esophageal perforation	4
Complication of thoracentesis/chest tube	4
Subdiaphragmatic infection	3
Spontaneous pneumothorax	1
Septicemia	1
Other causes	5

Modified from Bryant RE, Salmon CJ. Pleural empyema. Clin Infect Dis 1996;22(5):749.

fibrosis.[67] In the preantibiotic era, *Streptococcus pneumoniae* accounted for 60% to 70% of cases, *Streptococcus pyogenes* for 10% to 15% of cases, and *Staphylococcus aureus* for 5% to 10% of cases of empyema. *Streptococcus pneumoniae* now accounts for only 5% to 10% of cases, and many infections are mixed, with anaerobes present in 25% to 76% of empyemas either as sole organisms or in combination with other aerobic or facultative organisms.[68] Bacterial pathogens associated with nontuberculous pleural empyema are summarized in **Box 7**. Factors predisposing to aspiration such as altered mental status, alcoholism, and periodontal disease are common in patients with anaerobic infections of the pleura. Empyema complicating

Box 7 Common pathogens for nontuberculous pleural empyema
Anaerobic Bacteria:
Bacteroides fragilis group
Prevotella spp
Fusobacterium nucleatum
Peptostreptococcus
Microaerophilic streptococci
Aerobic Bacteria:
Streptococcus pneumoniae
Streptococcus pyogenes
Streptococcus milleri
Staphylococcus aureus
Enterobacteriaceae
Klebsiella pneumoniae
Pseudomonas aeruginosa
MRSA

hemothorax is often caused by *Staphylococcus*, whereas that associated with pneumothorax or hematogenous seeding of a serous effusion is often caused by aerobic gram-negative bacilli.[69] Immunocompromised patients are prone to pleural involvement with fungal, mycobacterial, or aerobic gram-negative bacillary infection.[65,70] Amoebic liver abscess is associated with pleural involvement in up to 15% to 20% of cases. Nocardia infections occur more frequently in patients with underlying conditions, such as organ transplantation, malignancy, diabetes mellitus, AIDS, and long-term use of steroids. Empyema caused by *Mycobacterium tuberculosis* is a rare disease in which pus is present in the pleural space and the predominant pleural cell is the polymorphonuclear leukocyte. Tuberculous empyema should be differentiated from tuberculous pleurisy, in which a lymphocytic effusion occurs from the immunologic response to tuberculous proteins.

Clinical Evaluation

Patients with bacterial pneumonia usually present with fever, shortness of breath, productive cough, and chest pain. Patients with anaerobic pleuropulmonary infection present with an indolent course and may show weight loss, fever, and chronic cough. A history of aspiration is often obtained and poor oral hygiene is often evident. The presence of persistent fever, chest pain, or leukocytosis despite the administration of appropriate antibiotics should suggest the presence of an empyema in patients with pulmonary or adjacent infection. Physical examination is remarkably nonspecific and reveals decreased breath sounds, dullness to percussion, and crackles over the affected area. Chronic empyemas may erode the chest wall and present with a spontaneous draining abscess, termed empyema necessitatis.[68]

Diagnosis

Chest radiograph and ultrasonography play an important role in the evaluation of empyema. As little as 25 mL of pleural fluid can elevate the hemidiaphragm radiographically, but blunting of the posterior costophrenic sulcus usually requires about 200 mL of fluid. The lateral decubitus chest film can detect as little as 5 mL of free pleural fluid.[71] Ultrasonography is particularly useful for detecting small amounts of pleural fluid, for easy identification of free or loculated pleural effusions, and for differentiating loculated effusions from solid masses. Ultrasonography also helps in diagnostic thoracentesis and pleural drainage. A chest CT scan with intravenous contrast is sometimes required for optimal evaluation of an empyema or loculated effusion. Thickening of the parietal pleura is suggestive of empyema.

An effusion should be sampled if the fluid is free flowing, is greater than 10 mm on a lateral decubitus film, or is loculated. Empyema fluid might appear purulent, bloody, or cloudy, with a very high white blood cell count (>50,000). Empyema fluid characteristically has a pH of less than 7.2, a glucose level of less than 40 mg/dL, and lactate dehydrogenase activity of at least 1000 IU/L.[72] Malodorous empyema fluid suggests the presence of anaerobic infection but is present in only about two-thirds of anaerobic empyemas. Most experts recommend drainage of the pleural space for a positive pleural fluid culture or Gram stain. However, only 61% of patients with established empyemas have a positive Gram stain. Although most patients with empyemas have a positive culture, the absence of growth does not mean that a pleural effusion does not require drainage.[73] A pleural fluid pH less than 7.2 indicates the need for drainage.[74] Spurious increase of empyema fluid pH values may occur in patients with urea-splitting *Proteus* infections.[75] The diagnosis of amoebic abscess with subdiaphragmatic rupture is suggested by the anchovy paste or chocolate appearance of pleural fluid. Approximately 98% of patients with pleural or pulmonary amebiasis have positive serologic tests for *Entamoeba histolytica.* Patients at risk of fungal empyema require appropriate smears and cultures of empyema fluid for detection of fungi. For patients at risk of nocardial infection of the lung and pleura, modified acid-fast stains of purulent secretions should be performed. Pleural tuberculosis can be confirmed by acid-fast smears of pleural fluid in fewer than one-quarter of cases but can be diagnosed by pleural biopsy and culture in more than 90% of patients.[76]

Treatment

Antibiotics
Effective therapy for an empyema requires control of infection, drainage of pus, and expansion of the lung. Initial empiric antimicrobial therapy should be based on the most likely pathogens, local antimicrobial susceptibility patterns, and all available results, including Gram stains. Most of the antibiotics adequately penetrate the pleural space except for aminoglycosides, which may be inactivated at low pleural fluid pH. Choices for initial empiric antibiotic therapy include a combination of a β-lactam and a β-lactamase inhibitor (amoxicillin/clavulanate, ampicillin/sulbactam, or piperacillin/tazobactam), a carbapenem (imipenem, ertapenem, or meropenem), or combination therapy with a third-generation cephalosporin (cefotaxime, ceftriaxone, or cefepime) and either clindamycin or metronidazole. These choices cover the most common pathogens associated with pleural empyema, including anaerobic organisms. Vancomycin should be added when infection with *Staphylococcus aureus* is suspected. The duration of antibiotic therapy for bacterial empyema depends on the sensitivity of the organism(s), response to initial therapy, extent of pulmonary parenchymal and pleural disease, adequacy of drainage, and host factors such as immune status. Prolonged antimicrobial therapy (4–6 weeks) may be necessary. Patients with pulmonary actinomycosis or nocardiosis may require 6 to 12 months of antimicrobial treatment.[77] Patients with tuberculous pleural disease should be treated with the same regimen and for the same duration as those with pulmonary tuberculosis. Patients infected with *Candida* species should receive an appropriate antifungal drug (fluconazole, caspofungin, or amphotericin B) for 2 weeks after the resolution of signs and symptoms of infection.[78] Amoebic empyema should be treated with pleural drainage and an appropriate antimicrobial agent. Metronidazole is considered the drug of choice and is administered for 10 days.

Drainage of empyema
In addition to antimicrobial therapy to control infection, drainage of pus is a major component of adequate treatment of pleural empyema. Repeated thoracentesis is rarely successful in such cases. Options for pleural drainage include tube thoracostomy, video-assisted thoracoscopic surgery (VATS), open decortication, and open thoracostomy. Tube thoracostomy (also known as chest tube) drainage is the least invasive option for drainage of empyema fluid. It is generally preferred over more invasive options for patients with uniloculated effusions and free-flowing fluid, but is also frequently used to drain multiloculated empyemas. Chest tubes are typically left in place until the drainage rate has decreased less than 50 mL/d and the empyema cavity has closed. Closed chest tube drainage without fibrinolytic therapy is successful in up to two-thirds of patients.[79] The most common reason for closed chest tube failure is pleural adhesions and intrapleural loculations that do not communicate with the chest tubes. When patients do not respond to chest tube drainage, a more definitive approach is needed.

Intrapleural administration of fibrinolytic agents (streptokinase, urokinase, and tissue plasminogen activator [TPA]) has been studied as a way to improve drainage of loculated parapneumonic effusions and empyemas. However, data are conflicting regarding the benefit of this approach.[80–83] A Cochrane review failed to show a reduction in death among patients who received fibrinolytic therapy. When surgical intervention was included as an end point, fibrinolytics reduced the risk of this specific outcome.[84] In a recent study, concomitant use of intrapleural DNase and TPA resulted in a greater decrease in radiographic pleural opacity, a lower rate of surgical referral, and a shorter hospital stay compared with placebo.[85] However, neither of the individual agents performed better than placebo.

Surgical intervention

Surgical options include thoracoscopy usually by VATS or full thoracotomy with decortication. VATS is most commonly used to debride multiloculated empyemas or uniloculated empyemas that fail to resolve with antibiotics and tube thoracostomy drainage, as an alternative to instillation of intrapleural fibrinolytics. VATS allows for minimally invasive debridement and drainage and can be followed by or converted to a thoracotomy if adequate pleural fluid drainage and lung expansion are not achieved. When visceral pleural fibrosis does not regress and limits reexpansion of the lung, a total pleurectomy/decortication may be required to achieve lung reexpansion.[86] Open thoracostomy involves a vertical incision through the chest wall with rib resection to permit open drainage at the inferior border of the empyema cavity. A chest tube is left in place; it is gradually advanced outward as the tract closes.

In summary, pulmonary infectious emergencies are responsible for significant morbidity and mortality, and frequently require treatment in Intensive Care Unit. Early aggressive treatment is required to effectively control these infections.

REFERENCES

1. Metlay JP, Fine MJ. Testing strategies in the initial management of patients with community-acquired pneumonia. Ann Intern Med 2003;138(2):109–18.
2. File TM Jr, Marrie TJ. Burden of community-acquired pneumonia in North American adults. Postgrad Med 2010;122(2):130–41.
3. Ortqvist A, Sterner G, Nilsson JA. Severe community-acquired pneumonia: factors influencing need of intensive care treatment and prognosis. Scand J Infect Dis 1985;17(4):377–86.
4. Leroy O, Santre C, Beuscart C, et al. A five-year study of severe community-acquired pneumonia with emphasis on prognosis in patients admitted to an intensive care unit. Intensive Care Med 1995;21(1):24–31.
5. Marrie TJ, Durant H, Yates L. Community-acquired pneumonia requiring hospitalization: 5-year prospective study. Rev Infect Dis 1989;11(4):586–99.
6. Torres A, Serra-Batlles J, Ferrer A, et al. Severe community-acquired pneumonia. Epidemiology and prognostic factors. Am Rev Respir Dis 1991;144(2):312–8.
7. Mandell LA, Wunderink RG, Anzueto A, et al. Infectious Diseases Society of America/American Thoracic Society consensus guidelines on the management of community-acquired pneumonia in adults. Clin Infect Dis 2007;44(Suppl 2): S27–72.
8. Kollef MH, Micek ST. Methicillin-resistant *Staphylococcus aureus*: a new community-acquired pathogen? Curr Opin Infect Dis 2006;19(2):161–8.
9. Francis JS, Doherty MC, Lopatin U, et al. Severe community-onset pneumonia in healthy adults caused by methicillin-resistant *Staphylococcus aureus* carrying the Panton-Valentine leukocidin genes. Clin Infect Dis 2005;40(1):100–7.
10. Fine MJ, Auble TE, Yealy DM, et al. A prediction rule to identify low-risk patients with community-acquired pneumonia. N Engl J Med 1997;336(4):243–50.

11. Lim WS, van der Eerden MM, Laing R, et al. Defining community acquired pneumonia severity on presentation to hospital: an international derivation and validation study. Thorax 2003;58(5):377–82.

12. Capelastegui A, Espana PP, Quintana JM, et al. Validation of a predictive rule for the management of community-acquired pneumonia. Eur Respir J 2006;27(1): 151–7.

13. van der Eerden MM, Vlaspolder F, de Graaff CS, et al. Comparison between pathogen directed antibiotic treatment and empirical broad spectrum antibiotic treatment in patients with community acquired pneumonia: a prospective randomised study. Thorax 2005;60(8):672–8.

14. Ruiz M, Ewig S, Marcos MA, et al. Etiology of community-acquired pneumonia: impact of age, comorbidity, and severity. Am J Respir Crit Care Med 1999; 160(2):397–405.

15. Woodhead MA, Macfarlane JT, McCracken JS, et al. Prospective study of the aetiology and outcome of pneumonia in the community. Lancet 1987;1(8534): 671–4.

16. Houck PM, Bratzler DW, Niederman M, et al. Pneumonia treatment process and quality. Arch Intern Med 2002;162(7):843–4.

17. Meehan TP, Fine MJ, Krumholz HM, et al. Quality of care, process, and outcomes in elderly patients with pneumonia. JAMA 1997;278(23):2080–4.

18. American Thoracic Society, Infectious Diseases Society of America. Guidelines for the management of adults with hospital-acquired, ventilator-associated, and healthcare-associated pneumonia. Am J Respir Crit Care Med 2005;171(4): 388–416.

19. Kollef MH, Shorr A, Tabak YP, et al. Epidemiology and outcomes of health-care-associated pneumonia: results from a large US database of culture-positive pneumonia. Chest 2005;128(6):3854–62.

20. Carratala J, Mykietiuk A, Fernandez-Sabe N, et al. Health care-associated pneumonia requiring hospital admission: epidemiology, antibiotic therapy, and clinical outcomes. Arch Intern Med 2007;167(13):1393–9.

21. Micek ST, Kollef KE, Reichley RM, et al. Health care-associated pneumonia and community-acquired pneumonia: a single-center experience. Antimicrob Agents Chemother 2007;51(10):3568–73.

22. Marrie TJ, Blanchard W. A comparison of nursing home-acquired pneumonia patients with patients with community-acquired pneumonia and nursing home patients without pneumonia. J Am Geriatr Soc 1997;45(1):50–5.

23. Meehan TP, Chua-Reyes JM, Tate J, et al. Process of care performance, patient characteristics, and outcomes in elderly patients hospitalized with community-acquired or nursing home-acquired pneumonia. Chest 2000;117(5):1378–85.

24. Palmer LB, Albulak K, Fields S, et al. Oral clearance and pathogenic oropharyngeal colonization in the elderly. Am J Respir Crit Care Med 2001;164(3):464–8.

25. Valenti WM, Trudell RG, Bentley DW. Factors predisposing to oropharyngeal colonization with gram-negative bacilli in the aged. N Engl J Med 1978;298(20): 1108–11.

26. El Solh AA, Pietrantoni C, Bhat A, et al. Indicators of potentially drug-resistant bacteria in severe nursing home-acquired pneumonia. Clin Infect Dis 2004; 39(4):474–80.

27. El-Solh AA. Health care-associated pneumonia. In: Sethi S, editor. Respiratory infections. 1st edition. New York: Informa Healthcare; 2010. p. 114–25.

28. Chastre J, Fagon JY. Ventilator-associated pneumonia. Am J Respir Crit Care Med 2002;165(7):867–903.

29. Mabie M, Wunderink RG. Use and limitations of clinical and radiologic diagnosis of pneumonia. Semin Respir Infect 2003;18(2):72–9.

30. Lauzier F, Ruest A, Cook D, et al. The value of pretest probability and modified clinical pulmonary infection score to diagnose ventilator-associated pneumonia. J Crit Care 2008;23(1):50–7.

31. Pugin J, Auckenthaler R, Mili N, et al. Diagnosis of ventilator-associated pneumonia by bacteriologic analysis of bronchoscopic and nonbronchoscopic "blind" bronchoalveolar lavage fluid. Am Rev Respir Dis 1991;143(5 Pt 1):1121–9.

32. Fagon JY, Chastre J, Wolff M, et al. Invasive and noninvasive strategies for management of suspected ventilator-associated pneumonia. A randomized trial. Ann Intern Med 2000;132(8):621–30.

33. Canadian Critical Care Trials Group. A randomized trial of diagnostic techniques for ventilator-associated pneumonia. N Engl J Med 2006;355(25):2619–30.

34. Gibot S, Cravoisy A, Levy B, et al. Soluble triggering receptor expressed on myeloid cells and the diagnosis of pneumonia. N Engl J Med 2004;350(5):451–8.

35. Chastre J, Wolff M, Fagon JY, et al. Comparison of 8 vs 15 days of antibiotic therapy for ventilator-associated pneumonia in adults: a randomized trial. JAMA 2003;290(19):2588–98.

36. Roupie E, Lepage E, Wysocki M, et al. Prevalence, etiologies and outcome of the acute respiratory distress syndrome among hypoxemic ventilated patients. SRLF Collaborative Group on Mechanical Ventilation. Société de Réanimation de Langue Française. Intensive Care Med 1999;25(9):920–9.

37. Brun-Buisson C, Minelli C, Bertolini G, et al. Epidemiology and outcome of acute lung injury in European intensive care units. Results from the ALIVE study. Intensive Care Med 2004;30(1):51–61.

38. Markowicz P, Wolff M, Djedaini K, et al. Multicenter prospective study of ventilator-associated pneumonia during acute respiratory distress syndrome. Incidence, prognosis, and risk factors. ARDS Study Group. Am J Respir Crit Care Med 2000;161(6):1942–8.

39. Bell RC, Coalson JJ, Smith JD, et al. Multiple organ system failure and infection in adult respiratory distress syndrome. Ann Intern Med 1983;99(3):293–8.

40. Chastre J, Trouillet JL, Vuagnat A, et al. Nosocomial pneumonia in patients with acute respiratory distress syndrome. Am J Respir Crit Care Med 1998;157(4 Pt 1): 1165–72.

41. Delclaux C, Roupie E, Blot F, et al. Lower respiratory tract colonization and infection during severe acute respiratory distress syndrome: incidence and diagnosis. Am J Respir Crit Care Med 1997;156(4 Pt 1):1092–8.

42. Meduri GU, Reddy RC, Stanley T, et al. Pneumonia in acute respiratory distress syndrome. A prospective evaluation of bilateral bronchoscopic sampling. Am J Respir Crit Care Med 1998;158(3):870–5.

43. Sutherland KR, Steinberg KP, Maunder RJ, et al. Pulmonary infection during the acute respiratory distress syndrome. Am J Respir Crit Care Med 1995;152(2): 550–6.

44. Baumann WR, Jung RC, Koss M, et al. Incidence and mortality of adult respiratory distress syndrome: a prospective analysis from a large metropolitan hospital. Crit Care Med 1986;14(1):1–4.

45. Richard Jean-Damien DD, Roux D. Pneumonia in ARDS. In: Sethi S, editor. Respiratory infections. New York: Informa Healthcare; 2009. p. 144–58.

46. Drakulovic MB, Torres A, Bauer TT, et al. Supine body position as a risk factor for nosocomial pneumonia in mechanically ventilated patients: a randomised trial. Lancet 1999;354(9193):1851–8.

47. Koeman M, van der Ven AJ, Hak E, et al. Oral decontamination with chlorhexidine reduces the incidence of ventilator-associated pneumonia. Am J Respir Crit Care Med 2006;173(12):1348–55.

48. Miano TA, Reichert MG, Houle TT, et al. Nosocomial pneumonia risk and stress ulcer prophylaxis: a comparison of pantoprazole vs ranitidine in cardiothoracic surgery patients. Chest 2009;136(2):440–7.

49. Rumbak MJ, Newton M, Truncale T, et al. A prospective, randomized, study comparing early percutaneous dilational tracheotomy to prolonged translaryngeal intubation (delayed tracheotomy) in critically ill medical patients. Crit Care Med 2004;32(8):1689–94.

50. Bartlett JG. Anaerobic bacterial infections of the lung and pleural space. Clin Infect Dis 1993;16(Suppl 4):S248–55.

51. Lorber B. Lung abscess. In: Mandell G, Bennett J, Dolin R, editors. Principles and practice of infectious diseases. 6th edition. Churchill Livingstone; 2005. p. 853–6.

52. Lorber B, Swenson RM. Bacteriology of aspiration pneumonia. A prospective study of community- and hospital-acquired cases. Ann Intern Med 1974;81(3):329–31.

53. Bartlett JG, Gorbach SL, Tally FP, et al. Bacteriology and treatment of primary lung abscess. Am Rev Respir Dis 1974;109(5):510–8.

54. Stark DD, Federle MP, Goodman PC, et al. Differentiating lung abscess and empyema: radiography and computed tomography. AJR Am J Roentgenol 1983;141(1):163–7.

55. Mansharamani N, Balachandran D, Delaney D, et al. Lung abscess in adults: clinical comparison of immunocompromised to non-immunocompromised patients. Respir Med 2002;96(3):178–85.

56. Bartlett JG. Diagnostic accuracy of transtracheal aspiration bacteriologic studies. Am Rev Respir Dis 1977;115(5):777–82.

57. Bandt PD, Blank N, Castellino RA. Needle diagnosis of pneumonitis. Value in high-risk patients. JAMA 1972;220(12):1578–80.

58. Levison ME, Mangura CT, Lorber B, et al. Clindamycin compared with penicillin for the treatment of anaerobic lung abscess. Ann Intern Med 1983;98(4):466–71.

59. Gudiol F, Manresa F, Pallares R, et al. Clindamycin vs penicillin for anaerobic lung infections. High rate of penicillin failures associated with penicillin-resistant *Bacteroides melaninogenicus*. Arch Intern Med 1990;150(12):2525–9.

60. Perlino CA. Metronidazole vs clindamycin treatment of anerobic pulmonary infection. Failure of metronidazole therapy. Arch Intern Med 1981;141(11):1424–7.

61. Levison ME. Anaerobic pleuropulmonary infection. Curr Opin Infect Dis 2001;14(2):187–91.

62. Herth F, Ernst A, Becker HD. Endoscopic drainage of lung abscesses: technique and outcome. Chest 2005;127(4):1378–81.

63. Lemmer JH, Botham MJ, Orringer MB. Modern management of adult thoracic empyema. J Thorac Cardiovasc Surg 1985;90(6):849–55.

64. Ali I, Unruh H. Management of empyema thoracis. Ann Thorac Surg 1990;50(3):355–9.

65. Smith JA, Mullerworth MH, Westlake GW, et al. Empyema thoracis: 14-year experience in a teaching center. Ann Thorac Surg 1991;51(1):39–42.

66. Bryant RE, Salmon CJ. Pleural empyema. Clin Infect Dis 1996;22(5):747–62.

67. Hott JW, Sparks JA, Godbey SW, et al. Mesothelial cell response to pleural injury: thrombin-induced proliferation and chemotaxis of rat pleural mesothelial cells. Am J Respir Cell Mol Biol 1992;6(4):421–5.

68. Septimus E. Pleural effusion and empyema. In: Mandell G, Bennett J, Dolin R, editors. Principles and practice of infectious diseases. 6th edition. Churchill Livingstone; 2005. p. 846–52.

69. Caplan ES, Hoyt NJ, Rodriguez A, et al. Empyema occurring in the multiply traumatized patient. J Trauma 1984;24(9):785–9.

70. Varkey B, Rose HD, Kutty CP, et al. Empyema thoracis during a ten-year period. Analysis of 72 cases and comparison to a previous study (1952 to 1967). Arch Intern Med 1981;141(13):1771–6.

71. Moskowitz H, Platt RT, Schachar R, et al. Roentgen visualization of minute pleural effusion. An experimental study to determine the minimum amount of pleural fluid visible on a radiograph. Radiology 1973;109(1):33–5.

72. Poe RH, Marin MG, Israel RH, et al. Utility of pleural fluid analysis in predicting tube thoracostomy/decortication in parapneumonic effusions. Chest 1991; 100(4):963–7.

73. Alfageme I, Munoz F, Pena N, et al. Empyema of the thorax in adults. Etiology, microbiologic findings, and management. Chest 1993;103(3):839–43.

74. Heffner JE, Brown LK, Barbieri C, et al. Pleural fluid chemical analysis in parapneumonic effusions. A meta-analysis. Am J Respir Crit Care Med 1995;151(6): 1700–8.

75. Pine JR, Hollman JL. Elevated pleural fluid pH in *Proteus mirabilis* empyema. Chest 1983;84(1):109–11.

76. Levine H, Metzger W, Lacera D, et al. Diagnosis of tuberculous pleurisy by culture of pleural biopsy specimen. Arch Intern Med 1970;126(2):269–71.

77. Peabody JW Jr, Seabury JH. Actinomycosis and nocardiosis. A review of basic differences in therapy. Am J Med 1960;28:99–115.

78. Rex JH, Walsh TJ, Sobel JD, et al. Practice guidelines for the treatment of candidiasis. Infectious Diseases Society of America. Clin Infect Dis 2000;30(4):662–78.

79. Miller KS, Sahn SA. Chest tubes. Indications, technique, management and complications. Chest 1987;91(2):258–64.

80. Davies RJ, Traill ZC, Gleeson FV. Randomised controlled trial of intrapleural streptokinase in community acquired pleural infection. Thorax 1997;52(5):416–21.

81. Diacon AH, Theron J, Schuurmans MM, et al. Intrapleural streptokinase for empyema and complicated parapneumonic effusions. Am J Respir Crit Care Med 2004;170(1):49–53.

82. Maskell NA, Davies CW, Nunn AJ, et al. U.K. Controlled trial of intrapleural streptokinase for pleural infection. N Engl J Med 2005;352(9):865–74.

83. Tokuda Y, Matsushima D, Stein GH, et al. Intrapleural fibrinolytic agents for empyema and complicated parapneumonic effusions: a meta-analysis. Chest 2006;129(3):783–90.

84. Cameron R, Davies HR. Intra-pleural fibrinolytic therapy versus conservative management in the treatment of adult parapneumonic effusions and empyema. Cochrane Database Syst Rev 2008;(2):CD002312.

85. Rahman NM, Maskell NA, West A, et al. Intrapleural use of tissue plasminogen activator and DNase in pleural infection. N Engl J Med 2011;365(6):518–26.

86. Chan DT, Sihoe AD, Chan S, et al. Surgical treatment for empyema thoracis: is video-assisted thoracic surgery "better" than thoracotomy? Ann Thorac Surg 2007;84(1):225–31.

Cardiac Emergencies
Infective Endocarditis, Pericarditis, and Myocarditis

Tin Han Htwe, MD[a], Nancy Misri Khardori, MD, PhD[b,c,*]

KEYWORDS

- Infective endocarditis • Pericarditis • Myocarditis • Congestive heart failure • Fever
- Leukocytosis

KEY POINTS

- Infective endocarditis is increasing in incidence.
- *Staphylococcus aureus* as a cause of endocarditis is becoming more common in both native valve and prosthetic valve endocarditis.
- After initial supportive care and presumptive antimicrobial therapy, the results of blood cultures and antimicrobial susceptibility should be used to optimize definitive therapy.
- Most cases of acute pericarditis and acute myocarditis are caused by viruses.

INTRODUCTION

Of all the medical specialties, cardiology has the most emergent situations. Noninfectious cardiac emergencies are appreciated and managed appropriately in the emergency department as well as the Intensive care unit. Although infectious cardiac emergencies have somewhat less dramatic presentations, they can lead to significant morbidity and mortality if not diagnosed early and managed appropriately. Because of the involvement of infectious agents in cardiac emergencies, there is a need for constant surveillance of common infectious agents and their resistance patterns to be able to presumptively treat life-threatening cardiac infections. When and if cultures do become available after 3 to 4 days, the selection of definitive antimicrobial therapy becomes much easier. This article focuses on the epidemiology, microbiology, and management of infective endocarditis (IE), pericarditis, and myocarditis. The emphasis on the changing microbiology of IE deserves special consideration. The treatment guidelines from The American Heart Association and the European Society of Cardiology are reviewed.

[a] Division of Infectious Diseases, Sentara Medical Group, 850 Kempsville Road, Norfolk, VA 23502-3979, USA; [b] Division of Infectious Diseases, Department of Internal Medicine, Eastern Virginia Medical School, 825 Fairfax Avenue, Norfolk, VA 23507, USA; [c] Department of Microbiology and Cell Biology, Eastern Virginia Medical School, 825 Fairfax Avenue, Norfolk, VA 23507, USA
* Corresponding author.
E-mail address: khardoNM@evms.edu

Med Clin N Am 96 (2012) 1149–1169
http://dx.doi.org/10.1016/j.mcna.2012.09.003
0025-7125/12/$ – see front matter © 2012 Published by Elsevier Inc.

IE

As the name implies, IE is the term used for infection of endocardial surface of the heart with formation of conglomerates made of bacteria and platelets (vegetations) on the heart valves, even though it can also involve septal defects and mural endocardium.[1]

A Paradigm Shift

In the western world, the incidence of IE has been reported to 1.7 to 11.2 per 100,000 populations per year. The American Heart Association estimates about 100,000 to 200,000 annual new cases in the United States each year. The percentage of acute IE cases has increased significantly compared with that in the preantibiotic era (20% vs 75%).[1,2]

In the past, IE was an indolent subacute illness occurring predominantly in patients with underlying valvular disease. However, in the last 25 years the disease paradigm has shifted to more acute presentation and lack of classical sings of infective endocarditis. IE carries significant morbidity and mortality despite advances in diagnostic, medical, and surgical interventions. IE-related in-hospital mortality ranges from 15% to 20% and 1 year mortality can be up to 40%.[1,2]

A prospective cohort study reviewed subjects admitted with a diagnosis of IE in 25 countries from June 2000 to September 2005. The results showed changing pattern of clinical presentation of IE and its microbiology. Most of the subjects with IE presented with an acute illness (<30 days) and *Staphylococcus aureus* was the most common pathogen. Mitral and aortic valves were most commonly involved. Predisposing factors for IE were the subject being an intravenous drug user (IVDU), degenerative valvular disease, and indwelling venous catheters. In-hospital mortality was approximately 18% and it was higher in subjects with older age, prosthetic valve endocarditis, mitral valve vegetations, paravalvular involvement, pulmonary edema, and staphylococcal causes. About 5% of subjects required surgical intervention. Early surgical intervention and viridan streptococcal causes had better outcomes. The most common complication was heart failure (32%), embolization (22%), stroke (17%), and intracardiac abscess (14%).[2]

Three successive population-based studies in France (1991, 1999, and 2008) showed no increase in overall incidence of infective endocarditis or streptococcal endocarditis after scaling down of the antibiotic prophylaxis for dental procedures. However, there was a marked rise in staphylococcal endocarditis with both native and prosthetic valves observed.[3]

This paradigm shift in the cause of IE is thought to be due to increasing medical comorbidities and more exposure to the health care environment.[4]

A recent study in the Czech Republic showed that the crude incidence of IE was 3.4 cases per 100,000 inhabitants per year. Vegetations were most frequently found on the aortic and mitral valves. The most common organism was *S aureus* (29.9%). Skin and soft tissue infections (13%) and hemodialysis catheter infections (8.2%) were common precursors to IE. Predisposing factors included remote cardiac surgery (19.4%) and degenerative valvular changes (11.9%). In-hospital mortality rate was 27.5%. Surgical intervention during antibiotic therapy was performed in 36 subjects (27.5%). Nearly 39% of total IE episodes (134) occurred in subjects with cardiac and noncardiac medical procedures and devices.[5]

A recent large cohort study at a university system in France followed 847 subjects with definite diagnosis of IE over 11 years (2000 to 2011). They reported a mortality rate of 22.5%, IE-related mortality was 15.9%. Sudden death over a 6-month period occurred in 2.7% of patients with IE treated medically. Sudden death was associated with diabetes mellitus, signs of heart failure at admission, and severe comorbidities. Most cases were caused by *Streptococcus* spp. Sudden death was caused by acute myocardial infarction (AMI), cardiac tamponade, perivalvular extension, myocardial abscess with free wall perforation, and malignant arrhythmia.[6]

MICROBIOLOGY

Gram-positive organisms remain the predominant cause of infective endocarditis. A retrospective Canadian study in 1996 reported the microbial causes of IE as *Streptococci* (43%), *Staphylococci* (30%), and *Enterococci* (5%). Gram-negative organisms accounted for 10% of native valve endocarditis. The most common organism in IDVUs was *S aureus* (40%), followed by *Pseudomonas aeruginosa* (13%) and polymicrobial causes (27%), and the remaining were culture negative. Early prosthetic valve endocarditis is caused mostly by coagulase-negative *Staphylococci* (CNS). The microbiological spectrum of late prosthetic valve endocarditis is broader and includes organisms that cause native valve endocarditis and those that cause early prosthetic valve endocarditis.[7]

Tricuspid valve is more commonly involved in IDVUs (73%). But left-sided IE with polymicrobial infection and systemic embolization are also on the rise in this population.[7,8]

A recent large international prospective cohort study showed *S aureus* to be the most common pathogen (31%), followed by *Streptococci* (17%) and CNS (11%) in IVDUs.[2]

A review of endocarditis in IVDUs describes polymicrobial infections composed of *S aureus*, *Streptococcus pneumoniae*, *P aeruginosa*, and mixed infections with *Candida* spp and other rare bacteria depending on the type of drugs abused. *P aeruginosa* infection is strongly associated with pentazocine-tripelennamine usage. *Candida* spp are associated with brown heroin dissolved in lemon juice. Human oral cavity normal flora such as *Haemophilus influenzae*, *Eikenella corrodens*, and *Streptococcus milleri* can play a role in IE related to intravenous (IV) drug use due to habitual cleaning of needles with saliva.[8]

The use of a cardiovascular implantable electronic device is another factor responsible for the increase in staphylococcal infections. *S aureus* and CNS caused 29% and 42% of IE in this subject population. The pathogenesis of infections related to the devices is the adherence and biofilm formation by *Staphylococci* and infections caused by small colony variant *S aureus*.[9–11]

IE caused by *S aureus* shows increasing incidence as well as mortality over the past 50 years.[12] The highest increase of staphylococcal IE in the United States is due to chronic hemodialysis access, more people with diabetes mellitus, and increased use of intravascular devices.[13,14]

Coagulase negative staphylococcal infections of prosthetic valves cause higher mortality and more virulent complications such as heart failure and valvular abscess formation.[15] More aggressive CNS strains such as *S lugdunensis* can cause severe IE of native valves resulting in fatal outcomes despite appropriate antimicrobial therapy and surgical intervention. Therefore, early surgical intervention must be considered, particularly for the *S lugdunensis* IE.[16]

A recent international collaborative study involving 2751 subjects in 61 hospitals in 28 countries reported that non–*Haemophilus aphrophilus*, *Actinobacillus actinomycetemcomitans*, *Cardiobacterium hominis*, *Eikenella corrodens*, and various species of *Kingella* (HACEK) gram-negative organisms are responsible for less than 2% cases of IE. The most common predisposing factor was health care–related infections (>50%), which included indwelling cardiac devices. Patients with prosthetic valves and IVDUs formed a minority of the group. *Escherichia coli* (29%) was the most common non-HACEK gram-negative organism, followed by *P aeruginosa* (22%).[17] IE caused by *P aeruginosa* was also reported in subjects on hemodialysis and renal transplant recipients with bacteremia.[18,19]

Candida endocarditis has high mortality rate and usually has a fatal outcome. Risk factors for IE caused by *Candida* spp are heroin use, immunosuppression, indwelling venous catheters, prosthetic valves, and recent cardiac surgery. *Candida albicans* (48%) is the most common species followed by *C parapsilosis* (21%), *C glabarata* (15%), *C tropicalis* (9%), and unspeciated *Candia* (6%). More than 50% of these infections were health care–associated.[20,21]

ACUTE CARDIOVASCULAR COMPLICATIONS

Acute cardiovascular complications of IE are usually related to vegetations. Vegetations in IE are composed of deposits of bacteria, fibrin, and platelets. They are usually found along the line of closure of a valve leaflet on the atrial surface of atrioventricular valves or on the ventricular surface of semilunar valves. Vegetations can be solitary or multiple. In acute IE, vegetations are more friable, softer, and tend to be necrotic and suppurative compared with those in subacute IE. Vegetations can cause destruction of heart structures with perforation of the valve leaflet or rupture of the chordae tendinae, interventricular septum, or papillary muscle. Valve ring abscesses can lead to fistula formation into the myocardium and pericardial space.

Myocardial abscesses, myocardial infarction, myocarditis are complications commonly associated with acute staphylococcal IE.

Mycotic aneurysms are often seen at bifurcation points of vessels, including the sinus of Valsalva; a ligated patent ductus arteriosus; and the splenic, coronary, pulmonary, superior mesenteric, and cerebral arteries. These develop during the acute phase of IE but remain dormant until they rupture and cause embolization. They are usually associated with streptococcal infections.[1]

Generally, IE presents with insidious onset of nonspecific vague symptoms that include malaise, generalized weakness, low-grade fever, and arthralgia. However, IE can present with serious and potentially fatal acute cardiovascular symptoms, including acute chest pain syndrome, acute decompensated congestive heart failure, malignant arrhythmia, and acute respiratory failure.

The most common serious presentation of *S aureus* IE is congestive heart failure, which can be an initial presentation or develop during the course of illness. In a retrospective survey, it was commonly reported with left-sided IE (49%) and rarely seen in right-sided IE (3%). Other rare but serious cardiovascular complications include myocardial abscesses (mostly in left-sided prosthetic valve IE), atrioventricular block, acute coronary syndrome, aortocavitary fistulous tract formation, and pericarditis.[12]

Mitral valve is more commonly involved than aortic valve in left-sided IE. Left-sided IE has a much higher mortality than right-sided IE (38% vs 17%) owing to an association with systemic embolization and multiorgan failure. Right-sided IE occurs in patients with IVDUs and vascular catheter-related bacteremia.[12]

AMI can occur in the setting of the acute phase of IE because of embolization of coronary arteries from the aortic valve vegetations, decreased blood flow from valve insufficiency, or blockage of coronary ostium by large vegetation. Most of the coronary embolization in patients with acute IE involves the left anterior descending artery. It can rarely cause transmural myocardial infarction. A case series of two subjects describes a young subject with AMI and *Lactobacillus jensenii* mitral valve vegetation complicated by left ventricular apical thrombus, which required anticoagulation. The second subject was a 40-year-old IVDU with patent foramen ovale and IE involving both mitral valve and tricuspid valve due to methicillin-susceptible *S aureus* (MSSA). IE was complicated by pulmonary septic emboli, pericardial and pleural effusion, multiple brain embolic abscesses, and later by pseudoaneurysm arising from the inferior septal wall of left ventricle that needed surgical repair. The authors reviewed 13 other documented cases of AMI in the setting of acute IE. Organisms involved were *Streptococci*, *Enterococci*, *Staphylococci*, and *Lactobacilli*.[22]

Treatment of AMI in this setting is controversial. Thrombolytic therapy is not recommended because of higher risk of intracerebral hemorrhagic complications. Urgent percutaneous coronary intervention is the preferred option but definitive treatment should be individualized.[22–25]

Sudden death can be caused by perforation of the free wall myocardial abscess of the left ventricle leading to hemopericardium, which is a rare complication of staphylococcal IE.[26]

In a retrospective multicenter review of 2055 cases of native aortic valve IE, periannular extension of infection occurred in 9.8% of subjects. The incidence of heart failure, ventricular septal defect, and third-degree atrioventricular block were higher in subjects with aortocavitary fistulization compared with nonruptured abscess. Most subjects (86%) required surgical intervention carrying in-hospitality mortality of 29%.[27]

The International Collaboration on Endocarditis Merged Database (ICE-MD) describes 311 subjects with aortic valve IE of which 22% had periannular abscess formation. *S aureus* was an independent risk factor for abscess formation.[28]

A subject with patent ductus arteriosus developed aortic valve IE, which extended to the sinus of Valsalva and pericardium, leading to pericarditis, cardiac tamponade, and systemic septic embolization.[29]

A case of endocarditis caused by group A *Streptococcus* presented with fever, pharyngitis, and acute renal failure due to glomerulonephritis without valvular vegetation and later developed heart failure. The subject had several peripheral stigmata of IE, which included Janeway lesions and splinter hemorrhages.[30]

Group A streptococcal endocarditis has been reported in association with IVDU and in children following varicella infections. It more commonly affects the right side of the heart with embolic phenomena.[31–34]

DIAGNOSIS
Clinical Symptoms and Signs

The most common presentation of IE is fever accompanied by nonspecific symptoms of chills, generalized weakness, arthralgia, and poor appetite. However, fever can be absent in the elderly, immunosuppressed patients, and in patients with prior antibiotic use. Acute IE presents with rapid progression of very high fever and embolic phenomena. Septic pulmonary emboli can present as acute respiratory failure with pleuritic chest pain and hemoptysis. Cardiovascular emboli and valvular dysfunction can present as acute chest pain mimicking AMI and heart failure. Acute abdominal pain can be seen in splenic infarct, and hematuria and acute renal failure occur with renal infarct and glomerulonephritis. Classic peripheral cutaneous signs are usually absent in acute IE, except embolic lesions involving the extremities.

Acute IE should be suspected in patients who are IVDUs, with new onset of murmur, intracardiac devices, indwelling vascular devices, positive blood cultures with organisms known to cause IE, underlying valvular diseases, embolic lesions of unknown source, immunocompromised conditions, previous history of IE, new conduction disturbances, peripheral organ abscesses, and focal and nonspecific neurologic deficits.

Clinical diagnosis of IE is usually based on modified Duke criteria.

Major criteria include[1] positive blood cultures with IE-related pathogens from (1) two separate blood cultures, (2) at least two positive blood cultures drawn more than 12 hours apart, (3) all of three blood cultures, (4) a majority of more than four separate blood cultures (first and last sample drawn a minimum of 1 hour apart),[2] or (5) echocardiographic evidence of IE. Minor criteria include fever, vascular and immunologic phenomena, predisposing heart conditions or IV drug use, and positive blood cultures not meeting the major criteria.

Definitive IE is defined as the presence of two major criteria, one major and two minor criteria, or five minor criteria.

Laboratory

Abnormalities in routine laboratory studies finding include elevated leukocyte count with left-shift C-reactive protein or sedimentation rate, anemia, and microscopic hematuria.

Microbiology

Three sets of blood cultures (each set should contain both aerobic and anaerobic bottles with at least 10 mL of blood in each bottle) should be drawn from peripheral sites before starting antimicrobial therapy in the first 24 hours. Cultures should not be delayed awaiting a fever spike. Obtaining blood samples from central venous catheters is not recommended. Negative blood cultures after 5 days of intubation need subculture on specialized media. Repeating blood cultures on day 1 and day 3 after starting antimicrobial therapy is recommended.

Echocardiography

Echocardiogram is the main stay of diagnosis in IE. It should be performed in less than 12 hours after presentation in patients suspected to have IE. Transesophageal echocardiogram (TEE) is more sensitive than transthoracic echocardiogram (TTE) for abscess and vegetation; however, cost and accessibility might be limiting factors. TTE should be performed in every suspected case of IE. TEE should be performed in patients with no abnormal finding on TTE when the clinical index of suspicion for IE is high, such as staphylococcal bacteremia, valve replacement, and patients with chronic hemodialysis access.

If initial TEE in patients with high probability of IE is negative or indeterminate, it should be repeated in 7 to 10 days. In addition to vegetation, echocardiogram can detect abscess, dehiscence of prosthetic valve, and dysfunction of a native valve.

TEE or TTE should be repeated during the course of treatment in the presence of persistent bacteremia, development of heart failure, or conduction abnormality.

A repeat TEE or TTE may be useful for detection of clinically silent complications, especially if the size of vegetation at the baseline is large. A repeat echocardiogram, usually TTE is recommended at the completion of treatment to establish new base line and to compare with initial findings.[1,21,35]

A prospective review of 103 subjects with S aureus bacteremia showed the superiority of TEE in the diagnosis of IE. The sensitivity of TTE versus TEE to detect IE in this subject population was 32% versus 100%. TEE detected evidence of IE in 19% of subjects with a negative and 21% of subjects with an indeterminate TTE.[36]

In a report of 19 cases of valvular perforation in acute IE, TEE had better diagnostic sensitivity (95%) versus 45% for TTE in detecting this complication.[37]

A recent review article recommend TEE in staphylococcal bacteremia in the setting of fever and prolonged bacteremia (>3 days); prosthetic valves or intracardiac devices; embolic or cutaneous manifestations; or relapse of staphylococcal bacteremia.[38]

About a quarter (25%) of vegetations seen on TEE in patients with left-sided IE are mobile and larger than 10 mm. They tend to produce new emboli after initiation of anti-microbial therapy. Vegetations produced by *Staphylococci* and non–viridan *Streptococci* are more likely to cause embolization.[39]

MANAGEMENT
Antimicrobial Therapy

The **Tables 1–4** list the antibiotic agents recommended for treatment of IE based on the organism grown and the type of valve involved.

Staphylococcal Infections

For IE caused by MSSA, nafcillin or cefazolin is the recommend therapy. Vancomycin is still the recommend therapy for IE caused by methicillin-resistant *S aureus* (MRSA) in the current guidelines. However, vancomycin failures have been reported with high minimum inhibitory concentrations (MICs) greater than 1 μg/mL.[21,35]

Daptomycin is a cyclic lipopeptide bactericidal antibiotic that is non-inferior to standard treatment with vancomycin plus low-dose gentamicin for *S aureus* bacteremia and right-sided endocarditis.[40,41]

A retrospective case control study showed that daptomycin offers better clinical and microbiological outcome in the treatment of MRSA blood stream infection with strains that have vancomycin MICs greater than 1 μg/mL.[42]

Addition of low-dose initial aminoglycoside to an anti–staphylococcal beta-lactam, vancomycin, or daptomycin has shown variable results.

Current guidelines recommend optional addition of gentamicin for first 3 to 5 days of treatment. However, a prospective cohort study showed that low-dose gentamicin therapy (1 mg/Kg every 8 hours) for first 4 days leads to nephrotoxicity and should not be used routinely.[43]

Table 1
Presumptive (initial) antibiotic therapy for native valve endocarditis and prosthetic valve endocarditis (>12 months)

Antimicrobial	Dosage	Duration
Vancomycin	30 mg/kg/24 h IV in 2 divided doses	4–6 wk
or		
Ampicillin-sulbactam	12 g/d in 4 divided doses	
or		
Ampicillin-clavulanate	Same as ampicillin-sulbactam	
plus		
Gentamicin	3 mg/kg/d in 2 or 3 divided doses	
Patients allergic or intolerant to penicillin:		4–6 wk
Vancomycin	30 mg/kg/24 h IV in 2 divided doses	
plus		
Gentamicin	Same as above	
plus		
Ciprofloxacin	1000 mg/d oral in 2 divided doses	
	or	
	800 mg IV in 2 divided doses	

Table 2 Presumptive (initial) antibiotic therapy for prosthetic valve endocarditis (<12 months)		
Antimicrobial	**Dosage**	**Duration**
Vancomycin plus	30 mg/kg/24 h IV in 2 divided doses	6 wk
Gentamicin plus	3 mg/kg/d in 2 or 3 divided doses	2 wk
Rifampin	1200 mg/d in 2 divided doses	

Vancomycin recommended trough is 10 to 15 mg/L and peak is 30 to 45 mg/L.

A study using animal pharmacodynamic modeling showed that addition of a single high-dose of gentamicin to vancomycin or daptomycin at the start of antimicrobial therapy clears bacteremia faster.[44]

Streptococcal Infections

For S pneumoniae and group A Streptococcus–associated IE caused by highly penicillin sensitive strains, 4 week of therapy with penicillin G or first-generation or third-generation cephalosporins is recommend. Vancomycin is recommended for penicillin allergic and/or intolerant patients.

For streptococcal pneumoniae strains that are relatively resistant to penicillin (MICs between 0.1 and 1 µg/mL) and highly resistant to penicillin (MICs >2 µg/mL), third-generation cephalosporins can still be used. With meningeal involvement, third-generation cephalosporins are recommended in all patients because of better penetration into central nervous system. For cefotaxime-resistant strains with MICs >2 µg/mL with meningeal involvement, addition of vancomycin and rifampin should be considered. Usual recommended duration for S pneumoniae IE is 4 weeks.

For IE due to Streptococcus Group A, B, C, G, and S milleri group, the addition of an aminoglycoside for first 2 weeks is recommended owing to increasing resistance to penicillin.[21,35]

P aeruginosa Infections

Treatment of IE caused by P aeruginosa can be challenging. In a study of 11 subjects with endocarditis caused by P aeruginosa, eight subjects were treated with antimicrobial combinations and three subjects with monotherapy with an aminoglycoside. Surgical intervention was needed in 55% of subjects. Postsurgical complication rates and in-hospital mortality rates were 73% and 36%, respectively. Surgery or antimicrobial treatment did not improve the outcome significantly.[17]

Treatment regimens for IE caused by P aeruginosa are based on clinical experience and no large clinical trial has been performed. American Heart Association guidelines recommend antipseudomonal beta-lactam antibiotics (cefepime, imipenem-cilastatin, ticarcillin, piperacillin, azlocillin, ceftazidime, or cefepime in full doses) with high-dose tobramycin (tobramycin (8 mg/kg/d IV). It is recommended to maintain peak and trough concentrations of 15 to 20 mg/L and 2 mg/L, respectively.[35]

Successful treatment with combination therapy with imipenem-cilastatin plus amikacin and imipenem-cilastatin plus ciprofloxacin has been reported in renal transplant recipients.[18]

Minimum recommended duration of treatment with the combination regimen is 6 weeks. Toxicity with this regimen is reported to be low. Successful treatment with initial combination followed by monotherapy has been reported.[35]

Table 3
Definitive (organism-based) antibiotic therapy for native valve endocarditis

Organisms	Antimicrobial Regime	Duration of Therapy
MSSA	Nafcillin or oxacillin 12 g/24 h IV in 4–6 equally divided doses	6 wk (2 wk for uncomplicated right-sided IE)
	Optional	
	Gentamicin (3 mg/kg/d in 2 or 3 divided doses)	3–5 d
	Patients unable to tolerate nafcillin or oxacillin (nonanaphylaxis)	
	Cefazolin 6 g/24 h IV in 3 equally divided	6 wk
	Optional	
	Gentamicin (same dose as mentioned above)	3–5 d
MRSA or Patients unable to tolerate oxacillin or nafcillin with anaphylactic conditions	Vancomycin 30 mg/kg/ 24 h IV in 2 equally divided doses	6 wk
Enterococci spp sensitive to penicillin, gentamicin, and vancomycin	Ampicillin sodium 12 g/24 h IV in 6 equally divided doses	4–6 wk
	or	
	Aqueous crystalline penicillin G 18–30 million U/24 h IV either continuously or in 6 equally divided doses	4–6 wk
	plus	
	Gentamicin (dose as mentioned above)	6 wk
	Patients unable to tolerate penicillin or ampicillin	
	Vancomycin (dose as mentioned above)	6 wk
	plus	
	Gentamicin (dose as mentioned above)	6 wk
Enterococci spp susceptible to penicillin, streptomycin, and vancomycin; and resistant to gentamicin	Ampicillin (dose as mentioned above)	4–6 wk (4 wk for patient with symptoms <3 mo)
	or	
	Aqueous crystalline penicillin G (dose as mentioned above)	
	plus	
	Streptomycin 15 mg/kg/ 24 h IV/IM in 2 equally divided doses	4–6 wk (4 wk for patient with symptoms <3 mo)
	Patients unable to tolerate penicillin or ampicillin	
	Vancomycin (dose as mentioned above)	6 wk
	plus	
	Streptomycin (dose as mentioned above)	6 wk
Enterococci strains resistant to penicillin and susceptible to aminoglycoside and vancomycin	Beta-lactamase–producing strain Ampicillin-sulbactam 12 g/24 h IV in 4 equally divided doses	6 wk (>6 wk for gentamicin resistant strains)
	plus	
	Gentamicin (dose as mentioned above)	6 wk
	Penicillin resistant strains	
	Vancomycin (dose as mentioned above)	
	plus	
	Gentamicin (dose as mentioned above)	

(continued on next page)

Table 3 (continued)		
Organisms	**Antimicrobial Regime**	**Duration of Therapy**
Enterococci strains resistant to penicillin, aminoglycoside, and vancomycin	*E faecium*, linezolid 1200 mg/24 h IV/PO in 2 equally divided doses or	Minimum 8 wk
	Quinupristin-dalfopristin 22.5 mg/kg/ 24 h IV in 3 equally divided doses	
	E faecalis imipenem/cilastatin 2 g/24 h IV in 4 equally divided doses plus	Minimum 8 wk
	Ampicillin (dose as mentioned above) or	Minimum 8 wk
	Ceftriaxone sodium 4 g/24 h IV/IM in 2 equally divided doses plus	Minimum 8 wk
	Ampicillin (dose as mentioned above)	Minimum 8 wk
Streptococcal strains Highly penicillin-susceptible viridians group *Streptococci* and *Streptococcus bovis*	Aqueous crystalline penicillin G (dose as mentioned above) or	4 wk
	Ceftriaxone sodium 2 g/24 h IV/IM in 1 dose or	4 wk
	Aqueous crystalline penicillin G (or) Ceftriaxone (doses as mentioned above) plus	4 wk
	Gentamicin (dose as mentioned) Patients unable to tolerate penicillin or ceftriaxone	2 wk
	Vancomycin (dose as mentioned above)	4 wk
Viridan group streptococci and *Streptococcus bovis* relatively resistant to penicillin (MIC >0.12 μg/mL and <0.5 μg/mL)	Aqueous crystalline penicillin G (dose as mentioned above) or	4 wk
	Ceftriaxone (dose as mentioned above) plus	4 wk
	Gentamicin (see above) Patients unable to tolerate penicillin or ceftriaxone	2 wk
	Vancomycin (see above)	4 wk
Viridan group *Streptococci* and *Streptococcus bovis* resistant to penicillin (MIC >0.5μg/mL)	Use the same regimen as for penicillin resistant *Enterococci* spp	—

Abbreviations: IM, intramuscular; MRSA, methicillin-resistant *S aureus*.

Combination therapy with fluoroquinolones and aminoglycosides has shown promising results in animal models and human cases but development antibiotic resistance is the limiting factor.[45]

In a rabbit model, left-sided IE caused by *P aeruginosa* showed better outcome with a combination of ceftazidime and amikacin compared with monotherapy with ceftazidime or aztreonam. Addition of amikacin to aztreonam did not make a statistically significant difference.[46]

Table 4
Definitive (organism-based) antibiotic therapy for prosthetic valve endocarditis

Microorganism	Antimicrobial Regime	Duration of Therapy
MSSA	Nafcillin or oxacillin 12 g/24 h IV in 6 equally divided doses	6 wk or longer
	or	
	Cefazolin 6 g/24 h IV in 3 equally divided doses	
	or	
	Penicillin G 24 million U/24 hr in 4–6 divided doses (for strains with MIC <0.1 μg/mL and non–beta-lactamase producing	6 wk or longer
	plus	
	Rifampin 900 mg/ 24 h IV/po in 3 equally divided doses	6 wk or longer
	plus	
	Gentamicin 3 mg/kg/ 24 h IV/IM in 2 or 3 equally divided doses	2 wk
MRSA (or) Penicillin allergic patients with anaphylactic conditions	Vancomycin 30 mg/kg/ 24 h in 2 divided doses	6 wk or longer
	plus	
	Rifampin 900 mg/24 h IV/PO in 3 equally divided doses	6 wk or longer
	plus	
	Gentamicin 3 mg/kg/ 24 h IV/IM in 2 or 3 equally divided doses	2 wk
Enterococci spp sensitive to penicillin, gentamicin and vancomycin	Ampicillin sodium 12 g/24 h IV in 6 equally divided	4–6 wk
	or	
	Aqueous crystalline penicillin G 18–30 million U/24 h IV either continuously or in 6 equally divided doses	4–6 wk
	plus	
	Gentamicin sulfate 3 mg/kg/ 24 h IV/IM in 3 equally divided doses	2 wk
	Patients unable to tolerate penicillin or ampicillin	
	Vancomycin (doses as mentioned above)	6 wk
	plus	
	Gentamicin (doses as mentioned above)	6 wk
Viridans group streptococci and Streptococcus bovis	Penicillin sensitive strains (MIC <0.12 μg/mL) Aqueous crystalline penicillin G (dose as mentioned)	6 wk
	or	
	Ceftriaxone 2 g/24H IM /IV	6 wk
	Optional	
	Gentamicin (dose as mentioned above)	2 wk
	Patients unable to tolerate penicillin or ampicillin	
	Vancomycin (dose as mentioned above)	6 wk
	Penicillin fully or relatively resistant strains (MIC >0.12 μg/mL)	
	Aqueous crystalline penicillin G (dose as mentioned above)	6 wk
	or	
	Ceftriaxone (dose as mentioned above)	6 wk
	plus	
	Gentamicin (dose as mentioned above)	6 wk
	Patients unable to tolerate penicillin or ceftriaxone	
	Vancomycin (dose as mentioned above)	6 wk

Adapted from AHA and ESC guidelines Habib G, Hoen B, Tornos P, et al. Guidelines on the prevention, diagnosis, and treatment of infective endocarditis. Eur Heart J 2009;30(19):2369–413; and Baddour LM, Wilson WR, Bayer AS, et al. Infective endocarditis: diagnosis, antimicrobial therapy, and management of complications. Circulation 2005;111(23):e394–434.

Candida Infections

European Society of Cardiology guidelines recommend amphotericin B for 6 to 8 weeks to treat IE caused by *Candida* spp. This should be followed by fluconazole for long-term suppression because of a high relapse rate.[21]

The most recent guidelines from Infectious Disease Society of America recommend primary therapy for *Candida* IE to be amphotericin B (liposomal or traditional) with or without addition of 5-flucytosine or an echinocandin. Step-down therapy with fluconazole is recommended after the susceptibility is available. Valve replacement is strongly recommended and lifelong suppression with fluconazole is recommended in poor surgical candidates.[47]

American Heart Association guidelines also recommend two phases of therapy. The initial phase is to control the candidemia with combination antifungal therapy for a minimum of 6 weeks and valve replacement. Suppression therapy is recommended for patients at risk for valve replacement. Valve replacement is strongly recommended in fungal endocarditis of prosthetic valves.[35]

In an international prospective study of IE caused by *Candida* spp (33 subjects), Amphotericin B was the most commonly used antifungal agent (59%), followed by fluconazole (44%) and echinocandins (37%). Combination therapy was used in only two cases. Mortality rates were similar between combination treatment (surgery and antifungal) and antifungal treatment alone (33.3% vs 27.8%).[20]

A case report of relapsing *C parapsilosis* endocarditis in an IVDU and review of 71 cases in the literature showed risk factors for *C parapsilosis* to be prosthetic valve endocarditis (57%), followed by the patients being an IVDU (20%). Amphotericin B was used to treat most cases (57%), caspofungin was used in 4.1%, and voriconzole in 2.7%. Thirty-eight percent of subjects received single-agent therapy, whereas 35% received combination treatment, and 22% received sequential treatment. Current guidelines recommend valve replacement in fungal endocarditis regardless of the type of valve.[48]

A case of prosthetic valve infective endocarditis due to *C glabrata* was successfully treated with a combination of fluconazole and caspofungin without surgical intervention. The patient was initially treated with a combination of fluconazole and IV amphotericin B but developed renal toxicity after a short period, after which the amphotericin B was discontinued. However, because of persistent fungemia, caspofungin was added to fluconazole at 6 weeks. This was followed by lifelong suppression with fluconazole.[49]

Surgical treatment

The indications for surgical intervention in IE[1] are (1) heart failure despite medical treatment and development of acute severe valvular regurgitation leading to pulmonary edema or cardiogenic shock[2]; (2) persistent infection locally with development of valvular abscess, insufficiency, or perforation and fistula formation; (3) infection systemically with uncontrolled fever and persistent bacteremia (7–10 days)[3]; or (4) fungal infections and infections caused by multidrug resistant organisms.[4] Large vegetations (>10 mm) and enlarging vegetations despite antimicrobial therapy to prevent embolization are also indications for surgical intervention.[21,35]

In a retrospective study of *S aureus* endocarditis, valve replacement significantly reduced the mortality in left-sided prosthetic valve endocarditis.[18]

Emergency surgical intervention for acute mitral valve endocarditis presenting with cardiogenic shock also improved outcome.[50] Timing of surgery for patients who have met the clinical and echocardiographic criteria for surgical intervention is still controversial. A recent Korean study showed that early preemptive surgery in subjects with acute left-sided native valve IE with severe valvular disease and large vegetations (10 mm or larger) causes significant reduction in embolization risk (one subject in surgery arm vs eight subjects treated medically). The subjects were taken for surgery within 48 hours of diagnosis.[51]

ACUTE PERICARDITIS
Introduction

Acute pericarditis is the inflammation of fibrous tissue layer surrounding the heart and base of great vessels. It usually presents as acute chest pain in adults. It is important to recognize the clinical syndrome because the complications of pericarditis can be as serious as cardiac tamponade or pericardial effusion leading to heart failure and death.

Diagnosis is based on characteristic chest pain and electrocardiographic changes with or without pericardial rub on auscultation. However, establishing the cause can be challenging because most cases turn out to be idiopathic despite extensive work-up.[52]

Causes and Incidence

Causes of acute pericarditis can be simply divided into infectious and noninfectious. Infectious causes are mostly viral (most commonly echovirus and coxsackieviruses A and B), accounting for 90% of cases (**Table 5**). Other causes include bacteria *S pneumoniae*, MRSA, and *Mycobacterium tuberculosis* in patients with HIV.[52]

Table 5	
Reported pathogens in acute infectious pericarditis	
Viruses	Coxsackievirus A and B
	Echovirus
	Hepatitis B, Hepatitis C
	Epstein- Barr virus
	Cytomegalovirus virus
	Adenovirus
	HIV
	HHV-6
	Parvovirus B19
	Influenza
	Measles
	Mumps
	Varicella
Bacteria	Gram-positive: *S aureus*, *S pneumoniae*, *S pyogenes*, *S agalactiae*, *Listeria* spp
	Gram-negative: *H influenzae*, *P aeruginosa*, and other species, *Neisseria meningitidis*, *E coli*, *Salmonella typhi*, *K pneumoniae*, *P miribalis*
	Mycoplasma spp, *Chlamydia* spp, *Legionella* spp, *Bordetella holmesii*
	Anaerobes: *Clostridium* spp, *Actinomyces* spp, *Bacteroides* spp, *Propionibacterium* spp
	Mycobacterium tuberculosis
Fungi	*Candida* spp, *Aspergillus* spp, *Blastomyces dermatitidis* immunocompromised patients
	Histoplasma capsulatum (in immunocompetent patients)
Parasites	*Echinococcus granulosus*
	Toxoplasma gondii

Data from Refs.[52–56]

Most cases of bacterial (purulent) pericarditis reported in the literature are caused by gram-positive organisms (64%), gram-negative organisms (27%), polymicrobial infections (2.3%), *Candida* spp (1.1%), *Aspergillus* spp (0.3%), and other miscellaneous species (4.4%). *S aureus* (56%) is the most common bacterial pathogen followed by *S pneumoniae* (33%). In the gram-negative group, *H influenzae* (45%) is the leading organsim.[56] *S aureus* pericarditis occurs mostly in patients with infective endocarditis.[57]

The incidence of pericarditis caused by *S pneumoniae* has decreased dramatically in recent years; however, it can still cause acute purulent pericarditis leading to cardiac tamponade, especially in immunosuppressed patients with underlying malignancy.[58] Other risk factors for purulent pericarditis in the postantibiotic era include recent thoracic surgery, chronic kidney disease, alcohol abuse, and rheumatoid arthritis.[56]

A triad of meningitis, pneumonia, and endocarditis (Austrian triad) complicated by suppurative pericarditis and cardiac tamponade has been reported in an immunocompetent patient.[59]

There are case reports of pericarditis caused by *Clostridium sordellii* in the pediatric population and *Listeria monocytogenes* and *Bordetella holmesii* in immunocompromised patients with malignancy.[60–62]

Tuberculous pericarditis is most commonly seen in developing countries, especially in Africa. HIV infection accounts for up to 85% of these cases.[63]

Clinical Presentation

The most common clinical presentation is acute onset of sharp stabbing retrosternal chest pain, which is pleuritic in nature, worsened by inspiration and supine position and relieved by sitting up and leaning forward. Pain radiates to one or both trapezius muscle ridges. Patients usually have high-grade fever.

The most salient clinical sign in pericarditis is high-pitched frictional rub that is most audible at the left parasternal border and best heard in the leaning-forward position at the end of expiration.

Tachycardia, hypotension, and pulsus paradoxus (a decrease in systolic arterial pressure of more than 10 mm Hg with inspiration) can be seen in cardiac tamponade, which is an indication for urgent echocardiogram and pericardiocentesis.[52]

Cardiac tamponade is more common in bacterial and neoplastic pericarditis compared with that caused by virus.[54]

Pericarditis has been reported in 21 cases in the past 40 years in patients diagnosed with infective endocarditis. The aortic valve was mostly involved and underlying medical comorbidities included diabetes mellitus type 2, and alcohol or substance abuse.[57]

Diagnosis

The characteristic electrocardiographic finding in pericarditis is widespread concave ST-segment elevation and PR-segment depression. Chest radiography can show cardiomegaly if the pericardial effusion is large enough (>250 mL). Echocardiography confirms the diagnosis and evaluates the extent of disease. In addition to leukocytosis, elevated sedimentation rate and serum C-reactive protein level, and elevated troponin levels are seen during initial work-up. HIV and antinuclear antibody testing is recommend. Serologic testing for other viruses does not alter management.

Pericardiocentesis is indicated in pericardial tamponade, recurrent pericarditis, and in patients who fail medical therapy for both diagnostic and therapeutic purposes.

The fluid should be sent for cell counts, triglycerides; cytology; and bacterial, fungal, and mycobacterial cultures. An elevated adenosine deaminase level and polymerase chain-reaction assay offer earlier diagnosis in patients with a high index of suspicion for *M tuberculosis* pericarditis. Thoracocentesis is recommended if there is associated pleural effusion.[52]

Management

Indications for hospitalization for acute pericarditis include fever, large pericardial effusion, suspected cardiac tamponade, immunosuppressed conditions, anticoagulation, and myocarditis with elevation of troponin.[54]

The mainstay for symptomatic treatment of pericarditis is nonsteroidal antiinflammatory agents (NSAIDs) and colchicine. The use of glucocorticosteroids in the treatment of acute pericarditis is controversial. In general, they are recommended for recurrent episodes and severe cases not relieved by NSAIDs and colchicine. Specific antimicrobial treatment should be tailored if and when an infectious agent is identified.[52]

Prognosis

Pericarditis generally is self-limited but complications, especially cardiac tamponade, can have poor outcome. Recurrence can occur in up to 24% of patients, which is common in the early course of the disease (2 weeks) but usually less severe in the initial episode.[54]

Purulent pericarditis carries a high mortality rate, especially if the diagnosis is delayed.

The mortality rate is also higher in patients with both purulent pericarditis and IE (60%).[63] Even in the setting of appropriate treatment, mortality is around 40%.[56]

Higher index of clinical suspicion, prompt intervention, and appropriate antimicrobial therapy improves prognosis.

MYOCARDITIS
Introduction

Myocarditis is the inflammation of myocardium due to infectious and noninfectious causes. It has variable clinical presentations mimicking other cardiac emergencies.

Presence of an inflammatory cellular infiltrate with or without associated myocyte necrosis on stained heart-tissue sections defines myocarditis based on the Dallas criteria. Fulminant lymphocytic myocarditis associated with preceding viral prodromal symptoms within a couple of weeks has good prognosis. On the other hand, acute lymphocytic (nonfulminant) myocarditis has more gradual onset of cardiovascular symptoms and is associated with poor prognosis.[64]

Causes

Infectious agents as well as drugs, toxins, and autoimmune disorders, including sarcoidosis, can cause myocarditis.

Viral infections are the most common cause of acute myocarditis, coxsackievirus B has been the most reported. Other viral causes include the influenza virus, cytomegalovirus, hepatitis C virus, and adenovirus and parvovirus B19.[64–67]

A large European prospective placebo-controlled multicenter study involving more than 3055 subjects showed viral cause in 11.8% of acute or chronic myocarditis subjects with reduced ejection fraction. The viruses included enterovirus 2.2%, cytomegalovirus 5.4%, and adenovirus 4.2%.[67]

Influenza virus infection is known to cause myocarditis in complicated cases, but the exact prevalence is not known. A pregnant patient was diagnosed with perimyocarditis during acute H1N1 influenza illness and fulminant myocarditis with a fatal outcome was reported in a pediatric patient during the 2009 H1N1 pandemic.[68]

Myocarditis can develop as a side effect of vaccination. Two reported cases of myocarditis following small pox immunization have been reported.[69]

Acute myopericarditis caused by dual infection with coxsackieviruses A and B has been reported.[70]

The most common virus detected was in myocarditis in a German study was parvovirus B19 followed by human herpes virus 6 (HHV-6) and both parvovirus B19 and HHV-6. Coxsackievirus B and Epstein- Barr virus were detected in one subject each.

Most subjects presented with chest pain followed by cardiac failure and malaise. Interestingly, subjects with parvovirus B19 had better outcomes even though intermittent myocardial infarct-like illness was common in first 4 weeks of illness. Patients with HHV-6 had worse prognoses and most subjects with dual infection with parvovirus B19 and HHV-6 did not improve at all. Dual infection and HHV-6 myocarditis tend to present with new onset heart failure and septal late gadolinium enhancement on cardiac MRI, and to develop chronic heart failure.[66]

Case reports of bacterial myocarditis include those caused by *Staphylococci* spp, *Streptococci* spp, and *Borrelia burgdoferi*.[71–74] Acute Lyme disease myocarditis has been present with atrioventricular block.[74]

Clinical Presentation

Clinical presentation of myocarditis includes acute or subacute onset of idiopathic cardiac failure following a viral-like illness or upper-respiratory infection, mild chest pain, respiratory distress, cardiogenic shock, malignant cardiac arrhythmia, and sudden death. Most commonly, it presents as cardiac failure with nonischemic dilated cardiomyopathy of acute or subacute onset. Preceding viral illness may or may not be present.[64]

Myocarditis can present as myopericarditis. In a study of acute pericarditis, myopericarditis was found in 14.6% of the subjects. Independently associated clinical features included arrhythmia and ST-segment elevation, male gender, age less than 40 years, and recent febrile illness.[75]

A recent case series found a distinct subset of young males (age 17–42) presenting with acute chest pain, ST-segment elevation, and elevated cardiac enzymes. This condition was preceded by viral-like illness except in one subject. This was not followed by development of Q wave and cardiac angiogram was normal. The outcome was favorable.[76]

Diagnosis

Endomyocardial biopsy is the gold standard for diagnosis of myocarditis but is not routinely performed. Recent studies suggest that noninvasive imaging such as cardiac MRI can be used to diagnose acute myocarditis, which shows as an abnormal signal in the affected area.[64]

Abnormal EKG findings are common in patients with myocarditis. In a German study, 77% of subject with biopsy proven myocarditis had abnormal EKG finding at presentation. The most common abnormal EKG finding was ST-segment abnormalities (69%), followed by bundle branch block (26%), and Q wave (8%); however, a normal EKG does not rule out myocarditis.[77]

Management

Management of acute myocarditis is supportive care for left ventricular dysfunction and arrhythmia control.[64,65] The use of glucocorticoids in acute phase of myocarditis is not recommended owing to harmful effects shown in animal models with coxsackievirus infection and lack of benefit in controlled trials. Cyclosporine for immunosuppressive therapy offered marginal benefit.[78,79]

Data from animal studies has shown beneficial effect of IV immunoglobulin. However, a placebo-controlled trial in humans did not show any benefit and IV immunoglobulin therapy is not routinely recommended in adults.[64,65]

Use of antivirals in myocarditis is controversial. The beneficial effect of interferon has been demonstrated in animal models, but controlled human studies did not support its use. Myocarditis usually presents a few weeks after the initial viral infection, but studies have shown that persistent presence of viral genome in myocardium is associated with poor outcome. A study showed a decrease or clearance of persistent viral genome in myocardium with interferon therapy in chronic myocarditis. The viruses treated were enterovirus, parvovirus B19, and adenovirus. Specific antiviral therapy with ganciclovir improved the outcome in cytomegalovirus myocarditis. If a bacterial pathogen is revealed or suspected, antibacterial therapy should be instituted.[64,65]

SUMMARY

Cardiac infections presenting as emergencies include complications of infective endocarditis, including congestive heart failure, chordae tendinae rupture, cardiac arrhythmias, and embolic phenomenon; acute pericarditis, including cardiac tamponade; and acute myocarditis presenting with malignant cardiac arrhythmias or congestive heart failure. Most of these emergent infectious disease manifestations of the cardiovascular system have a good prognosis if diagnosed early and managed appropriately. Newer diagnostic modalities and combined treatment guidelines are available from the European Society of Cardiology and the American Heart Association.

REFERENCES

1. Fowler V Jr, Scheld W, Bayer A. Endocarditis and intravascular infections. In: Mandell GL, Bennett J, Dolin R, editors. Mandell, Douglas, and Bennett's principles and practice of infectious diseases. 7th edition. Philadelphia: Elsevier Churchill Livingstone; 2010. p. 1067–112.
2. Murdoch DR, Corey GR, Hoen B, et al. Clinical presentation, etiology, and outcome of infective endocarditis in the 21st century: the International Collaboration on Endocarditis-Prospective cohort study. Arch Intern Med 2009;169(5): 463–73.
3. Duval X, Delahaye F, Alla F, et al. Temporal trends in infective endocarditis in the context of prophylaxis guideline modifications: three successive population-based surveys. J Am Coll Cardiol 2012;59(22):1968–76.
4. Wang A. The changing epidemiology of infective endocarditis: the paradox of prophylaxis in the current and future eras. J Am Coll Cardiol 2012;59(22):1977–8.
5. Dzupova O, Machala L, Baloun R, et al. Incidence, predisposing factors, and aetiology of infective endocarditis in the Czech Republic. Scand J Infect Dis 2012;44(4):250–5.
6. Thuny F, Hubert S, Tribouilloy C, et al. Sudden death in patients with infective endocarditis: findings from a large cohort study. Int J Cardiol 2012. [Epub ahead of print].
7. Sandre RM, Shafran SD. Infective endocarditis: review of 135 cases over 9 years. Clin Infect Dis 1996;22(2):276–86.
8. Sousa C, Botelho C, Rodrigues D, et al. Infective endocarditis in intravenous drug abusers: an update. Eur J Clin Microbiol Infect Dis 2012. [Epub ahead of print].

9. Sohail M, Uslan D, Khan A, et al. Microbiology and pathogenesis of cardiovascular implantable electronic device infections. Mayo Clin Proc 2008;83(Issue 1):46–53.

10. Nagpal A, Baddour LM, Sohail MR. Microbiology and pathogenesis of cardiovascular implantable electronic device infections. Circ Arrhythm Electrophysiol 2012; 5(2):433–41.

11. Gandhi T, Crawford T, Riddell J 4th. Cardiovascular implantable electronic device associated infections. Infect Dis Clin North Am 2012;26(1):57–76.

12. Fernández Guerrero ML, González López JJ, Goyenechea A, et al. Endocarditis caused by *Staphylococcus aureus*: a reappraisal of the epidemiologic, clinical, and pathologic manifestations with analysis of factors determining outcome. Medicine (Baltimore) 2009;88(1):1–22.

13. Cabell CH Jr, Jollis JG, Peterson GE, et al. Changing patient characteristics and the effect on mortality in endocarditis. Arch Intern Med 2002;162:90–4.

14. Fowler VG Jr, Miro JM, Hoen B, et al. *Staphylococcus aureus* endocarditis: a consequence of medical progress. JAMA 2005;293:3012–21.

15. Lalani T, Kanafani ZA, Chu VH, et al. Prosthetic valve endocarditis due to coagulase-negative staphylococci: findings from the International Collaboration on Endocarditis Merged Database. Eur J Clin Microbiol Infect Dis 2006;25(6):365–8.

16. Hoovels L, Munter P, Colaert J, et al. Three cases of destructive native valve endocarditis caused by *Staphylococcus lugdunensis*. Eur J Clin Microbiol Infect Dis 2005;24:149–52.

17. Morpeth S, Murdoch D, Cabell CH, et al. Non-HACEK gram-negative bacillus endocarditis. Ann Intern Med 2007;147:829–35.

18. Nasim A, Baqi S, Akhtar SF. *Pseudomonas aeruginosa* endocarditis in renal transplant recipients. Transpl Infect Dis 2012;14(2):180–3. http://dx.doi.org/10.1111/j.1399-3062.2011.00667.x.

19. Hassan KS, Al-Riyami D. Infective endocarditis of the aortic valve caused by pseudomonas aeruginosa and treated medically in a patient on haemodialysis. Sultan Qaboos Univ Med J 2012;12(1):120–3.

20. Baddley JW, Benjamin DK Jr, Patel M, et al. *Candida* infective endocarditis. Eur J Clin Microbiol Infect Dis 2008;27(7):519–29.

21. Habib G, Hoen B, Tornos P, et al. Guidelines on the prevention, diagnosis, and treatment of infective endocarditis. Eur Heart J 2009;30(19):2369–413.

22. Khan F, Khakoo R, Failinger C. Managing embolic myocardial infarction in infective endocarditis: current options. J Infect 2005;51(3):e101–5.

23. Voss F, Bludau HB, Haller C. Mitral valve endocarditis: an uncommon cause of myocardial infarction. Z Kardiol 2003;92(8):686–8.

24. Koike S, Takayama S, Furihata A, et al. Infective endocarditis causing acute myocardial infarction by compression of the proximal left coronary artery due to a mycotic aneurysm of the sinus of Valsalva. Jpn Circ J 1991;55(12):1228–32.

25. Ural E, Bldirici U, Kahraman G, et al. Coronary embolism complicating aortic valve endocarditis: treatment with successful coronary angioplasty. Int J Cardiol 2007;119(3):377–9.

26. Anguera I, Quaglio G, Ferrer B, et al. Sudden death in *Staphylococcus aureus*–associated infective endocarditis due to perforation of a free-wall myocardial abscess. Scand J Infect Dis 2001;33(8):622–5.

27. Anguera I, Miro JM, Evangelista A, et al. Periannular complications in infective endocardities involving native aortic valves. Am J Cardiol 2006;98(9):1254–60.

28. Anguera I, Miro JM, Cabell CH, et al. Clinical characteristics and outcome of aortic endocarditis with periannular abscess in the international collaboration on endocarditis merged database. Am J Cardiol 2005;96(7):976–81.

29. Satoh T, Nishida N. Patent ductus arteriosus with infective endocarditis at age 92. Intern Med 2008;47(4):263–8.
30. Branch J, Suganami Y, Kitagawa I, et al. A rare case of group a streptococcal endocarditis with absence of valvular vegetation. Intern Med 2010;49(15): 1657–61.
31. Barg NL, Kish MA, Kauffman CA, et al. Group a streptococcal bacteremia in intravenous drug abusers. Am J Med 1985;78:569–74.
32. Winterbotham A, Riley S, Kavanaugh-McHugh A, et al. Endocarditis caused by group a beta-hemolytic streptococcus in an infant: case report and review. Clin Infect Dis 1999;29:196–8.
33. Tyrrell GJ, Lovgren M, Kress B, et al. Varicella-associated invasive group a streptococcal disease in alberta, Canada–2000–2002. Clin Infect Dis 2005;40: 1055–7.
34. Ramirez CA, Naraqi S, McCulley DJ. Group a beta-hemolytic streptococcus endocarditis. Am Heart J 1984;108:1383–6.
35. Baddour LM, Wilson WR, Bayer AS, et al. Infective endocarditis: diagnosis, antimicrobial therapy, and management of complications. Circulation 2005;111(23): e394–434.
36. Fowler VG Jr, Li J, Corey GR, et al. Role of echocardiography in evaluation of patients with *Staphylococcus aureus* bacteremia: experience in 103 patients. J Am Coll Cardiol 1997;30(4):1072–8.
37. De Castro S, Cartoni D, d'Amati G, et al. Diagnostic accuracy of transthoracic and multiplane transesophageal echocardiography for valvular perforation in acute infective endocarditis: correlation with anatomic findings. Clin Infect Dis 2000;30(5):825–6.
38. Palraj BR, Sohail MR. Appropriate use of echocardiography in managing *Staphylococcus aureus* bacteremia. Expert Rev Anti Infect Ther 2012;10(4):501–8.
39. Hill EE, Herijgers P, Claus P, et al. Clinical and echocardiographic risk factors for embolism and mortality in infective endocarditis. Eur J Clin Microbiol Infect Dis 2008;27(12):1159–64.
40. Fowler VG Jr, Boucher HW, Corey GR, et al. Daptomycin versus standard therapy for bacteremia and endocarditis caused by *Staphylococcus aureus*. N Engl J Med 2006;355:653–65.
41. Rehm SJ, Boucher H, Levine D, et al. Daptomycin versus vancomycin plus gentamicin for treatment of bacteraemia and endocarditis due to staphylococcus aureus: subset analysis of patients infected with methicillin-resistant isolates. J Antimicrob Chemother 2008;62(6):1413–21.
42. Moore CL, Osaki-Kiyan P, Haque NZ, et al. Daptomycin versus vancomycin for bloodstream infections due to methicillin-resistant staphylococcus aureus with a high vancomycin minimum inhibitory concentration: a case-control study. Clin Intect Dis 2012;54(1):51–8.
43. Cosgrove SE, Vigliani GA, Fowler VG Jr, et al. Initial low-dose gentamicin for staphylococcus aureus bacteremia and endocarditis is nephrotoxic. Clin Infect Dis 2009;48(6):713–21.
44. Tsuji BT, Rybak MJ. Short-course gentamicin in combination with daptomycin or vancomycin against *Staphylococcus aureus* in an in vitro pharmacodynamic model with simulated endocardial vegetations. Antimicrob Agents Chemother 2005;49(7):2735–45.
45. Bayer AS, Hirano L, Yih J. Development of beta-lactam resistance and increased quinolone MICs during therapy of experimental *Pseudomonas aeruginosa* endocarditis. Antimicrob Agents Chemother 1988;32:231–5.

46. Pefanis A, Giamarellou H, Karayiannakos P, et al. Efficacy of ceftazidime and aztreonam alone or in combination with amikacin in experimental left-sided *Pseudomonas aeruginosa* endocarditis. Antimicrob Agents Chemother 1993;37: 308–13.

47. Pappas PG, Kauffman CA, Andes D, et al. Clinical practice guidelines for the management of candidiasis. Clin Infect Dis 2009;48(5):503–35.

48. Garzoni C, Nobre VA, Garbino J. *Candida parapsilosis* endocarditis: a comparative review of the literature. Eur J Clin Microbiol Infect Dis 2007;26:915–26.

49. Lye D, Hughes A, O'Brien D, et al. *Candida glabrata* prosthetic valve endocarditis, treated successfully with fluconazole plus caspofungin without surgery: a case report and literature review. Eur J Clin Microbiol Infect Dis 2005;24: 753–5.

50. Gelsomino S, Maessen JG, van der Veen F, et al. Emergency surgery for native mitral valve endocarditis: the impact of septic and cardiogenic shock. Ann Thorac Surg 2012;93(5):1469–76.

51. Kang DH, Kim YJ, Kim SH, et al. Early surgery versus conventional treatment for infective endocarditis. N Engl J Med 2012;366(26):2466–73.

52. Lange RA, Hillis LD. Clinical practice. Acute pericarditis. N Engl J Med 2004; 351(21):2195–202.

53. Rahman A, Liu D. Pericarditis—clinical features and management. Aust Fam Physician 2011;40(10):791–6.

54. Tingle LE, Molina D, Calvert CW. Acute pericarditis. Am Fam Physician 2007; 76(10):1509–14.

55. Imazio M, Spodick DH, Brucato A, et al. Controversial issues in the management of pericardial diseases. Circulation 2010;121(7):916–28.

56. Parikh SV, Memon N, Echols M, et al. Purulent pericarditis: report of 2 cases and review of the literature. Medicine (Baltimore) 2009;88(1):52–65.

57. Katz LH, Pitlik S, Porat E, et al. Pericarditis as a presenting sign of infective endocarditis: two case reports and review of the literature. Scand J Infect Dis 2008; 40(10):785–91.

58. Tatli E, Buyuklu M, Altun A. An unusual complication of pneumococcal pneumonia: acute tamponade due to purulent pericarditis. Int J Cardiol 2007;119(1): e1–3.

59. Vindas-Cordero JP, Sands M, Sanchez W. Austrian's triad complicated by suppurative pericarditis and cardiac tamponade: a case report and review of the literature. Int J Infect Dis 2009;13(1):e23–5.

60. Chaudhry R, Verma N, Bahadur T, et al. *Clostridium sordellii* as a cause of constrictive pericarditis with pyopericardium and tamponade. J Clin Microbiol 2011;49(10):3700–2.

61. Nei T, Hyodo H, Sonobe K, et al. First report of infectious pericarditis due to *Bordetella holmesii* in an adult patient with malignant lymphoma. J Clin Microbiol 2012;50(5):1815–7.

62. Delvallée M, Ettahar N, Loïez C, et al. An unusual case of fatal pericarditis due to *Listeria monocytogenes*. Jpn J Infect Dis 2012;65(4):312–4.

63. Ntsekhe M, Mayosi BM. Tuberculous pericarditis with and without HIV. Heart Fail Rev 2012. [Epub ahead of print].

64. Cooper L. Myocarditis. N Engl J Med 2009;360:1526–38.

65. Knowlton K, Savoia M, Oxman M. Myocarditis and pericarditis. In: Mandell GL, Bennett J, Dolin R, editors. Mandell, Douglas, and Bennett's principles and practice of infectious diseases. 7th edition. vol. 1. Philadelphia: Elsevier Churchill Livingstone; 2010. p. 1153–71.

66. Mahrholdt H, Wagner A, Deluigi CC, et al. Presentation, patterns of myocardial damage, and clinical course of viral myocarditis. Circulation 2006;114:1581–90.

67. Hufnagel G, Pankuweit S, Richter A, et al. The European Study of Epidemiology and Treatment of Cardiac Inflammatory Diseases (ESETCID). First epidemiological results. Herz 2000;25:279–85.

68. Babamahmoodi F, Davoodi A, Ghasemian R, et al. Report of two rare complications of pandemic influenza a (H1N1). J Infect Dev Ctries 2012;6(2):204–7.

69. Sharma U, Tak T. A report of 2 cases of myopericarditis after Vaccinia virus (smallpox) immunization. WMJ 2011;110(No 6):291–4.

70. Lee WS, Lee KJ, Kwon JE, et al. Acute viral myopericarditis presenting as a transient effusive-constrictive pericarditis caused by coinfection with coxsackieviruses A4 and B3. Korean J Intern Med 2012;27(2):216–20.

71. LeLeiko RM, Bower DJ, Larsen CP. MRSA-associated bacterial myocarditis causing ruptured ventricle and tamponade. Cardiology 2008;111(3):188–90.

72. Raev D. Acute staphylococcal myocarditis masquerading as an acute myocardial infarction. Int J Cardiol 1997;60(1):95–8.

73. Boruah P, Shetty S, Kumar SS. Acute streptococcal myocarditis presenting as acute ST-elevation myocardial infarction. J Invasive Cardiol 2010;22(10): E189–91.

74. Horowitz HW, Belkin RN. Acute myopericarditis resulting from Lyme disease. Am Heart J 1995;130(1):176–8.

75. Imazio M, Cecchi E, Demichelis B, et al. Myopericarditis versus viral or idiopathic acute pericarditis. Heart 2008;94:498–501.

76. Costantini M, Oreto G, Albanese A, et al. Presumptive myocarditis with ST-Elevation myocardial infarction presentation in young males as a new syndrome. Clinical significance and long term follow up. Cardiovasc Ultrasound 2011;9:1.

77. Deluigi C, Ong P, Hill S, et al. ECG findings in comparison to cardiovascular MR imaging in viral myocarditis. Int J Cardiol 2011. http://dx.doi.org/10.1016/j.ijcard.2011.07.090.

78. Parrillo JE, Cunnion RE, Epstein SE, et al. A prospective, randomized, controlled trial of prednisone for dilated cardiomyopathy. N Engl J Med 1989;321(16): 1061–8.

79. Mason JW, O'Connell JB, Herskowitz A, et al. A clinical trial of immunosuppressive therapy for myocarditis. The myocarditis treatment trial investigators. N Engl J Med 1995;333(5):269–75.

Intra-abdominal and Pelvic Emergencies

Sushma Singh, MD[a], Nancy Misri Khardori, MD, PhD[a,b,*]

KEYWORDS

- Intra-abdominal emergencies • Pelvic emergencies • Intra-abdominal infections
- Peritonitis

KEY POINTS

- The presence of peritoneal reflections and mesenteric attachments leads to compartmentalization of the intraperitoneal space and the potential of spreading exudates to sites distant from the source.
- Intra-abdominal infections can masquerade as a fever of obscure origin or as dysfunction of neighboring organs, such as lower lobe pneumonia related to a subphrenic abscess or an abscess causing small bowel obstruction.
- The most common features of an intra-abdominal infectious process are diffuse or localized pain and fever.

INTRA-ABDOMINAL INFECTIONS

Introduction

The abdominal/pelvic cavity has been labeled as a Pandora's box. The diversity in intra-abdominal/pelvic infections is more than any other organ system. The peritoneal cavity has a large surface area extending from the undersurface of the diaphragm to the pelvic floor. The peritoneal cavity is a closed space in males. In females, the free ends of the fallopian tubes open into the peritoneal cavity. Because of the presence of many dependent recesses, pouches, and paracolic gutters in the peritoneal cavity, loculation followed by abscess formation is common. The presence of peritoneal reflections and mesenteric attachments leads to compartmentalization of the intraperitoneal space and the potential of spreading exudates to sites distant from the source. In addition, abscesses can form in the intra-abdominal/pelvic organs, such as the liver, spleen, pancreas, and ovaries/fallopian tubes.[1]

[a] Division of Infectious Diseases, Department of Internal Medicine, Eastern Virginia Medical School, 825 Fairfax Avenue, VA 23507, USA; [b] Department of Microbiology and Cell Biology, Eastern Virginia Medical School, 825 Fairfax Avenue, Norfolk, VA 23507, USA
* Corresponding author. Division of Infectious Diseases, Department of Internal Medicine, Eastern Virginia Medical School, 700 West Olney Road, Norfolk, VA 23507.
E-mail address: nkhardori@gmail.com

Med Clin N Am 96 (2012) 1171–1191
http://dx.doi.org/10.1016/j.mcna.2012.09.002
0025-7125/12/$ – see front matter © 2012 Published by Elsevier Inc.

medical.theclinics.com

Several clinical scenarios can end up in intra-abdominal abscesses. The common causes include penetrating abdominal trauma, abdominal surgery, diverticulitis, appendicitis, pancreatitis, biliary disease, perforated viscus, and primary peritonitis. Intra-abdominal infections can masquerade as fever of obscure origin or as dysfunction of neighboring organs, such as lower lobe pneumonia related to a subphrenic abscess or an abscess causing small bowel obstruction.[2] An urgent surgical intervention is the mainstay of management of serious intra-abdominal infections.[3]

The most common features of an intra-abdominal infectious process are diffuse or localized pain and fever. However, the presentation can be atypical in the elderly and in the immunocompromised host; therefore, the index of suspicion for a significant intra-abdominal process should be high in these patients even though they are afebrile. It is also important to remember that the pain from an abdominal process can be referred to a distant site, such as gall bladder pain referred to the right shoulder.

The causes of intra-abdominal pain are listed in **Boxes 1** and **2** (reviewed from[4,5]).

SECTION A: PERITONITIS
Acute Peritonitis

Because of the large surface area, dependent recesses, pouches, and paracolic gutters created by reflections of the peritoneal membrane, it is highly likely to get infected from diverse sources. Inflammation of the peritoneum, diffuse or localized, can result from infections; irritating chemicals (like bile); carcinomatosis; foreign-body reaction, such as talc peritonitis; connective tissue disorders, such as systemic lupus erythematosus; and diseases of unknown cause, such as familial Mediterranean fever.

Infectious peritonitis is categorized as primary, secondary, or tertiary. In primary peritonitis, there is no known intra-abdominal or distant source. In secondary peritonitis, an intra-abdominal process, such as a ruptured appendix or a perforated peptic ulcer, is the cause. Tertiary peritonitis is defined as late-stage disease whereby the infection persists or recurs after treatment of secondary peritonitis. In such cases, microbiological diagnosis is difficult because it is usually associated with the presence of low-grade pathogens (eg, coagulase-negative staphylococci) or nosocomial pathogens. The direct correlation of such culture results with the ongoing infectious process is difficult.[6]

Box 1
Gastrointestinal causes

1. Esophageal: gastroesophageal reflux disease, esophagitis (candida, herpes simplex virus, eosinophilic), perforation, spasm

2. Gastric: foreign-body ingestion, peptic ulcer disease, acute gastritis

3. Biliary: acute cholecystitis, cholangitis, gall bladder or common bile duct stone

4. Hepatic: hepatitis (viral, alcoholic, autoimmune), pyogenic liver abscess, hepatocellular carcinoma causing hemorrhage/infarct

5. Pancreatic: acute or chronic pancreatitis, pancreatic cancer

6. Small bowel: small bowel obstruction, mass, celiac disease

7. Large bowel: diverticulitis, acute appendicitis, inflammatory bowel disease, volvulus, obstruction either by malignancy or ileus, constipation

> **Box 2**
> **Nongastrointestinal causes**
>
> 1. Respiratory: pneumonia, pneumothorax, pulmonary embolism
>
> 2. Cardiac: myocardial infarction, especially inferior wall; endocarditis; myocarditis; pericarditis; and heart failure causing hepatic congestion
>
> 3. Vascular: mesenteric ischemia (intestinal angina), aortic dissection, and abdominal aortic aneurysm rupture
>
> 4. Splenic: infarct
>
> 5. Urinary system: nephrolithiasis, urinary tract infection, acute pyelonephritis, perinephric abscess, urinary retention
>
> 6. Peritoneal: primary bacterial peritonitis and secondary peritonitis
>
> 7. Female reproductive system: ectopic pregnancy, pelvic inflammatory disease, endometriosis, ovarian malignancy, and torsion
>
> 8. Others: acute intermittent porphyria, hypercalcemia, hyperthyroidism, hyperparathyroidism, incarcerated hernia, herpes zoster, heavy metal poisoning, hemolytic anemia, and psychiatric disorders

Primary Peritonitis/Spontaneous Bacterial Peritonitis

Spontaneous bacterial peritonitis (SBP) is the most frequent and life-threatening infection in patients with cirrhosis. It is defined by the presence of more than 250 polymorphonuclear cells (PMN) per microliter in ascitic fluid in the absence of an intra-abdominal focus of infection or malignancy.[7] Among hospitalized patients with cirrhosis and ascites, SBP is diagnosed in 10% to 30%.[8] The risk of SBP is increased in patients with cirrhosis with a low ascitic fluid protein level (1 g/dL or lower) and in patients with gastrointestinal hemorrhage. In a small number of patients, the ascitic fluid has bacteria but no PMN. Such cases may be an early stage peritonitis, with PMN appearing 2 to 3 days later, or bacteria may simply have translocated without causing infection. Cirrhosis complicated by SBP has a bad prognosis, with a 1-year mortality of 31% to 93%. The in-hospital mortality of a first episode is 10% to 50%.[7]

Pathophysiology

Except for a small number of cases caused by transient bacteremia, most cases of SBP are caused by translocation of bacteria from the gastrointestinal tract. Bacterial translocation in cirrhosis occurs because of (1) alterations in gut microbiota, (2) increased intestinal permeability, and (3) impaired peritoneal immunity.[9]

Microbiology

Most cases of SBP (>90%) are monomicrobial. Enteric organisms are the most common, accounting for 69% of pathogens. *Escherichia coli* is the most frequently recovered pathogen, followed by *Klebsiella pneumoniae*, *Streptococcus pneumoniae*, other streptococcal species, and enterococci.[10] Peritonitis caused by *Mycobacterium tuberculosis*, *Neisseria gonorrhoeae*, *Chlamydia trachomatis*, or *Coccidioides immitis* is uncommon and usually the result of a disseminated infection or sometimes spread from the adjacent foci of infection.

Recently, enterococci have been grown in 11% to 35% of cases of SBP. Prior antibiotic therapy and nosocomial acquisition were shown to be independent risk factors for enterococcal SBP. The 90-day survival was worse in enterococcal SBP (12%) compared with nonenterococcal (50%) infection.[11]

The frequent use of primary antibiotic prophylaxis and multiple hospitalizations and procedures has led to an increase in multiresistant organisms in SBP. **Fig. 1**A, B shows the distribution of pathogens in community-acquired and nosocomial SBP (see **Fig. 1**).[12]

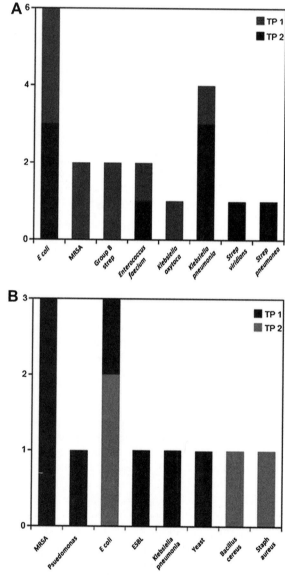

Fig. 1. (*A*) Microorganisms seen in community acquired spontaneous bacterial peritonitis (SBP). (*B*) Microorganisms seen in hospital acquired SBP. TP, Treatment period; MRSA, Methi-cillin-resistant Staphylococcus aureus; ESBL, Extended-spectrum beta-lactamase. (*Reproduced from* Jafferbhoy HM et al. Spontaneous bacterial peritonitis prophylaxis in the era of health-care associated infection. Gut. November 2012,Vol 61;No. 11: 1644–5; with permission.)

Clinical manifestations

Typically, patients present with fever, abdominal pain, nausea, vomiting, and diarrhea and have diffuse and rebound abdominal tenderness on examination. Bowel sounds are hypoactive or absent. However, atypical presentations are common with insidious onset and the absence of findings of peritoneal irritation. In stable patients with chronic liver disease, SBP should always be in the differential diagnosis when decompensation occurs.

Occasionally, gonococcal perihepatitis (Fitz-Hugh–Curtis syndrome) and tuberculous peritonitis present as insidious-onset primary peritonitis.

Diagnosis

Paracentesis is the diagnostic method of choice for SBP with the presence of PMN at greater than 250 PMN per microliter. However, a cutoff of 500 PMN per microliter is reported to have the best specificity.[7] It is important to use a large volume (10–20 mL) of ascitic fluid for cultures and preferably inoculate them at the bedside. These fluids increase the yield of the cultures because the number of bacteria in the ascitic fluid is usually low.

In typical SBP, cultures are positive and the PMN count is greater than 250/μL. When the cultures are positive and the PMN count is less than 250/μL, the syndrome is called bacterascites. In contrast, ascitic fluid with negative culture but a higher PMN of 500/μL or more is called culture negative neutrophilic ascites (CNNA). CNNA and SBP are managed identically. Bacterascites formed of SBP can be self-limited and managed with careful observation and repeat paracentesis after 48 hours.[2]

Treatment

Cefotaxime and similar third-generation cephalosporin antibiotics are as efficacious as the combination of ampicillin plus an aminoglycoside for presumptive therapy for primary bacterial peritonitis.[13] Alternate choices include broad-spectrum penicillins (eg, ticarcillin and piperacillin); carbapenems (eg, imipenem, meropenem, doripenem, and ertapenem); β-lactam/β-lactamase combinations (eg, piperacillin-tazobactam, ticarcillin-clavulanate, and ampicillin-sulbactam); and the newer fluoroquinolones, such as levofloxacin and moxifloxacin. A 5-day therapy has been shown to be effective; however, most patients are treated for 10 to 14 days.[14]

Prevention

Primary prophylaxis using trimethoprim-sulfamethoxazole (TMP-SMX) or oral fluoroquinolones has been commonly used in recent years. The recurrence rate after the first episode of SBP is 43% in 6 months and 69% in 1 year. Primary prophylaxis is recommended in patients with cirrhosis who have had upper gastrointestinal bleeding and/or have ascitic fluid albumin less than 1.5 g/L. Norfloxacin 400 mg/d, ciprofloxacin 750 mg/wk, and TMP-SMX (one double strength dose given once daily for 5 days each week) are the agents used commonly and are equally efficacious.

Of note is the finding that a *Clostridium difficile* infection is more common in patients receiving quinolones for prophylaxis.[12]

A retrospective review of 404 patients with cirrhosis and ascites showed that rifaximin caused a 72% reduction in SBP compared with no antibiotic prophylaxis. Rifaximin also increased the time to transplant survival.[15]

Secondary Peritonitis

Secondary peritonitis is caused by spillage of a gastrointestinal or genitourinary microorganism in to the peritoneal cavity because of a breach in the mucosal barrier, such as perforated appendicitis, perforated diverticulitis, cholecystitis, and perforated peptic ulcer.

Microbiology

In contrast to primary peritonitis, most cases of secondary peritonitis are polymicrobial. The pathogens in secondary peritonitis are a reflection of existing gastrointestinal flora. The common pathogens are members of Enterobacteriaceae (*E coli, Proteus mirabilis, K pneumoniae*); various streptococci and enterococci; and anaerobic organisms, such as the *Bacteroides fragilis* group, *Peptococci*, and *Peptostreptococci*. Bacteremia commonly caused by *E coli, Bacteroides* spp, or both occurs in 20% to 30% of patients.[16]

Clinical manifestation and diagnosis

Clinical manifestations include fever, abdominal pain and tenderness, abdominal distention, and leukocytosis. Free air under the diaphragm may be seen on a plain radiograph of the abdomen in the presence of a perforated viscus. A computed tomography (CT) scan usually shows free fluid or gas in the peritoneum, which, in association with a compatible clinical picture, confirms the diagnosis.

Management

Prompt surgical intervention is required in patients with a perforated viscus or intra-abdominal abscess for source control, debridement, and the prevention of recurrent soilage.

Table 1 lists the likely pathogens, first-line agents, and alternate agents for the antimicrobial therapy for secondary peritonitis and other intra-abdominal infections. The spectrum of activity should include aerobic and anaerobic gram-negative bacilli as well as gram-positive pathogens, like enterococci.[17]

SECTION B: INTRA-ABDOMINAL ABSCESSES
Intraperitoneal Abscess

Anatomy

Intraperitoneal abscesses locate themselves to the site of the primary disease and progress in the direction of dependent peritoneal drainage. Appendicitis is associated with right lower quadrant and pelvic abscesses, and colonic diverticulitis is associated with left lower quadrant and pelvic abscesses. Pancreatitis causes abscesses within the lesser sac.

A case series of 267 patients with intra-abdominal abscesses revealed the location to be in the subphrenic space in about 50%, more than half of which were in the left perihepatic space.[18,19]

Microbiology

The predominant bacteria in intra-abdominal infections are gram-negative aerobic and anaerobic bacilli, streptococci, and enterococci. The most common isolates in most series are the *B fragilis* group and *E coli*.[20,21]

Intra-abdominal abscesses are often polymicrobial, with at least 5 to 6 organisms isolated in most series. The presence of anaerobic bacteria is assumed even though they may not grow in culture.[22] The presence of certain organisms in abscesses can indicate the area of origin of infection; for example, *Citrobacter* species strongly suggests a biliary or upper gastrointestinal source; *Staphylococcus aureus* suggests hematogenous source. An *S aureus* intra-abdominal abscess, particularly in retroperitoneal or perinephric locations, is also associated with vertebral osteomyelitis.

A perforation of the colon is likely to lead to the presence of *Candida* species in the abscess in addition to bacteria.

In patients who have received prior antibiotic therapy, the changed enteric flora to the selection processes can be seen in abscesses. In such situations, more resistant enteric bacteria, *Enterococcus faecium*, are more likely.[23] This phenomenon is clearly demonstrated by a case report of abdominal abscess caused by recently described NDM-1–producing *K pneumoniae* in Spain after receiving treatment of appendicitis in India.[24]

Pathogenesis

A breach in the normal gastrointestinal mucosal defense barrier is the initial event that allows entry of the gastrointestinal flora into the peritoneal cavity. This breach can be macroscopic, such as perforations, or microscopic, leading to transmigration of microorganisms. A diffuse peritonitis is followed by localization, usually in the pelvis, perihepatic spaces, and paracolic gutters. In addition, abscesses may develop around diseased organs, such as periappendiceal, pericholecystic, and perinephric abscesses. Penetrating trauma caused by stabbing, gunshots, motor vehicular accidents, other trauma, or surgical interventions also leads to intra-abdominal/pelvic abscess formation.

Clinical manifestation and diagnosis

The general clinical features of an intra-abdominal abscess include those seen in other acute infectious processes, such as intermittent high-grade fever, shaking, and chills, with abdominal pain and tenderness over the involved area. In undiagnosed patients, hypotension and septic shock may be presenting features. Unfortunately, this acute course is modified by prior antibiotics and may lead to misdiagnosis.[25] The presence of leukocytosis with or without left shift is common; however, in the elderly, left shift may be present without the leukocytosis.

Plain radiography is helpful in locating the abscess in about 50% of patients.[26] The findings include free air in the peritoneal cavity, air-fluid levels caused by loculated abscess, displaced loops of bowel by an abscess, and the so-called soap-bubble appearance, loss of the normal psoas shadow.[2]

Ultrasound and CT are much more sensitive and specific than plain radiography.[27] Ultrasonography is a noninvasive and readily available technique that is helpful in determining the size, shape, consistency, and anatomic relationship of intra-abdominal abscesses. The limitations of ultrasound are interference by overlying gas-filled viscera, ileus, postoperative wounds, and the presence of drains. The CT scan is now considered the radiographic method of choice for the evaluation of intra-abdominal abscesses, with specificity and sensitivity exceeding 90%. Contrast material is commonly administered orally and intravenously to better define the size and location of the abscess. The superiority of the CT scan lies in its ability to detect extraluminal gas, which is highly suggestive of an abscess.[28]

At this point, magnetic resonance imaging has not been shown to add significantly to the diagnostic value of the CT scan.

Treatment

The mainstay of treatment of any intra-abdominal abscess is drainage either surgical or percutaneous. The mortality rate in undrained abdominal abscesses ranges between 45% and 100%.[29,30] The advantage of percutaneous drainage lies in its noninvasive nature compared with surgical intervention. Ultrasound- or CT-guided drainage makes it even safer.

Table 1
Antimicrobial treatment of various intra-abdominal infections

Infections	Common Microorganism	First-Line Antimicrobial Therapy	Second-Line Antimicrobial Therapy in Case of Allergy/Intolerance
1. Intra-abdominal abscesses and secondary peritonitis[a]	Gram negative aerobic and anaerobic bacilli, streptococci, enterococci (most common E coli and B fragilis group)	β-lactam/β-lactamase inhibitor combinations, like ampicillin-sulbactam, ticarcillin-clavulanic acid, piperacillin-tazobactam or Carbapenem, like imipenem, meropenem, doripenem or Tigecycline	Fluoroquinolones, like moxifloxacin, levofloxacin, and ciprofloxacin, plus metronidazole or Aztreonam plus metronidazole
2. Intra-abdominal infection/secondary peritonitis with history of previous hospitalization or antibiotic exposure[a]	Aforementioned organisms plus Pseudomonas aeruginosa, S aureus, vancomycin-resistant enterococci	Carbapenems plus aminoglycoside plus vancomycin or linezolid	Aforementioned agents plus aminoglycoside and vancomycin or linezolid
3. Cholecystitis and cholangitis	Gram-negative aerobic and anaerobic bacilli, streptococci, Enterococci, salmonella	β-lactam/β-lactamase inhibitor combinations, like ampicillin-sulbactam, ticarcillin-clavulanic acid, piperacillin-tazobactam or Carbapenem, like imipenem, meropenem, doripenem or Tigecycline	Fluoroquinolones plus metronidazole

4.	Pyelonephritis and perinephric abscesses	Enteric gram-negative bacteria, including, E coli, K pneumonia, P mirabilis	Fluoroquinolones, like levofloxacin, ciprofloxacin / or / β-lactam/β-lactamase inhibitor combinations, like piperacillin-tazobactam / or / Third-generation cephalosporin, like ceftriaxone	Aminoglycoside, like gentamycin, tobramycin / or / Trimethoprim/sulfamethoxazole
5.	Infectious colitis			
		C difficile	Oral metronidazole / or / Oral vancomycin (in severe cases can use oral vancomycin with IV metronidazole)	Fidaxomicin (recently FDA approved) / or / Rifaximin / or / Fecal transplant
		Salmonella (non-typhi)	Fluoroquinolones, like ciprofloxacin, levofloxacin, moxifloxacin / or / Third-generation cephalosporins, like ceftriaxone	Trimethoprim/sulfamethoxazole / or / Macrolide, like azithromycin
		Campylobacter	Macrolides like erythromycin	Fluoroquinolones like ciprofloxacin (increasing resistance documented)
		Entamoeba histolytica	Metronidazole or tinidazole followed by paromomycin or diloxanide furoate or iodoquinol	

Abbreviation: FDA, Food and Drug Administration.

a In case of perforated viscus antifungal therapy with either fluconazole or echinocandins should be considered for Candida spp.

Ultrasound provides real-time imaging and it is the method of choice for the relatively superficially located and unilocular abscesses, where there is little risk of transgressing a vascular structure, bowel, or pleural cavity. The combined use of fluoroscopy and ultrasound allows precise positioning of the drainage catheter with an increase in both the safety and effectiveness of the procedure. Ultrasound is particularly useful for transrectal or transvaginal drainage procedures.[31] Successful drainage is indicated by improvement in the clinical picture and collapse of the abscess cavity on repeat scanning. However, complications can occur, such as hemorrhage, spillage, fistula formation, and inadequate drainage of the abscess through the catheter caused by viscosity of the pus. Surgical intervention is indicated for these complications.

The concomitant use of early, aggressive, and appropriate antimicrobial therapy, after taking initial blood cultures, improves the outcome in abdominal abscesses, especially in patients who present with sepsis syndrome. While awaiting culture results, the presumptive antibiotic choices are the same as for acute peritonitis (ie, polymicrobial coverage for aerobic and anaerobic gram negative bacilli [see **Table 1**]). Several recent randomized controlled trials have shown that conservative antibiotic treatment of acute appendicitis without abscess formation is comparable with early surgical intervention. However, a recurrence rate of 14% within 12 months was observed.[32,33]

RETROPERITONEAL ABSCESSES

The source of retroperitoneal infections is either an organ contained outside the peritoneum or retroperitoneal extension, such as in retrocecal appendicitis, perforated duodenal ulcers, pancreatitis, and diverticulitis. The large area and rather nondiscrete boundaries of the retroperitoneum allow some retroperitoneal abscesses to become large before being recognized.[34]

In addition to systemic signs of infection and pain, erythema may be observed around the umbilicus (similar to the Cullen sign seen in retroperitoneal hemorrhage) or flank (Gray Turner sign seen in retroperitoneal hemorrhage). The diagnostic imaging modality of choice is the CT scan, which may demonstrate stranding of the retroperitoneal soft tissues and/or unilocular or multilocular collections.[34] Treatment is usually percutaneous drainage and broad-spectrum antimicrobial therapy, as in the case of intra-abdominal abscesses (see **Table 1**).

VISCERAL ABSCESSES
Liver Abscess

Pyogenic liver abscess can develop by the extension of biliary tract infection, portal bacteremia from intra-abdominal septic foci, and systemic bacteremia. Less common causes include direct extension from a contiguous site of infection, complication of abdominal surgery, trauma, complication of hepatocellular carcinoma, or percutaneous transhepatic biliary drainage procedures in patients with cancer and obstructive jaundice.[35–37]

Like the intra-abdominal abscesses, liver abscesses are usually polymicrobial. A liver abscess caused by S aureus is usually associated with bacteremia.

Fever, chills, abdominal pain, and leukocytosis are common in patients with liver abscesses. A liver abscess can rupture and cause acute peritonitis and sepsis syndrome. A CT scan is the most optimal diagnosis modality. In the presence of epidemiologic risk factors, an amoebic liver abscess caused by Entamoeba histolytica should be included in the differential diagnosis. Amoebic liver abscess is usually solitary and confined to the right lobe of the liver. Serologic studies are highly sensitive and specific.

Treatment is usually percutaneous drainage along with broad-spectrum antibiotic therapy, as in acute peritonitis and intra-abdominal abscess (see **Table 1**). If metronidazole is not a part of the chosen regimen, it should be added in patients with suspicion of amoebic liver abscess.

Splenic Abscess

Splenic abscesses are often a result of bacteremia. The risk factors include hemoglobinopathy, splenic infarction, trauma, and immunosuppression. Fever and chills and left upper quadrant pain are common manifestations. CT scan and ultrasonography are equally useful. Percutaneous drainage and antimicrobial therapy should both be used unless drainage is considered unsafe.[38] Initial antibiotic therapy should include vancomycin for *S aureus* (both methicillin susceptible and resistant) and broad-spectrum gram-negative agents, like piperacillin plus tazobactam, meropenem, and doripenem. Once the organism causing bacteremia is identified, therapy should be directed to the pathogen based on susceptibility result.

SECTION C: GALL BLADDER AND BILIARY TRACT INFECTION
Acute Cholecystitis

Acute inflammation of the gallbladder is most commonly caused by the obstruction of the cystic duct from gallstones or biliary sludge and occurs in 1% to 3% of people with symptomatic gallstones.

Pathogenesis
Obstruction leads to increased intraluminal pressure with compromise of blood supply and lymphatic drainage, which, along with the presence of supersaturated bile lead, to acute inflammation. Infection complicates 20% to 50% of acute cholecystitis cases. Complications that follow infection include gangrenous cholecystitis, emphysematous cholecystitis (a life-threatening complication in elderly patients with diabetes), gallbladder empyema, pyogenic liver abscess, and bacteremia.

Acalculous cholecystitis accounts for a minority (<15%) of patients with acute cholecystitis. It is usually seen in critically ill patients, such as severe trauma, burns, sepsis syndrome, immunosuppression, extensive surgery, and human immunodeficiency virus infection. It is difficult to diagnose, and the mortality rate is high.[39,40]

Acute gangrenous cholecystitis is a medical and surgical emergency estimated to complicate about a fourth of cases of acute cholecystitis. The mortality rate for this complication is 15% to 40%.[41] Gangrenous cholecystitis occurs in elderly men with cardiovascular disease, patients with diabetes, those with multiple medical comorbidities, and trauma. It is thought to arise from acute cholecystitis complicated by infection, inflammation, bile stasis, and ischemia leading to gall bladder necrosis and perforation[42] Asymmetric gallbladder wall thickening, absence of gallbladder stones, impairment of gallbladder wall perfusion on color Doppler, and air within the gallbladder wall are all suggestive of acute gangrenous cholecystitis. The treatment is urgent cholecystectomy. Percutaneous cholecystostomy is an alternative in severely ill patients with significant surgical risk.[43]

Clinical manifestation and diagnosis
The most common presentation is pain in the right upper quadrant with or without radiation to the infrascapular region, which is continuous in nature as compared with biliary colic. The presence of a Murphy sign (tenderness on palpation of gallbladder

fossa exacerbated by deep inspiration), with or without a palpable mass, is highly suggestive of biliary tract disease. In addition, systemic signs of infection, fever, tachycardia, and leukocytosis are common. Alkaline phosphatase and bilirubin are only elevated when common bile duct is obstructed.[44]

Imaging studies

Cholescintigraphy (hepatobiliary iminodiacetic acid [HIDA] scanning) has a sensitivity of 96% for the diagnosis of acute cholecystitis compared with 81% for ultrasonography and 85% for magnetic resonance imaging. The specificity for the 3 diagnostic modalities is 90%, 83%, and 81%, respectively. The CT scan has a sensitivity of 94% and specificity of 59%. These data make the HIDA scan the imaging modality of choice for acute cholecystitis.[45]

Microbiology

Bacterial cultures from the bile and surgical sites in patients with acute cholecystitis and acute cholangitis typically yield the members of the normal intestinal flora, which include aerobic and anaerobic gram-negative bacilli and enterococci. Parasites can cause relapsing cholangitis in Asia.[46]

Treatment

Treatment is aimed at the removal of obstruction, either surgically or endoscopically, such as endoscopic retrograde cholangiopancreatography (ERCP). Percutaneous drainage is used for patients who are not stable for a surgical or endoscopic approach. The presumptive antimicrobial therapy is directed against polymicrobial enteric flora and is similar to that in peritonitis and intra-abdominal abscess (see **Table 1**).

Acute Cholangitis

Cholangitis refers to inflammation and/or infection of the common bile duct. Obstruction of the common bile duct leads to biliary stasis, which favors the growth of bacteria and increased pressure predisposes to bacteremia. Bacteria may then ascend along the biliary tract (hence, the terms ascending and suppurative cholangitis).

Acute cholangitis is suggested by Charcot triad of the right upper quadrant or epigastric abdominal pain, fever or chills (or both), and jaundice, which is reported in 50% to 70% of patients. The addition of hypotension and altered mental status to Charcot triad constitute Reynolds pentad, which is seen in less than 14% of patients with ascending cholangitis.[47]

In addition to leukocytosis, routine laboratory studies show cholestatic liver function tests with elevations in alkaline phosphatase, γ-glutamyl transpeptidase, and bilirubin (particularly conjugated bilirubin). Amylase and transaminases may also be elevated. Treatment consists of the decompression of the biliary tract and antibiotic therapy in addition to supportive measures. Antibiotic choices are the same as for other intra-abdominal infections (see **Table 1**). ERCP is the procedure of choice for biliary decompression and is successful in 90% of the cases. Despite the advances in diagnosis and management, acute cholangitis continues to be associated with high mortality.[48]

SECTION D: INFECTIOUS COLITIS
Infectious Colitis

Inflammation of colonic mucosa can be caused by inflammatory bowel disease (IBD), ischemia/necrosis, irradiation, or infection. Infectious causes of colitis are diverse. A recent study from the National Commission for Digestive Diseases reported that the rate of age-adjusted hospitalizations from gastrointestinal infections increased by 92.8% between 1979 (76.1 per 100 000) and 2004 (146.7 per 100 000).[49] Infectious colitis is defined as bacterial invasion and infiltration into the mucosa resulting in an acute inflammation leading to the disruption of the mucosal barrier. The presence of mucus, red blood cells, and white blood cells in the stool is a correlate of mucosal inflammation.

Common causes of infectious colitis include nontyphoid *Salmonella* (NTS), *Shigella*, *Campylobacter*, enterohemorrhagic *E coli* (EHEC), *E histolytica*, *C difficile*, and *Cytomegalovirus*.[50]

Salmonella

Salmonella enterocolitis is characterized by fever, cramping, abdominal pain, and diarrhea that start 8 to 48 hours after ingestion of an infectious dose. Symptoms generally last for 3 to 5 days. The source of infection is usually contaminated food. In addition to colitis, ulcerations of the colonic mucosa with erosion and crypt abscess formation can occur. *Salmonella* usually involves the small bowel. Colonic involvement results in blood and white blood cells in the stool. *Salmonella enterica* serovar typhimurium is the most common serotype causing food-borne gastroenteritis in the United States.[50]

Major food sources are contaminated meat and poultry products. In 2 recent food-borne outbreaks of NTS reported in the United States, contaminated imported jalapeno and serrano peppers from Mexico in 2008 and peanut butter in 2009 were the source.[51] IBD, as a late complication following Salmonella or Campylobacter infection, is reported in a population-based cohort study.[52] Most cases of salmonella enteritis/colitis do not require antimicrobial therapy. Severely ill patients and those with risk factors for developing extraintestinal spread should be treated with fluoroquinolones or third-generation cephalosporins.

Shigella

Shigellosis as a cause of infectious colitis is responsible for 10% to 20% of cases worldwide. More than 200 million infections and 650 000 deaths are reported each year are.[53] *Shigella* species produce a potent toxin (Shiga toxin) with enterotoxic, cytotoxic, and neurotoxic properties. They are invasive pathogens causing acute bloody dysentery with abdominal pain and systemic manifestations of fever, malaise, and headache. The incubation period is usually less than 72 hours but may range from 6 hours to 9 days.

Antibiotic treatment of shigella infections is recommended for most cases. It causes marked symptomatic improvement within 48 hours and reduces the average duration of illness to 3 days. Consequently, antibiotic treatment also reduces the period of presence of *Shigella* in the stool and, therefore, secondary transmission.[54]

Shigella dysentery is complicated by Reiter syndrome after 2 to 5 weeks of illness in up to 10% of patients. Patients with histocompatibility antigen HLA-B27 are at the highest risk.

Campylobacter

Campylobacter causes 14% of infectious diarrhea worldwide. In a recent study from Sweden, *Campylobacter jejuni* was isolated in 56% patients with colitis.[55] *C jejuni* and *Campylobacter coli* are the most prevalent species causing enteric infections. The sources of infection include contaminated water, raw milk, and uncooked meat and poultry. In contrast to *Salmonella* and *Shigella*, *Campylobacter* lacks plasmid-promoting bacterial invasion and classical enterotoxins. *C jejuni* disrupts the mucosal barrier by invading and replicating in infected epithelial cells via Toll-like receptors (TLR-2 and TLR-4). *Campylobacter* infection increases the risk of postinfectious irritable bowel syndrome and is associated with IBD.[56] The sequelae of *Campylobacter* infection also include reactive arthritis and Guillain-Barré syndrome.

Most patients with mild to moderate *C jejuni* enterocolitis do not need antibiotic treatment. Antibiotic therapy is beneficial for severely ill patients. Macrolides and fluoroquinolones are the antibiotics of choice. However, increasing resistance to fluoroquinolones is being reported.

EHEC

EHEC is one of the common causes of infectious colitis in the Western world, including the United States. EHEC (serotype O157) producing a Shiga-like toxin is estimated to account for 15% to 36% of bloody diarrhea and 75% to 90% of hemolytic uremic syndrome (HUS) in North America. HUS develops in 8% of EHEC infections.[57]

The usual incubation period after ingestion of contaminated food or water is 3 to 4 days. The common sources of infection include undercooked beef, raw milk, or other products contaminated by the intestinal contents of cattle. Contaminated water is a less likely source of infection. The symptoms are abdominal cramps and watery diarrhea followed by bloody diarrhea. HUS and thrombocytopenia can occur 2 to 4 days after the onset of diarrhea, especially in children younger than 5 years and in older adults, respectively.[1] Antibiotic therapy has not been shown to be effective for disease caused by EHEC and may increase the frequency of HUS.

E histolytica

E histolytica causes diarrhea/dysentery in developing countries of Central and South America, Africa, and the Indian subcontinent. An estimated 40 000 to 100 000 people die annually of amebiasis, making this disease only second to malaria as a cause of death from parasitic diseases.[58]

E histolytica cysts are ingested, resist the gastric acid pH, and undergo digestion of the capsule in the small bowel. The released trophozoites cause invasion of the colonic mucosa and produce shallow, flask-shaped, undermining ulcers. The trophozoites may then seed the liver via the portal vein with possible extension to the diaphragm, lung, or pericardium. Dissemination is more common in patients with malnutrition, during late pregnancy, and patients on steroid and cytotoxic medications. Asymptomatic cyst carriage has been reported in 1% to 5% of the population in the Southern United States. The presence of trophozoites in the stool is diagnostic of infection.

A commercially available enzyme-linked immunosorbent assay (ELISA) is able to identify *E histolytica* antigens in stool.[59] Serologic methods are also available for diagnosis. The molecular diagnostic techniques are in research at this time.

The mainstay of treatment is nitroimidazole derivatives, such as metronidazole, tinidazole, and ornidazole, for amoebic colitis as well as amoebic liver abscess. Surgical drainage is avoided in uncomplicated cases. A luminal active agent, such as diloxanide furoate, paromomycin, and iodoquinol, is used to eradicate colonization by the cysts.

C difficile

C difficile is an anaerobic spore forming gram-positive bacillus commonly found in the environment. *C difficile* infection (CDI) is defined as the presence of diarrhea (≥3 unformed stools in a 24-hour period) and toxin A or B (or both) or toxigenic *C difficile* in the stool. Pseudomembranous colitis associated with CDI is defined by characteristic colonoscopic and/or histopathologic findings.[60] CDI is now the most common cause of hospital-acquired diarrhea in industrialized countries. Antibiotic use is a major contributing factor to the increased incidence of CDI.

The source of infection is person-to-person fecal-oral transmission. Transmission is enhanced by environmental contamination, infected fomites, and carriage on the hands of health care workers. Disruption of the normal bowel flora with overgrowth of *C difficile* and toxin production is responsible for the pathogenesis of CDI. The two potent toxins, toxin A (enterotoxin) and toxin B (cytotoxin), lead to colonic mucosal disruption, inflammation, and CDI.[61] In addition to antibiotics, chemotherapeutic agents, solid-organ or bone marrow transplantation, inflammatory bowel disease (IBD) leads to increased colonization by *C difficile* spores. Prolonged hospitalization, advanced age, and immunosuppression are other risk factor for CDI.

Historically, use of lincosamides (clindamycin) has been associated with CDI. However, most antibiotics, except vancomycin, have been reported as the agents used before the development of CDI. Cephalosporins that have no antimicrobial activity against *C difficile* and newer fluoroquinolones with a broader spectrum of activity against gastrointestinal flora are now commonly associated with CDI. In addition, the newer strain of *C difficile*, North American pulsed-field gel electrophoresis type 1 (designated as NAP1), is resistant to fluoroquinolones. The extensive use of fluoroquinolones in the community is thought to have contributed to the emergence of this hypervirulent strain producing the binary toxin.[62]

Most patients with CDI have a history of antibiotic exposure in the preceding 8 weeks and/or the presence of other risk factors. Clinical illness ranges from mild to moderate diarrhea to fulminant pseudomembranous colitis and toxic megacolon, which could be fatal. The usual symptoms are watery diarrhea with mucus and abdominal cramping. More severe illness causes high-grade fever, nausea, and dehydration. Leukocytosis and leukemoid reaction are commonly seen and may be the only clues to the presence of CDI. Recurrences of CDI are common and may be caused by relapse or reinfection.

The diagnosis of CDI is confirmed by the detection of toxin A and/or B in the stool. This test should be performed only on diarrheal stool. The sensitivity of currently available ELISA ranges from 63% to 94%, but positive predictive value is low.[60]

Stool culture for *C difficile* is cumbersome, has a long turnaround time, and may be positive even in the absence of toxin production. Glutamine dehydrogenase is present in both toxigenic and nontoxigenic *C difficile*. Enzyme immunoassay for glutamine dehydrogenase has a sensitivity of 85% to 95% and a specificity of 89% to 99%.[60] However, the test does not differentiate between toxigenic and nontoxigenic strains, as is true for the culture. Because of the high negative predictive value, this test is used in a 2-step algorithm in conjunction with an enzyme immunoassay that detects toxins.

The recent Food and Drug Administration (FDA) approval of a polymerase chain reaction (PCR) for toxigenic *C difficile* has a rapid turnaround time and sensitivity of about 94%. It may be positive in asymptomatic patients colonized with toxigenic *C difficile* strains.

Oral metronidazole and oral vancomycin have been the mainstay of therapy for CDI. Although there is no difference in cure rates between oral metronidazole and oral vancomycin in patients with mild disease, oral vancomycin demonstrated superiority in patients with severe disease. The likely explanation is that the secretion of metronidazole into the colonic mucosa and lumen is impaired in severe disease because of poor blood flow.[63] Hence, the Infectious Diseases Society of America's (IDSA) guidelines recommend the use of oral vancomycin as the first-line therapy in patients with severe disease, defined as those with a white blood cell count of more than 15 000 per microliter, serum creatinine level more than 1.5 times the premorbid level, hypotension, shock, ileus, and toxic megacolon. Fecal transplant has been shown to be effective for treating recurrent CDI. Recently, Fidaxomicin, a macrocyclic antibiotic, has been approved by the FDA for the treatment of CDI. Louie and colleagues[64] conducted a randomized double-blind trial comparing the efficacy of oral Fidaxomicin 200 mg 3 times daily for 10 days with oral vancomycin 125 mg 4 times a day for 10 days in the treatment of CDI. Cure rates of CDI with Fidaxomicin were noninferior to those achieved with oral vancomycin. However, Fidaxomicin (7.8%) significantly decreased the recurrence rate of CDI compared with vancomycin (25.5%) in patients with non–BI/NAP1/PCR ribotype 027 strains. Emergent colectomy may be life saving in patients with fulminant CDI, including toxic megacolon, peritonitis, and colonic perforation.[65]

SECTION E: PYELONEPHRITIS AND PERINEPHRIC ABSCESS
Acute Pyelonephritis

Acute pyelonephritis is a clinical syndrome characterized by flank pain and/or tenderness and fever, often associated with dysuria, urgency, and frequency of urination. These symptoms can also be seen with renal calculi or renal infarction. However, acute pyelonephritis is differentiated by pyuria and significant bacteriuria.[1]

Pathogenesis
Ascending infection from the urethra to the bladder and up the ureter to the kidney allows the bacteria to establish infection. The mucosa of the bladder has antibacterial properties that eliminate organisms through mucus trapping and a polymorphonuclear leukocyte response. In addition, the normal urine has a low pH, low osmolarity, high urea concentration, and high organic acid content, all of which inhibit bacterial growth. Obstructive uropathy from many causes promote the bacterial growth and infection. A silent infection of the kidney is present in 30% of patients with lower urinary tract infection (UTIs) symptoms. Hematogenous infections may produce focal abscesses or areas of pyelonephritis within a kidney with positive urine cultures. Hematogenous spread is usually seen with relatively virulent organisms, like S aureus or S typhi.

In severe pyelonephritis, the kidney is enlarged with raised yellowish abscesses on the surfaces.

Clinical manifestations and diagnosis
Symptoms of pyelonephritis range from mild (ie, low-grade fever with low backache and costovertebral angle tenderness) to severe (ie, high-grade fever, shaking chills, nausea, vomiting, and dehydration).[66] Leukocytosis is seen in both mild and severe forms. Pyuria and bacteriuria are easily demonstrable on urine microscopy and gram stain. Blood stream infection may complicate the course of acute pyelonephritis. Bacteremia from pyelonephritis is seldom associated with the more serious sequelae of gram-negative infections, which lead to septic shock, disseminated intravascular coagulation, or both. Emphysematous pyelonephritis is a particularly severe form of pyelonephritis associated with production of gas in renal and perinephric tissues and is seen exclusively in patients with diabetes. Acute papillary necrosis resulting in obstructive uropathy can lead to severe pyelonephritis, which is also seen in patients with diabetes.

Ultrasound and CT scan of the abdomen demonstrate perinephric stranding or intrarenal abscesses. Urine and blood cultures guide definitive antimicrobial therapy.

Microbiology
More than 95% of UTIs including pyelonephritis are caused by a single bacterial species. E coli is the most common infecting organism in acute pyelonephritis.[67] Obstructive uropathy caused by structural abnormalities or neurogenic bladder is associated with infections caused by other gram-negative bacteria (Proteus, Pseudomonas, Klebsiella, Enterobacter spp), enterococci, and staphylococci. Repeated

courses of antimicrobial therapy and frequent instrumentation ultimately contribute to the infection by bacteria resistant to multiple antibiotics. *Corynebacterium urealyticum*, a gram-positive, urea-splitting, slow-growing bacillus, is an important nosocomial pathogen causing complications, like mucosal encrustations and struvite stones, especially in renal transplant recipients. It is highly resistant to antimicrobials, although usually sensitive to glycopeptides.[68] In patients with indwelling catheters, *Candida* spp often colonize the catheter, which sometimes leads to true infection.

Treatment
Mild to moderate illness responds well to orally administered antimicrobial agents. Intravenous antimicrobial therapy becomes necessary in patients who do not tolerate oral therapy. Gram stain of the urine, especially with the predominant organism, may help choose presumptive antimicrobial therapy.

Oral ciprofloxacin (500 mg twice daily) for 7 days (or levofloxacin 750 mg daily for 5 days), with or without an initial 400-mg dose of intravenous ciprofloxacin, is often used as a first-line therapy. This practice may not be safe in communities where the resistance of community-acquired uropathogens to fluoroquinolones exceeds 10%.[69] Multiple studies, including a prospective multicenter trial conducted in Sweden, have demonstrated that the 7-day regimen of ciprofloxacin is successful and safer than the 14-day regimen.[70] IDSA guidelines recommend an initial intravenous dose of a long-acting parenteral antimicrobial, such as 1 g of ceftriaxone, or a consolidated 24-hour dose of an aminoglycoside for a front-line therapy for pyelonephritis if the prevalence of fluoroquinolones resistance in the community exceeds 10%.

Patients requiring hospitalization are treated initially with an intravenous antimicrobial regimen, such as a fluoroquinolone; an aminoglycoside, with or without ampicillin; an extended-spectrum cephalosporin or extended-spectrum penicillin, with or without an aminoglycoside; or a carbapenem. The choice between these agents should be based on local resistance surveillance data. Definitive therapy is guided by and tailored from susceptibility results.[69]

Perinephric Abscess

Perinephric abscess is an uncommon complication of acute pyelonephritis. The most common predisposing factors are urinary tract calculi/obstruction and diabetes mellitus. Most of them are caused by ascending UTI with the usual uropathogenic organisms. Occasionally, bacteremia, especially caused by *S aureus*, can lead to a hematogenous perinephric abscess. Rarely contiguous spread from a neighboring site of infection, such as the colon or overlying rib, can lead to perinephric abscess. The usual presentation is insidious, with fever, weight loss, night sweats, and anorexia associated with flank or back pain. Symptoms referring to the urinary tract are often lacking. Physical examination reveals costovertebral angle tenderness and sometimes the abscess can be palpable.[2] The index of suspicion for perinephric abscess should be high in patients with a febrile illness and unilateral flank pain who have not responded to appropriate therapy for acute pyelonephritis.

In addition to leukocytosis and anemia, signs of renal inflammation, such as pyuria or proteinuria, are seen on urinalysis. Abdominal ultrasound and CT scan are very helpful for early diagnosis. The most common CT scan findings include thickening of the Gerota fascia, renal enlargement, focal parenchymal inflammation, and fluid and/or gas in and around the kidney.

In patients with a clinical or radiographic suspicion of perinephric abscess, needle aspiration under ultrasonographic or CT guidance is safe and diagnostic. A percutaneously introduced small catheter provides immediate decompression and continuous drainage.[71] Early recognition of perinephric abscess by abdominal ultrasound or CT scan followed by prompt percutaneous drainage and antimicrobial therapy has significantly improved the prognosis. Surgical intervention is indicated only when percutaneous drainage is contraindicated or fails. Presumptive broad-spectrum parenteral antimicrobial therapy, as discussed earlier in acute pyelonephritis, should be started before or immediately after drainage. The results of blood, urine, and drainage cultures should be used to determine definitive antimicrobial therapy. It is important to treat the underlying cause for obstruction and to intensively manage diabetes.

Nephrectomy is reserved for emphysematous pyelonephritis, patients with diffusely damaged renal parenchyma, or patients with refractory sepsis as an urgent intervention for survival.

REFERENCES

1. Levison ME, Bush LM. Intra-Abdominal Infection. Mandell, Douglas and Bennett's Principles and Practice of Infectious Disease, 7th edition. Section F; Chapter 71:1011.
2. Liles WC, Dellinger EP. Infectious diseases; The Clinician's Guide to Diagnosis, Treatment and Prevention online version. Sept 2009; Infectious syndromes: chapter on Intra-Abdominal abscesses.
3. Ranji SR, Goldman LE, Simel DL, et al. Do opiates affect the clinical evaluation of patients with acute abdominal pain? JAMA 2006;296(14):1764–74.
4. Cartwright SL, Knudson MP. Evaluation of acute abdominal pain in adults. Am Fam Physician 2008;77(7):971–8.
5. Lyon C, Clark DC. Diagnosis of acute abdominal pain in older patients. Am Fam Physician 2006;74(9):1537–44.
6. Nathens AB, Rotstein OD, Marshall JC. Tertiary peritonitis: clinical features of a complex nosocomial infection. World J Surg 1998;22:158–63.
7. Wiest R, Krag A, Gerbes A. Spontaneous bacterial peritonitis: recent guidelines and beyond. Gut 2012;61(2):297–310.
8. Mowat C, Stanley AJ. Spontaneous bacterial peritonitis— diagnosis, treatment and prevention. Aliment Pharmacol Ther 2001;15:1851–9.
9. Wiest R, Garcia-Tsao G. Bacterial translocation (BT) in cirrhosis. Hepatology 2005;41:422–33.
10. Wilcox CM, Dismukes WE. Spontaneous bacterial peritonitis: a review of pathogenesis, diagnosis and treatment. Medicine (Baltimore) 1987;66:447–56.
11. Reuken PA, Pletz MW, Baier M, et al. Emergence of spontaneous bacterial peritonitis due to enterococci - risk factors and outcome in a 12-year retrospective study. Aliment Pharmacol Ther 2012;35(10):1199–208.
12. Jafferbhoy HM, Miller MH, Gashau W, et al. Spontaneous bacterial peritonitis prophylaxis in the era of healthcare associated infection. Gut 2012.
13. Soared-Weiser K, Paul M, Beegs M. Evidence based case report. Antibiotic treatment for spontaneous bacterial peritonitis. BMJ 2002;324:100–3.
14. Runyon BA, McHutchison JG, Antillon MR, et al. Short-course versus long-course antibiotic treatment of spontaneous bacterial peritonitis: a randomized controlled study of 108 patients. Gastroenterology 1991;100:1737–42.
15. Hanouneh MA, Hanouneh IA, Hashash JG, et al. The role of rifaximin in the primary prophylaxis of spontaneous bacterial peritonitis in patients with liver cirrhosis. J Clin Gastroenterol 2012;46(8):709–15.
16. Wilson SE, Hopkins JA. Clinical correlates of anaerobic bacteriology in peritonitis. Clin Infect Dis 1995;20(Suppl 2):S251.

17. Blot S, De Waele JJ, Vogelaers D. Essentials for selecting antimicrobial therapy for intra-abdominal infections. Drugs 2012;72(6):e17–32.
18. Patterson HC. Left subphrenic abscess. Am Surg 1977;43:430–3.
19. Saini S, Kellum JM, O'Leary MP, et al. Improved localization and survival in patients with intra-abdominal abscesses. Am J Surg 1983;145:136–42.
20. Brook I, Frazier EH. Aerobic and anaerobic microbiology in intra-abdominal infections associated with diverticulitis. J Med Microbiol 2000;49:827.
21. Swenson RM, Lorber B, Michaelson TC, et al. The bacteriology of intra-abdominal infections. Arch Surg 1974;109:398.
22. Altemeier WA, Culbertson WR, Fullen WD, et al. Intra- abdominal abscesses. Am J Surg 1973;125:70–9.
23. Samuelsson A, Isaksson B, Jonasson J, et al. Changes in the aerobic faecal flora of patients treated with antibiotics for acute intra-abdominal infection. Scand J Infect Dis 2012;25:1–8.
24. Oteo J, Domingo-García D, Fernández-Romero S. Abdominal abscess due to NDM-1-producing Klebsiella pneumoniae in Spain. J Med Microbiol 2012;61: 864–7.
25. Milne GA, Geere IW. Chronic subphrenic abscess: the missed diagnosis. Can J Surg 1977;20:162–5.
26. Connell TR, Stephens DH, Carlson HC, et al. Upper abdominal abscess: a continuing and deadly problem. AJR Am J Roentgenol 1980;134:759–65.
27. Mueller PR, Simeone JF. Intra-abdominal abscesses: diagnosis by sonography and computed tomography. Radiol Clin North Am 1983;21:425–43.
28. Gupta H, Dupuy DE. Advances in imaging of the acute abdomen. Surg Clin North Am 1997;77:1245.
29. Montgomery RS, Wilson SE. Intraabdominal abscesses: image-guided diagnosis and therapy. Clin Infect Dis 1996;23:28–36.
30. Branum GD, Tyson GS, Branum MA, et al. Hepatic abscess. Changes in aetiology, diagnosis, and management. Ann Surg 1990;212(6):655–62.
31. Men S, Akhan O, Köroğlu M. Percutaneous drainage of abdominal abscess. Eur J Radiol 2002;43(3):204–18.
32. Styrud J, Eriksson S, Nilsson I, et al. Appendectomy versus antibiotic treatment in acute appendicitis: a prospective multicenter randomized controlled trial. World J Surg 2006;30:1033–7.
33. Vons C, Barry C, Maitre S, et al. Amoxicillin plus clavulanic acid versus appendicectomy for treatment of acute appendicitis: an open-label, non-inferiority, randomised controlled trial. Lancet 2011;377:1573–9.
34. Seymour NE, Bell RL. Abdominal Wall, Omentum, Mesentery, and Retroperitoneum. In: Brunicardi FC, Andersen DK, Billiar TR, et al, editors. Schwartz's Principles of Surgery. 9th ed. New York: McGraw-Hill; 2010.
35. Johannsen EC, Sifri CD, Madoff LC. Pyogenic liver abscesses. Infect Dis Clin North Am 2000;14:547.
36. Winkelstein JA, Marino MC, Johnston RB Jr, et al. Chronic granulomatous disease: report on a national registry of 368 patients. Medicine (Baltimore) 2000;79:155.
37. Lublin M, Bartlett DL, Danforth DN, et al. Hepatic abscess in patients with chronic granulomatous disease. Ann Surg 2002;235:383.
38. Thanos L, Dailiana T, Papaioannou G, et al. Percutaneous CT-guided drainage of splenic abscess. AJR Am J Roentgenol 2002;179:629.
39. Indar AA, Beckingham IJ. Acute cholecystitis. BMJ 2002;325(7365):639–43.
40. Shapiro MJ, Luchtefeld WB, Kurzweil S, et al. Acute acalculous cholecystitis in the critically ill. Am Surg 1994;60:335–9.

41. Ralls PW, Halls J, Lapin SA, et al. Prospective evaluation of the sonographic Murphy sign in suspected acute cholecystitis. J Clin Ultrasound 1982;1:113–5.

42. Merriam LT, Kanaan SA, Dawes LG, et al. Gangrenous cholecystitis: analysis of risk factors and experience with laparoscopic cholecystectomy. Surgery 1999; 126:680–5.

43. Stefanidis D, Bingener J, Richards M, et al. Gangrenous cholecystitis in the decade before and after the introduction of laparoscopic cholecystectomy. JSLS 2005;9:169–73.

44. Yokoe M, Takada T, Strasberg SM, et al. New diagnostic criteria and severity assessment of acute cholecystitis in revised Tokyo guidelines. J Hepatobiliary Pancreat Sci 2012;19(5):578–85.

45. Kiewiet JJ, Leeuwenburgh MM, Bipat S, et al. A systematic review and meta-analysis of diagnostic performance of imaging in acute cholecystitis. Radiology 2012;264(3):708–20.

46. Marcos LA, Terashima A, Gotuzzo E. Update on hepatobiliary flukes: fascioliasis, opisthorchiasis and clonorchiasis. Curr Opin Infect Dis 2008;21: 523–30.

47. Wada K, Takada T, Kawarada Y, et al. Diagnostic criteria and severity assessment of acute cholangitis: Tokyo guidelines. J Hepatobiliary Pancreat Surg 2007;14:52–8.

48. Sharma BC, Agarwal DK, Baijal SS, et al. Endoscopic management of acute calculous cholangitis. J Gastroenterol Hepatol 1997;12:874–6.

49. Everhart JE, Ruhl CE. Burden of digestive diseases in the United States part II: lower gastrointestinal diseases. Gastroenterology 2009;136:741–54.

50. Navaneethan U, Giannella RA. Infectious colitis. Curr Opin Gastroenterol 2011; 27:66–71.

51. Maki DG. Coming to grips with foodborne infection: peanut butter, peppers and nationwide salmonella outbreaks. N Engl J Med 2009;360:949–53.

52. Gradel KO, Nielsen HL, Schønheyder HC, et al. Increased short- and long term risk of inflammatory bowel disease after Salmonella or Campylobacter gastroenteritis. Gastroenterology 2009;137:495–501.

53. Lindberg AA, Pal T. Strategies for development of potential candidate Shigella vaccines. Vaccine 1993;11:168–79.

54. Prince Christopher RH, David KV, John SM, et al. Antibiotic therapy for Shigella dysentery. Cochrane Database Syst Rev 2010;(1):CD006784.

55. Ternhag A, Torner A, Svensson A, et al. Short- and long-term effects of bacterial gastrointestinal infections. Emerg Infect Dis 2008;14:143–8.

56. Marshall JK, Thabane M, Garg AX, et al. Eight year prognosis of postinfectious irritable bowel syndrome following waterborne bacterial dysentery. Gut 2010; 59:605–11.

57. Edelman R, Karmali MA, Fleming PA. Summary of the International Symposium and Workshop on Infections due to Verocytotoxin (Shiga-like toxin)–producing Escherichia coli. J Infect Dis 1988;157:1102–4.

58. Stanley SL Jr. Amoebiasis. Lancet 2003;361:1025–34.

59. Haque R, Mollah NU, Ali IK, et al. Diagnosis of amebic liver abscess and intestinal infection with the TechLab Entamoeba histolytica II antigen detection and antibody tests. J Clin Microbiol 2000;38:3235–9.

60. Cohen SH, Gerding DN, Johnson S, et al, Society for Healthcare Epidemiology of America, Infectious Diseases Society of America. Clinical practice guidelines for Clostridium difficile infection in adults: 2010 update by the Society for Healthcare Epidemiology of America (SHEA) and the Infectious Diseases Society of America (IDSA). Infect Control Hosp Epidemiol 2010;31(5):431–55.

61. Moudgal V, Sobel JD. Clostridium difficile colitis: a review. Hosp Pract (Minneap) 2012;40(1):139–48.
62. McDonald LC, Killgore GE, Thompson A, et al. An epidemic, toxin gene-variant strain of Clostridium difficile. N Engl J Med 2005;353(23):2433–41.
63. Zar FA, Bakkanagari SR, Moorthi KM, et al. A comparison of vancomycin and metronidazole for the treatment of Clostridium difficile-associated diarrhea, stratified by disease severity. Clin Infect Dis 2007;45(3):302–7.
64. Louie TJ, Miller MA, Mullane KM, et al, OPT-80-003 Clinical Study Group. Fidaxomicin versus vancomycin for Clostridium difficile infection. N Engl J Med 2011; 364(5):422–31.
65. Lamontagne F, Labbé AC, Haeck O, et al. Impact of emergency colectomy on survival of patients with fulminant Clostridium difficile colitis during an epidemic caused by a hypervirulent strain. Ann Surg 2007;245(2):267–72.
66. Pinson AG, Philbrick JT, Lindbeck GH. Fever in the clinical diagnosis of acute pyelonephritis. Am J Emerg Med 1997;15:148.
67. Ronald A. The etiology of urinary tract infection: traditional and emerging pathogens. Am J Med 2002;113(Suppl 1A):14S–9S.
68. Lopez-Medrano F, Garcia-Bravo M, Morales JM, et al. Urinary tract infection due to Corynebacterium urealyticum in kidney transplant recipients: an underdiagnosed etiology for obstructive uropathy and graft dysfunction-results of a prospective cohort study. Clin Infect Dis 2008;46:825–30.
69. Gupta K, Hooton TM, Naber KG, et al. International clinical practice guidelines for the treatment of acute uncomplicated cystitis and pyelonephritis in women: a 2010 update by the Infectious Diseases Society of America and the European Society for Microbiology and Infectious Diseases. Clin Infect Dis 2011;52(5): e103–20.
70. Sandberg T, Skoog G, Hermansson AB, et al. Ciprofloxacin for 7 days versus 14 days in women with acute pyelonephritis: a randomised, open-label and double-blind, placebo-controlled, non-inferiority trial. Lancet 2012;380(9840): 484–90.
71. Gerzof SG, Gale ME. Computed tomography and ultrasonography for diagnosis and treatment of renal and retroperitoneal abscesses. Urol Clin North Am 1982;9: 185–93.

Necrotizing Soft-Tissue Infections

Praveen K. Mullangi, MD[a],*, Nancy Misri Khardori, MD, PhD[b]

KEYWORDS

- Fasciitis • Myonecrosis • Flesh eating bacteria • Soft-tissue infection

KEY POINTS

- Necrotizing soft-tissue infection (NSTI) is a life-threatening, surgical, and medical emergency.
- A high index of suspicion is important for early recognition and in instituting prompt therapy without delay.
- Delay in surgical debridement and treatment is associated with increased mortality.
- Early diagnosis, aggressive surgical debridement, aggressive supportive care, and optimal presumptive antibiotic therapy significantly improve morbidity and mortality associated with NSTIs.

Skin and soft-tissue infections account for about 10% of hospitalizations in North America.[1] Most of these are superficial and are treatable with antibiotics and local care, and patients recover quickly. However, deeper infections can be life threatening, and require a high index of suspicion and the need for a combined medical and surgical intervention.

Cellulitis is an acute, spreading, pyogenic inflammation of the dermis and subcutaneous tissue. Necrotizing soft-tissue infection (NSTI), on the other hand, is an infection of the deeper subcutaneous tissues and fascia, characterized by extensive pain, rapidly spreading necrosis, and gangrene of the skin and underlying structures. NSTIs by definition include the presence of devitalized or necrotic tissue as part of their pathophysiology. There is fulminant tissue destruction and gangrenous changes leading to systemic signs of toxicity, high morbidity, and high mortality. NSTIs are infrequent, but highly lethal infections. The presence of devitalized or necrotic tissue provides growth medium for bacteria, and prevents the delivery of host cellular and humoral defense mechanisms and antimicrobial agents.[2] Ambroise Pare, the father of French surgery, described an infective process similar to present-day necrotizing fasciitis; however, Joseph Jones, a confederate surgeon, has been credited as the

[a] Division of Infectious Diseases, Springfield Clinic, 301 North 8th Street, Springfield, IL 62701, USA; [b] Department of Internal Medicine, Division of Infectious Diseases, Eastern Virginia Medical School, Norfolk, Virginia
* Corresponding author.
E-mail address: pmullangi@springfieldclinic.com

Med Clin N Am 96 (2012) 1193–1202
http://dx.doi.org/10.1016/j.mcna.2012.08.003
0025-7125/12/$ – see front matter © 2012 Elsevier Inc. All rights reserved.

medical.theclinics.com

first to describe the clinical manifestations of necrotizing fasciitis.[3] The incidence of NSTI in the United States is estimated to be between 500 and 1500 cases per year.[4] The overall published mortality of NSTI from 67 studies of NSTI with a total of 3302 patients is 23.5%.[2]

A variety of terms has been used to describe the NSTIs including phagedena, hospital gangrene, progressive bacterial synergistic gangrene (Meleney gangrene), Fournier gangrene, and hemolytic streptococcal gangrene.[5] Given the rapidity of progression and the fulminant nature of these infections, the organisms causing these infections have been commonly referred to as flesh-eating bacteria. NSTIs include a wide spectrum of presentations, including necrotizing forms of cellulitis, fasciitis, and myositis depending on the area and depth of involvement. Blood supply to the fascia is typically more tenuous than that of the muscle or healthy skin, making the fascia more vulnerable to infectious process.

Various aerobic and anaerobic pathogens can cause NSTIs either alone or in combination, and differ from the pathogens that cause nonnecrotizing soft-tissue infections. Most NSTIs are polymicrobial in nature, and average around 4.4 organisms per infection in one study.[2,6] When only one pathogen was isolated as a cause of NSTI, *Streptococcus* species was the most common pathogen isolated in about 39% of patients, followed by *Staphylococcus aureus*, isolated in about 30% of patients.[2]

Most commonly, the source of these infections is skin trauma or an underlying lesion (an ulcer or fissured toe). Exposure history may suggest the specific pathogen; for example, seawater exposure (*Vibrio vulnificus*); freshwater exposure (*Aeromonas hydrophila*); aquacultured fish (*Streptococcus iniae*); butcher, clam handler, or veterinarian (*Erysipelothrix rhusiopathiae*).[7] In more than 20% of patients with NSTI, the etiology is unknown and the patients are considered to have idiopathic NSTI.[3,8,9]

Necrotizing soft-tissue infections are also classified into two distinct entities based on bacteriology.[10] Type I infection involves at least one anaerobic species (*Bacteroides*, *Clostridium*, or *Peptostreptococcus*) is isolated in combination with one or more facultative anaerobic Streptococci (other than Group A) and members of the Enterobacteriaceae (eg, *Escherichia coli*, *Enterobacter*, *Klebsiella*, and *Proteus*).

Type II infection is caused by Group A streptococcal infection or other β-hemolytic streptococcal infection, either alone or in combination with other pathogens, most commonly *S aureus*.

Necrotizing fasciitis caused by community-associated methicillin-resistant *S aureus* as a monomicrobial infection has also been reported.[11]

GROUP A STREPTOCOCCAL INFECTIONS

Streptococcus pyogenes is the only species within the group of Group A, β-hemolytic streptococci. *S pyogenes* cause a wide variety of infections such as pharyngitis, erysipelas, scarlet fever, which are milder infections, to the more severe, rapidly invasive, necrotizing skin and soft-tissue infections. The only known reservoir for group A streptococcal infections (GAS) in nature is the skin and mucous membranes of the human host. On a global scale, GAS is an important cause of morbidity and mortality primarily in less developed countries, with more than 500,000 deaths per year. The importance of GAS infections in the United States was reinforced at the end of the twentieth century by a resurgence of severe invasive GAS infections (eg, streptococcal toxic shock syndrome and necrotizing fasciitis), with high morbidity and mortality.

S pyogenes are gram-positive, nonmotile, non–spore-forming, catalase-negative, aerobic organisms, occurring as pairs or as short to moderate-sized chains in clinical specimens, but form long chains when grown in broth media enriched with serum or blood. On blood agar plates, S pyogenes appears as white to gray colonies surrounded by zones of complete (β) hemolysis. The organism is enveloped in a hyaluronic acid capsule that serves as an accessory virulence factor in retarding phagocytosis by polymorphonuclear leukocytes and macrophages of the host.[12]

Hyaluronic acid capsule in GAS is a poor immunogen, as it is chemically similar to that found in human connective tissue. Antibodies to GAS hyaluronic acid have not been demonstrated in humans. M protein is the major somatic virulence factor of group A streptococci. Strains rich in this protein are resistant to phagocytosis by polymorphonuclear leukocytes, multiply rapidly in fresh human blood, and are capable of initiating disease. In the nonimmune host, M protein exerts its antiphagocytic effect by inhibiting activation of the alternative complement pathway on the cell surface. Strains that do not express M protein are avirulent. Acquired human immunity to streptococcal infection is based on the development of opsonic antibodies directed against the antiphagocytic moiety of M protein. Such immunity is type specific and quite durable, lasting for several years.

Other factors that play a role in pathogenesis of infections are: DNases (DNases A, B, C, and D), which cause degradation of deoxyribonucleic acid; hyaluronidase, an enzyme that degrades hyaluronic acid found in the ground substance of connective tissue; streptokinase, which promotes the dissolution of clots by catalyzing the conversion of plasminogen to plasmin; and streptococcal pyrogenic exotoxin B (SpeB), a potent protease and C5a peptidase that cleaves the human chemotaxin C5a at the PML binding site. These enzymatic agents serve to facilitate the liquefaction of pus and the spread of streptococci through tissue planes, which is a characteristic of streptococcal cellulitis and necrotizing fasciitis, and interfere with ingestion and killing by phagocytosis.

Streptococcal pyrogenic exotoxins (Spe) are a family of bacterial superantigens associated with streptococcal toxic shock syndrome, necrotizing fasciitis, and other severe infections. Superantigens are potent immunostimulators that are able to bind simultaneously to the major histocompatibility complex (MHC) class II molecules and the T-cell receptor, which results in activation of a large number of T cells expressing specific V-β subsets of the T-cell repertoire.[12] Superantigen activation of T cells leads to increased secretion of proinflammatory cytokines.

Clinical Manifestations

Predisposing factors for NSTIs due to S pyogenes are minor cuts, splinters, penetrating injuries, varicella lesions, burns, surgical procedures, childbirth, and muscle strain.[13] The initial lesion is mild erythema at the site of injury, which over the next 24 to 72 hours undergoes a rapid evolution with pronounced inflammation. The first cutaneous clue to streptococcal necrotizing fasciitis is diffuse swelling, followed by the appearance of bullae filled with clear fluid. There is rapid progression of bulla to hemorrhagic or violaceous color suggestive of dermal necrosis.[1,14,15] There are marked systemic symptoms, with early onset of shock and organ failure. The patient with streptococcal gangrene appears perilously ill, with high fever and extreme prostration.

Treatment

Prompt, aggressive surgical exploration and debridement of suspected deep-seated streptococcal infection is mandatory. Broad-spectrum antimicrobial therapy to provide polymicrobial coverage should be instituted initially. Once the streptococcal cause is confirmed, high-dose penicillin and clindamycin is appropriate. All strains of group A streptococci remain sensitive to penicillin. Clindamycin suppresses exotoxin and M protein production by group A streptococci, thereby preventing toxin production.

CLOSTRIDIAL INFECTIONS

Clostridia are anaerobic, gram-positive rods that are capable of forming endospores. Growth of *Clostridium perfringens* on blood agar plates is rapid, with colonies often detected within 12 to 16 hours of inoculation. Colonies are yellowish to gray and opaque, with irregular borders, and exhibit a characteristic double zone of hemolysis with an inner zone of β hemolysis surrounded by an outer zone of partial hemolysis. Clostridia are ubiquitous in nature, being found in soil and sediments and as members of the intestinal microflora of humans and animals. Clostridial myonecrosis (gas gangrene) is a life-threatening muscle infection that develops most commonly following a traumatic injury that is contaminated by clostridial spores. Traumatic contaminated wounds with vascular compromise lead to an anaerobic environment that is ideal for proliferation of Clostridia. Traumatic injury accounts for 70% of gas gangrene cases, and about 80% of these are caused by *C perfringens*.[16] Clostridial gas gangrene can also occur in the absence of trauma via hematogenous seeding of skeletal muscle, which is caused by *Clostridium septicum* and usually occurs in association with colonic neoplasms.[17] Other pathogens include *Clostridium novyi*, *Clostridium histolyticum*, *Clostridium bifermentans*, *Clostridium tertium*, and *Clostridium fallax*.

Many extracellular toxins are produced by clostridial species, of which only α- and θ-toxin have been implicated in the pathogenesis. α-Toxin, a lecithinase, is a hemolytic toxin that causes damage to cell membranes. In gas gangrene, muscle necrosis is severe and polymorphonuclear leukocytes (PMNs) are notably absent from infected tissues, which is in contrast to soft-tissue infections caused by other organisms, where there is significant influx of PMNs.[18] α-Toxin stimulates platelet aggregation and upregulates adherence molecules on PMNs and endothelial cells. This upregulation leads to a vascular occlusive state, reducing the blood flow to the muscle and leading to an anaerobic state favorable for clostridial infections.[19,20]

Clinical Manifestations

Clostridial myonecrosis generally begins within 24 to 72 hours after traumatic injury or surgery, depending on the size of the inoculum and the extent of the vascular compromise. Initial symptoms may include sudden onset of severe pain in the absence of obvious physical findings, suggesting a deep tissue infection. Pain is likely related to toxin-mediated ischemia. Following a penetrating trauma to the skin there is an initial redness at the site of the wound, followed by a rapidly spreading brown to purple discoloration of the skin. The progression of gas gangrene is rapid, and within hours of the initial symptoms gas may be detected within the underlying tissues. Bullae may develop on the overlying tense skin and may be filled with clear, red, blue, or purple fluid. Discharge has a characteristic "mousy" odor.[21] Gram stain of the discharge often reveals the typical gram-positive boxcar-shaped rods characteristic of *C perfringens*. Given the proischemic properties of the clostridial toxins, wounds from clostridial infections do not bleed easily. Fever is often minimal during the early stages of disease, but progression to full-blown sepsis with hypotension and multiorgan failure develops rapidly. Gas in the wound is a relatively late finding and by the time crepitus is appreciated, the patient may be near death.[22] Positive blood cultures may be noted in about 15% of patients, and even this is a late finding.

Treatment

Rapid diagnosis of clostridial myonecrosis is critical for proper therapeutic intervention. Mortality rates associated with gas gangrene approach 60%, and are highest in cases involving the abdominal wall and lowest in cases involving the extremities.[22] The most important part of therapy for clostridial myonecrosis is prompt surgical debridement of infected tissues. Penicillin remains the most commonly used antibiotic. Other agents used for treating clostridial myonecrosis include metronidazole, clindamycin, and carbapenems, although resistance to clindamycin has been reported.

AEROMONAS INFECTIONS

Aeromonas are gram-negative, nonsporulating, aerobic rods that usually are β-hemolytic on blood agar. *Aeromonas* species are oxidase positive, and this test distinguishes these organisms from the oxidase-negative Enterobacteriaceae. Aeromonas are ubiquitous inhabitants of fresh and brackish water; they have also been recovered from chlorinated tap water, including hospital water supplies. Aeromonas are isolated with increasing frequency in warmer months, and have been associated with diarrheal disease and are also reported as a cause of traveler's diarrhea in travelers returning from Asia, Africa, and Latin America. Aeromonas occasionally cause soft-tissue infections and sepsis, especially in immunocompromised hosts. Most Aeromonas soft-tissue infections are caused by *Aeromonas hydrophila*. *A hydrophila* wound infections can manifest as 3 major syndromes: cellulitis, myonecrosis, and ecthyma gangrenosum.[1] Infections typically occur on the extremities following traumatic aquatic injury or trauma followed by exposure to fresh water. Aeromonas soft-tissue infections can develop after exposure to soil-associated injuries. There was a reported outbreak of *A hydrophila* wound infections in participants of a mud football competition in Australia.[23] Aeromonas soft-tissue infections have also been reported as a complication of the use of medicinal leeches in surgery.[24,25] *Aeromonas* species are normal inhabitants of the foregut of leeches. Leeches lack the requisite proteolytic enzymes and are dependent on the symbiotic *Aeromonas* to digest the blood meal. Studies have shown a 2.5% to 14% incidence of Aeromonas infections following leech therapy, and it seems that this wide variation is based on the way the leeches are handled and is also based on the use of prophylactic antibiotics with leech therapy.[25,26]

Clinical Manifestations

Aeromonas can cause mild to severe infections. Cellulitis is the most frequently encountered form of soft-tissue infection. Cellulitis develops within 8 to 48 hours following trauma, and systemic signs are common.[27] Cellulitis is characterized by intense redness and induration at the site of injury. Suppuration and necrosis around the wound are frequent, and surgical debridement is often necessary. Myonecrosis and ecthyma are less commonly seen and typically found in immunocompromised hosts (eg, chronic liver disease, underlying malignancy).[28] Myonecrosis with bullous lesions is characterized by liquefaction and gangrene of muscles, with gas formation and crepitus resembling gas gangrene.[23] This form of disease requires aggressive surgical debridement and antimicrobial therapy.

Treatment

The clinically relevant *Aeromonas* species are resistant to penicillin and ampicillin but are usually susceptible to third-generation cephalosporins, aztreonam, and carbapenems. Most *Aeromonas* strains produce β-lactamases.

Fluoroquinolones are highly active against *Aeromonas* species, although the existence of nalidixic acid–resistant strains containing mutations in the *gyrA* gene raise concern that fluoroquinolone resistance could easily develop. Aminoglycosides are usually active, with resistance to tobramycin being more common than resistance to other aminoglycosides.[29]

DIAGNOSIS

Although early identification, debridement, and treatment of NSTIs are crucial, it is difficult to establish the diagnosis of NSTIs. It is worth considering patient factors that increase the risk of NSTIs, such as injectable drug use, obesity, chronic debilitating comorbidities such as diabetes, peripheral vascular disease, immunosuppression, malignancy, and cirrhosis.[30,31] Clinical characteristics that help in identification of NSTIs include tense edema, pain disproportionate to the appearance, skin discoloration, blisters/bullae, necrosis, and crepitus. The sensitivity of these findings is low and they are present in only 10% to 40% of patients with NSTIs.[5] Unexplained tachycardia, marked left shift, and an elevated creatine phosphokinase level are also important clues to the diagnosis of necrotizing fasciitis, and their presence in the right setting should prompt surgical inspection of the deep tissues. To complicate matters further, prior use of antibiotics and nonsteroidal anti-inflammatory drugs may mask or confound some of these findings, making it difficult to establish the diagnosis of NSTIs. Given the difficulty in establishing an early diagnosis, a wide array of diagnostic tools has been tested to diagnose NSTIs accurately and expeditiously.

Imaging studies such as plain radiography, ultrasonography, computed tomography (CT), and magnetic resonance imaging (MRI) have been used. Plain radiography can only help to identify subcutaneous gas. CT and MRI can identify other causes such as deep-seated abscesses, fascial thickening, and muscle involvement. These findings are very specific and helpful when present, but not sensitive in the screening of patients with NSTIs.

Examination of a frozen-section biopsy specimen from the compromised site has been studied. When performed early in the course of infection, it has been shown to avoid the delay in diagnosis and is associated with comparatively decreased mortality.[32]

As some of these tests are limited by availability and cost, the LRINEC (Laboratory Risk Indicator for Necrotizing Fasciitis) score was developed, which is based on routine, commonly available laboratory investigations. This score can stratify patients into high, moderate, and low risk categories for NSTIs based on total white blood cell count, hemoglobin, sodium, creatinine, glucose, and C-reactive protein. An LRINEC score of 6 or more should raise the suspicion of necrotizing fasciitis, and a score of 8 or more is strongly predictive of NSTI.[31] Patients with intermediate and high risk (score >6) had a positive predictive value of 92% and a negative predictive value of 96% (**Table 1**).[32]

The "finger test" is a bedside procedure whereby a 2-cm incision is made down to the deep fascia under local anesthesia and gentle probing with the index finger is performed. Lack of bleeding, presence of characteristic "dishwater pus," and lack of tissue resistance to blunt finger are features of a positive finger test suggestive of necrotizing fasciitis.[33] Measurement of compartment pressure may also be useful, and if pressures are greater than 40 mm Hg, immediate fasciotomy is indicated.[34] Once NSTI is confirmed, the incision is extended and additional debridement is performed.

Table 1
LRINEC (laboratory risk indicator for necrotizing fasciitis) score

	LRINEC Score
C-reactive protein	
<150	0
>150	4
WBC count (cells/mm^3)	
<15	0
15–25	1
>25	2
Hemoglobin (g/dL)	
>13.5	0
11–13.5	1
<11	2
Sodium (mmol/L)	
≥135	0
<135	2
Creatinine (mg/dL)	
≤1.6	0
>1.6	2
Glucose (mg/dL)	
≤180	0
>180	1

LRINEC score: ≤5, low risk; 6–7, intermediate risk; ≥8, high risk.
Modified from Wong HC, Khin WL, Heng SK, et al. The LRINEC (Laboratory Risk Indicator for Necrotizing Fasciitis) score: a tool for distinguishing necrotizing fasciitis from other soft tissue infections. Crit Care Med 2004;32:1535–41.

MANAGEMENT

Treatment of NSTI involves the principles of source control, antimicrobial therapy, supportive care, and monitoring. Whenever NSTI has been confirmed, surgical debridement is indicated. The impact of early and complete debridement has been shown to affect the patient outcome in NSTIs. Mortality has been found to be significantly lower with early and aggressive debridement.[6,9,33] Repeat debridements should be performed at intervals of 24 to 48 hours until no further necrosis or infected tissue is seen. Clinical presentation of all NSTIs is fairly similar, and time should not be wasted on identifying the possible causative pathogen. Surgical debridement should not be delayed, and broad-spectrum antibiotics should be initiated at the earliest opportunity to cover gram-positive, gram-negative, and anaerobic organisms. Acceptable regimens include ampicillin-sulbactam or piperacillin-tazobactam plus clindamycin plus ciprofloxacin and vancomycin. Other options are carbapenems such as imipenem/cilastatin or meropenem plus metronidazole, or clindamycin plus vancomycin. Clindamycin is added to reduce toxin production and has also been shown to decrease cytokine production.[35] Antibiotic therapy may be de-escalated and pathogen directed, based on cultures after surgical debridement and once the patient is stable.

Intravenous immune globulin (IVIG) has also been used in the treatment of NSTIs, despite the controversial benefit. IVIG contains neutralizing antibodies against some streptococcal superantigens and clostridial toxins. One Canadian study showed IVIG to be beneficial if the NSTI is associated with Group A streptococcal infection in patients who have developed streptococcal toxic shock syndrome.[36] IVIG has been shown to neutralize bacterial mitogenicity and to reduce T-cell production of interleukin-6 and tumor necrosis factor α.[37]

The role of hyperbaric oxygen therapy (HBO) in the treatment of NSTIs has been debated. HBO (100% oxygen at 3 atm) has been recommended for perioperative use in clostridial myonecrosis, as in vitro studies have shown it to inhibit bacterial growth and toxin production.[23,38] The rationale for the use of HBO in other NSTIs includes reversal of tissue hypoxia, enhanced neutrophil function, a direct toxic effect on select bacteria, and enhanced activity of certain antimicrobial agents.[38] Evidence to support the use of HBO is limited because of only small retrospective studies and the lack of availability of HBO at all centers. However, HBO may hasten wound closure.[6] Therefore the role of HBO therapy remains adjunctive to combined surgical and medical intervention.

PREDICTORS OF MORTALITY

Advanced age, the presence of 2 or more associated comorbidities (diabetes mellitus, peripheral vascular disease, chronic liver disease, cancer), and a delay from admission to operation of more than 24 hours have been shown to affect survival adversely.[5] In one study, the body surface area involved with infection (as expressed in burns) had a correlation with survival advantage. Truncal and perineal locations of infection incurred the greatest mortality.[6]

SUMMARY

NSTI is a life-threatening, surgical, and medical emergency. Clinical presentation, at least in the initial phase, can be misleading. Various studies have shown that delay in surgical debridement is associated with increased mortality. A high index of suspicion is important in early recognition and in instituting prompt therapy without delay. Early diagnosis, aggressive surgical debridement, aggressive supportive care, and optimal presumptive antibiotic therapy significantly improve morbidity and mortality associated with NSTIs.

REFERENCES

1. Vinh CD, Embil MJ. Rapidly progressive soft tissue infections. Lancet Infect Dis 2005;5:501–13.
2. May AK. Skin and soft tissue infections. Surg Clin North Am 2009;89(2):403–20.
3. Childers BJ, Potyondy LD, Nachreiner R, et al. Necrotizing fasciitis: a fourteen-year retrospective study of 163 consecutive patients. Am Surg 2002;68(2):109–16.
4. Anaya DA, Dellinger EP. Necrotizing soft tissue infection: diagnosis and management. Clin Infect Dis 2007;44(5):705–10 [Epub 2007 Jan 22].
5. Wong CH, Chang HC, Pasupathy S, et al. Necrotizing fasciitis: clinical presentation, microbiology, and determinants of mortality. J Bone Joint Surg Am 2003;85(8):1454–60.
6. Elliott DC, Kufera JA, Myers RA. Necrotizing soft tissue infections. Risk factors for mortality and strategies for management. Ann Surg 1996;224(5):672–83.
7. Swartz N. Cellulitis. N Engl J Med 2004;350:9.
8. Singh G, Ray P, Sinha SK, et al. Bacteriology of necrotizing infections of soft tissues. Aust N Z J Surg 1996;66(11):747–50.

9. Anaya DA, McMahon K, Nathens AB, et al. Predictors of mortality and limb loss in necrotizing soft tissue infections. Arch Surg 2005;140(2):151–7 [discussion: 158].

10. Stevens LD, Baddour ML. UpToDate: necrotizing soft tissue infections. 2012.

11. Miller LG, Perdreau-Renington F, Rieg G, et al. Necrotizing fasciitis caused by community-associated MRSA in Los Angeles. N Engl J Med 2005;352:1445.

12. Mandell GL. Mandell, Douglas, and Bennett's principles and practice of infectious diseases. 7th edition. Streptococcus pyogenes; 2009. Chapter 198.

13. Stevens DL. Invasive group A streptococcus infections. Clin Infect Dis 1992; 14(1):2–11.

14. Green RJ, Dafoe DC, Raffin TA. Necrotizing fasciitis. Chest 1996;110(1):219–29.

15. Chapnick EK, Abter EL. Necrotizing soft-tissue infection. Infect Dis Clin North Am 1996;10:835–55.

16. Awad MM, Bryant AE, Stevens DL, et al. Virulence studies on chromosomal alpha-toxin and theta-toxin mutants constructed by allelic exchange provide genetic evidence for the essential role of alpha-toxin in *Clostridium perfringens*-mediated gas gangrene. Mol Microbiol 1995;15:191.

17. DiNubile MJ, Lipsky BA. Complicated infections of skin and skin structures: when the infection is more than skin deep. J Antimicrob Chemother 2004;53:37–50.

18. Stevens LD, Bryant A. 2012 UpToDate: clostridial myonecrosis.

19. Bryant AE, Chen RY, Nagata Y, et al. Clostridial gas gangrene I. Cellular and molecular mechanisms of microvascular dysfunction induced by exotoxins of *Clostridium perfringens*. J Infect Dis 2000;182:799.

20. Bryant AE, Chen RY, Nagata Y, et al. Clostridial gas gangrene II. Phospholipase C-induced activation of platelet gpIIbIIIa mediates vascular occlusion and myonecrosis in *Clostridium perfringens* gas gangrene. J infect Dis 2000;182:808.

21. Mandell GL, Mandell, Douglas, and Bennett's principles and practice of infectious diseases, 7th edition 2009. Chapter 246. Gas gangrene and other Clostridium.

22. Nichols RL, Florman S. Clinical presentations of soft-tissue infections and surgical site infections. Clin Infect Dis 2001;33(Suppl 2):S84–93.

23. Vally H, Whittle A, Cameron S, et al. Outbreak of *Aeromonas hydrophila* wound infections associated with mud football. Clin Infect Dis 2004;38:1084–9.

24. Mackay DR, Manders EK, Saggers GC, et al. Aeromonas species isolated from medicinal leeches. Ann Plast Surg 1999;42:275–9.

25. Sartor C, Limouzin-Perotti F, Legré R, et al. Nosocomial infections with *Aeromonas hydrophila* from leeches. Clin Infect Dis 2002;35(1):E1–5 [Epub 2002 Jun 4].

26. Whitaker IS, Josty IC, Hawkins S, et al. Medicinal leeches and the microsurgeon: a four-year study, clinical series and risk benefit review. Microsurgery 2011;31(4):281–7.

27. Gold WL, Salit IE. *Aeromonas hydrophila* infections of skin and soft tissue: report of 11 cases and review. Clin Infect Dis 1993;16(1):69–74.

28. Ko WC, Lee HC, Chuang YC, et al. Clinical features and therapeutic implications of 104 episodes of monomicrobial *Aeromonas* bacteremia. J Infect 2000;40(3):267–73.

29. Vila J, Marco F, Soler L, et al. In vitro antimicrobial susceptibility of clinical isolates of *Aeromonas caviae*, *Aeromonas hydrophila* and *Aeromonas veronii* biotype *sobria*. J Antimicrob Chemother 2002;49(4):701–2.

30. Wong CH, Khin LW, Heng KS, et al. The LRINEC (Laboratory Risk Indicator for Necrotizing Fasciitis) score: a tool for distinguishing necrotizing fasciitis from other soft tissue infections. Crit Care Med 2004;32(7):1535–41.

31. Wall DB, Klein SR, Black S, et al. A simple model to help distinguish necrotizing fasciitis from nonnecrotizing soft tissue infection. J Am Coll Surg 2000;191(3): 227–31.

32. Stamenkovic I, Lew PD. Early recognition of potentially fatal necrotizing fasciitis: the use of frozen-section biopsy. N Engl J Med 1984;310:1689–93.
33. Andreasen TJ, Green SD, Childers BJ. Massive infectious soft-tissue injury: diagnosis and management of necrotizing fasciitis and purpura fulminans. Plast Reconstr Surg 2001;107(4):1025–35.
34. Bisno LA, Stevens LS. Streptococcal infections of skin and soft tissues. N Engl J Med 1996;334(4):240–5.
35. Stevens LD, Bisno LA, Chambers FH, et al. Practice guidelines for the diagnosis and management of skin and soft-tissue infections. Clin Infect Dis 2005;41:1373–406.
36. Kaul R, McGeer A, Low DE, et al. Population-based surveillance for group-A streptococcal necrotizing fasciitis: clinical features, prognostic indicators, and microbiologic analysis of seventy-seven cases. Ontario Group A Streptococcal study. Am J Med 1997;103:18–24.
37. Kaul R, McGeer A, Norrby-Teglund A, et al. Intravenous immunoglobulin therapy for streptococcal toxic shock syndrome—a comparative observational study. The Canadian Streptococcal Study Group. Clin Infect Dis 1999;28(4):800–7.
38. Rabinowitz PR, Caplan SE. Hyperbaric oxygen. In Mandell, Douglas, and Bennett's principles and practice of infectious diseases, 7th edition. Chapter 43.

Sepsis Syndrome, Bloodstream Infections, and Device-Related Infections

Mayar Al Mohajer, MD[a],*, Rabih O. Darouiche, MD[a,b,c,d]

KEYWORDS

- Sepsis • Septic shock • Bloodstream infection • Central line infection
- Device infection • Cardiac implantable electronic device • Cerebrospinal fluid shunt
- Prosthetic joint

KEY POINTS

- Early diagnosis and timely management of sepsis are imperative.
- Catheters should be removed in most cases of catheter-related bloodstream infections, especially when the infection is caused by *Staphylococcus aureus, Pseudomonas aeruginosa*, or *Candida* species.
- Transesophageal echocardiography should be performed in bacteremic patients with cardiac implantable electronic devices.
- Infected cerebrospinal shunts should be replaced temporarily with external ventricular drains and treated with antibiotics before reinsertion of new cerebrospinal shunts.
- Two-stage surgical replacement and intravenous antibiotics are the preferred management of prosthetic joint infections.

Disclosure: Dr Al Mohajer reports no financial disclosure or conflict of interest. Dr Darouiche coinvented the impregnation of devices with minocycline and rifampin and fully assigned his rights to his employer Baylor College of Medicine, which executed a licensing agreement with Cook and TyRx Pharma.

[a] Michael E. DeBakey VA Medical Center, Baylor College of Medicine, 1709 Dryden, Suite 5.82a, Houston, TX 77030, USA; [b] Department of Medicine, Baylor College of Medicine, 1333 Moursund Avenue, Suite A221, Houston, TX 77030, USA; [c] Department of Surgery, Baylor College of Medicine, 1333 Moursund Avenue, Suite A221, Houston, TX 77030, USA; [d] Department of PM&R, Baylor College of Medicine, 1333 Moursund Avenue, Suite A221, Houston, TX 77030, USA
* Corresponding author. Section of Infectious Diseases, Baylor College of Medicine, 1 Baylor Plaza, Houston, TX 77030.
E-mail address: mohajer@bcm.edu

Med Clin N Am 96 (2012) 1203–1223
http://dx.doi.org/10.1016/j.mcna.2012.08.008
0025-7125/12/$ – see front matter © 2012 Elsevier Inc. All rights reserved.

SEPSIS SYNDROME
Definitions

The term systemic inflammatory response syndrome (SIRS) has been used to describe physiologic changes in response to infectious or noninfectious events such as pancreatitis, burns, or trauma (**Fig. 1**).[1] The 1991 American College of Chest Physicians/Society of Critical Care Medicine Consensus Conference established definition criteria for SIRS, sepsis, and septic shock (**Table 1**).[1]

The 2001 International Sepsis Definitions Conference broadened the classification of SIRS/sepsis to include hyperglycemia, increased C-reactive protein (CRP) or procalcitonin, hyperlactatemia, decreased capillary refill, and hemodynamic instability or organ dysfunction.[2] The study investigators stressed that the clinician should go to the bedside, identify a myriad of symptoms, and then declare if the patient does look septic and have some criteria regardless of whether a source of infection is obvious. The criteria published in both 1991 and 2001 were criticized for having suboptimal performance,[3,4] because they both have high sensitivity but suffer from low specificity. The 2001 criteria had a slightly higher sensitivity but decreased specificity compared with the 1991 definitions. One study suggested that the 1991 criteria should not be used for clinical definition of sepsis because they fail to characterize this complex disease.[4]

Epidemiology

The population-adjusted incidence of sepsis has increased over the past few decades, mostly because of an increase in age and immunosuppression.[5,6] In a 1994 study, the estimated hospital-wide incidence was 2 cases per 100 admissions or 2.8 per 1000 patient-days.[6] However, the current incidence of sepsis syndrome in the United States is 240 per 100,000 people, whereas the incidence of severe sepsis is between 51 and 95 patients per 100,000 people. Sepsis is more common in men and among nonwhite persons.[7] The incidence and mortality of sepsis and severe sepsis are higher in the winter because of respiratory infections.[8]

Gram-negative bacteria were the most common cause of sepsis until the mid-1980s, when they were surpassed by gram-positive organisms. The occurrence of fungal sepsis has been on the increase as well.[5] Although less prominent, viruses

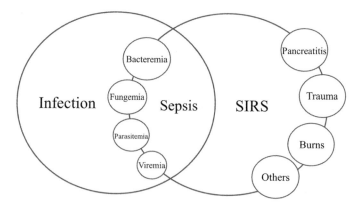

Fig. 1. The term systemic inflammatory response syndrome (SIRS) has been used to describe physiologic changes in response to infectious or noninfectious events such as pancreatitis, burns or trauma. (*Adapted from* ACCP/SCCM consensus conference: definitions for sepsis and organ failure and guidelines for the use of innovative therapies in sepsis. Crit Care Med 1992;20:865; with permission.)

Table 1
Definitions of SIRS and variations of sepsis and MODS

SIRS	Two or more of the following: Fever (>38°C) or hypothermia (<36°C) Tachycardia (heart rate >90 beats/min) Tachypnea (respiratory rate >20 breaths/min or hyperventilation ($Paco_2$ <32 mm Hg) Leukocytosis (WBC >12,000 cells/mm^3), leukopenia (WBC <4000 cells/mm^3) or bandemia (>10%)
Sepsis	SIRS in the presence of suspected or documented infectious process
Severe sepsis	Sepsis with organ dysfunction: Abrupt change in mental status Cardiac dysfunction Acute lung injury Lactic acidosis Thrombocytopenia or disseminated intravascular coagulopathy Decreased urinary output, increased creatinine, or significant edema Decreased capillary refill time Mottled skin Ileus Hyperbilirubinemia Hyperglycemia in the absence of diabetes Increased procalcitonin or C-reactive protein
MODS	Dysfunction in 1 or more organ requiring an intervention to maintain hemostasis
Septic shock	Severe sepsis plus: Systolic blood pressure <60 mm Hg despite fluid challenge or requiring low-dose vasopressors
Refractory septic shock	Septic shock requiring higher dose of vasopressors Dopamine >15 μg/kg/min or Norepinephrine or epinephrine >0.25 μg/kg/min

Abbreviations: MODS, multiple-organ dysfunction syndrome; $Paco_2$, partial pressure of carbon dioxide, arterial; WBC, white blood cells.

Adapted from ACCP/SCCM consensus conference: definitions for sepsis and organ failure and guidelines for the use of innovative therapies in sepsis. Crit Care Med 1992;20:866; with permission.

and parasites can also cause sepsis.[1] More patients with sepsis are being diagnosed with severe sepsis (25.6% in 1993 vs 43.8% in 2003).[9] Sepsis is the tenth leading cause of death in the United States.[7] There has been a marked increase in overall mortality caused by sepsis that is attributed, at least in part, to an increasing incidence of sepsis.[5,7] In 1 study, the in-hospital sepsis-related mortality doubled from 21.9 per 100,000 population in 1979 to 43.9 per 100,000 in 2000.[5] Conversely, survival rates of sepsis have been improving, mainly because of improved survival in gram-negative sepsis.[7] Death is more common in older patients, women, and blacks.[7,9] One study estimated the fatality rate of SIRS, sepsis, severe sepsis, and septic shock to be 7%, 16%, 20%, and 46%, respectively.[10] Moreover, sepsis incurs a huge financial burden, with annual cost exceeding 17 billion dollars in the United States.[11]

Pathogenesis

The ideal physiologic and immunologic host response is to eliminate pathogens, then resume homeostasis shortly afterward.[12] The innate immune system recognizes pathogens as foreign, which leads to the release of various inflammatory cytokines, phagocytosis, and bacterial killing. Proinflammatory and antiinflammatory mediators play a role in this response,[13] and sepsis results from dysregulation of these mechanisms.[12–14] The role of different factors in the pathogenesis of sepsis is presented in **Table 2**.

Cellular injury and immune dysregulation can lead to organ-specific effects. Hypotension is the hallmark of septic shock[1] and is usually related to excessive production of nitric oxide,[15] endotoxin release, and, to a lesser degree, decreased vasopressin secretion.[16] Other cardiovascular-related effects include myocardial dysfunction,[17] decreased vascular vasoconstriction in splanchnic organs,[18] a decrease in the number in functional capillaries and diffuse endothelial activation.[19] Pulmonary injury is manifested by pulmonary edema and hypoxemia caused by ventilation-perfusion

Table 2
Role of various factors in the pathogenesis of sepsis

Factors	Role in Sepsis
Bacterial endotoxin	Complement activation Triggering of coagulation and fibrinolytic pathways
Proinflammatory cytokines (TNF-α, interferon γ, IL-1, IL-2, and IL-6)	Clinical syndrome of SIRS (fever, tachycardia, and tachypnea)
Antiinflammatory cytokines (IL-4 and IL-10)	Concomitant septic immunosuppression and evasion of pathogens
Complement activation	Tissue injury and necrosis (membrane-attack complex and cell-bound ligands including C4b and C3b) Influx and activation of inflammatory cells (anaphylatoxins C5a and C3a)
Leukocyte recruitment dysfunction	Tissue damage by overwhelming activation Increased susceptibility to infections by decreased recruitment
CSMs (CD80, CD86, and PD-L1)	CD80/86 binding to CD28 causes T-cell activation and proliferation PD-L1:PD-1 interaction leads to T-cell anergy and apoptosis
Rapid lymphocytic apoptosis	Associated with the severity of sepsis symptoms and outcome
Delayed neutrophil apoptosis	Tissue damage by continuous release of soluble toxic products
Increased cell necrosis	Allows leakage of proteolytic enzymes
Coagulation dysfunction	Thrombin activates PARs on platelets and endothelial cells
Excessive nitric oxide production	Hypotension and decreased perfusion to organs
Zinc deficiency	Enhanced inflammation, infection spread, lung injury, and mortality
Increased tryptophan	Arterial vessel relaxation and hypotension
Genetic polymorphism	Various TLR and IL production genes are associated with poorer outcome

Abbreviations: CSMs, costimulatory molecules; IL, interleukin; PARS, protease-activated receptors; PD-L, programmed death ligand; TLR, toll-like receptor; TNF, tumor necrosis factor.

mismatch.[20] Sepsis can also lead to increased intestinal permeability of bacteria and toxins as well as liver, renal, central nervous system, and endocrine dysfunction.[21,22]

Diagnosis

The diagnosis of sepsis requires the presence of SIRS and identification of an infection source.[23] In some patients, the source of infection can easily be identified as wound infection, cellulitis, purpura fulminans, or a purulent discharge from urine, cerebrospinal fluid (CSF), peritoneal, or pleural cavity.[21] Imaging may disclose pulmonary infiltrates, intra-abdominal fluid collection, or thickened colon wall as infectious foci. Microbiologic analysis of fluid, blood, urine, and tissue is vital for pathogen identification. However, positive cultures may not yield microbial growth before 6 to 48 hours. Cultures are negative in about 30% of patients diagnosed with sepsis, especially those with previous antibiotic exposure and others infected by nonbacterial organisms or exposed to toxic agents.[1,21]

Numerous studies showed an advantage when using molecular methods in early identification of infectious source. Multiplex real-time polymerase chain reaction (PCR) analysis of blood samples provided early detection (within 6 hours) of specific pathogens in patients with SIRS.[24] The test had higher sensitivity than blood culture (39.9% vs 20.3%) and affected therapeutic decision-making but not mortality.[24] In situ hybridization is another method that can provide early organism-targeted therapy and impart a higher sensitivity than blood culture.[25]

Multiple investigational biomarkers of sepsis have been evaluated, without much success.[21] Although high levels of procalcitonin level were reported in septic patients,[26] 1 meta-analysis showed that procalcitonin could not correctly differentiate sepsis from nonseptic SIRS because both the sensitivity and specificity were 71%.[27] Routine use of procalcitonin has been discouraged.[21,27] Specific procalcitonin algorithms for low-acuity, moderate-acuity, and high-acuity patients have been proposed to limit unnecessary antibiotic use.[28]

Table 3 shows the role of other biomarkers in sepsis. Combining multiple biomarkers might be superior to the use of a single biomarker.[29] Plasma protein profiling using mass spectrometry is another tool that can help differentiate between patients with infectious versus noninfectious SIRS.[30]

Management

The International Surviving Sepsis Campaign Guidelines Committee published recommendations for the management of sepsis.[31] Early goal-directed resuscitation within 6 hours after recognition of sepsis symptoms is the cornerstone of therapy.[31] Intravenous antimicrobial should be started within 1 hour after obtaining cultures.[31] Late administration of antibiotics (>1 hour) is associated with increased mortality in patients with severe sepsis or septic shock.[32] The use of appropriate initial antibiotics is crucial because multiple studies showed that inappropriate initial choice of antibiotics can lead to poor outcomes.[33,34] Selection of antimicrobials should be based on multiple factors, including the patient's previous antibiotics exposure, allergies or drug intolerance, underlying conditions, clinical diagnosis, Gram stain findings, and antibiotics susceptibility pattern at the community and the local health care facility.[23,35]

Third-generation or fourth-generation cephalosporins, carbapenems, β-lactam/β-lactamase inhibitor combinations are proper initial choices in immunocompetent adults with no previous antibiotic exposure.[35] Vancomycin should be added in environments with high prevalence of methicillin-resistant *Staphylococcus aureus* (MRSA).[35] The use of combination therapy against gram-negative organisms versus monotherapy is controversial.[36,37] Although combination therapy can be more

Table 3
Role of biomarkers in sepsis

Biomarker	Clinical Usefulness
PCT	Possible role in the diagnosis of sepsis Sensitivity 71%, specificity 71% Useful in limiting antibiotic use
Lactic acid	Higher levels correlate with mortality
TREM1	Possible role in the diagnosis of sepsis Sensitivity 53%–96%; specificity 86%–89% Higher levels correlate with mortality
sCD14-ST	Possible role in the diagnosis of sepsis Higher levels correlate with disease severity
CD64 and CD64/CD16 ratio	Possible role in the diagnosis of sepsis Increased expression correlates with disease severity and mortality
suPAR	Low diagnostic value Higher levels correlate with organ dysfunction and disease severity
Angiopoietin 1	Lower levels correlate with mortality
Angiopoietin 2	Higher levels correlate with mortality
PSP/reg	Higher levels correlate with mortality

Abbreviations: PCT, procalcitonin; PSP/reg, pancreatic stone protein/regenerating protein; sCD14-ST, soluble CD14 subtype (presepsin); suPAR, soluble urokinase-type plasminogen activator receptor; TREM 1, triggering receptor expressed on myeloid cells.

adequate for empiric coverage and help prevent emergence of resistance, it is associated with increased drug toxicity, higher rate of superinfection, and additional cost.[36]

Two separate meta-analyses showed no benefit of combination therapy in patients with gram-negative bacteremia or sepsis,[38,39] whereas other studies reported that combination therapy in bacterial septic shock is associated with lower mortality and shrunken stay in the intensive care unit (ICU).[40,41] In a recent study, moxifloxacin did not offer additional benefit when added to meropenem in patients with severe sepsis.[37] The choice of combination therapy versus monotherapy should be based on the clinical status of the patient and potential occurrence of resistant organisms.[36] Antifungals should be empirically given in selected cases such as *Candida* colonization, previous use of broad-spectrum antibiotics for a long duration, prolonged ICU stay, total parenteral nutrition, presence of vascular access devices, mucositis, gastrointestinal perforation, or persistent fever in neutropenic patients.[35]

Source control is imperative in many cases of sepsis such as necrotizing fasciitis, gas gangrene, severe peritonitis, cholangitis, mesenteric ischemia, abscesses, walled-off pancreatic necrosis, severe *Clostridium difficile* infection, empyema, or urinary obstruction.[23,42] A percutaneous approach is preferred over a surgical procedure when possible. Intravascular devices should be removed if they are suspected to be the infection source.[23]

The response to antimicrobials should be reassessed within 48 to 72 hours, and therapy should be adjusted or stopped based on clinical response and microbiologic findings.[35] Recombinant human activated protein C is no longer available for the treatment of severe sepsis or septic shock, because recent data failed to show a decrease in mortality.[43] **Table 4** shows other interventions recommended for the management of sepsis.

Table 4
Management of sepsis

Initial resuscitation	Assess airway with intubation for high-risk patients Assess breathing, administer oxygen, and maintain low tidal volume if mechanical ventilation is used Assess circulation and administer fluid, vasopressors, inotropes, and transfusion as indicated (goals: MAP >65 mm Hg, CVP 8–12 mm Hg, hematocrit >30%, and $Scvo_2$ >70%)
Intravenous antibiotics	Administer antibiotics within 1 h and after obtaining cultures Assess the response to antibiotics within 48–72 h
Source control	Establish the source quickly (within 6 h if possible) Implement source control measures (abscess draining or tissue debridement) Remove intravascular devices if they are suspected to be the source
Blood product use	Give red blood cells when hemoglobin decreases to 7 g/dL in most cases Give platelets when counts are less than 5000/mm^3
Mechanical ventilation	Maintain a target tidal volume of 6 mL/kg Maintain plateau pressure ≤30 mm Hg Maintain head of bed elevation (45°) Use a weaning protocol and SBT regularly
Sedation and neuromuscular blockade	Use sedation protocols with daily interruption or lightening Avoid neuromuscular blocking agents if possible
Steroid use	Consider early steroid use in patients with severe septic shock requiring vasopressors
Glucose control	Use intravenous insulin to maintain glucose <180 mg/dL in hyperglycemic patients
Renal replacement	Use either intermitted hemodialysis or CVVH
Deep vein thrombosis prophylaxis	Use LMWH or low-dose UFH unless contraindicated
Stress ulcer prophylaxis	Use H_2 blockers or proton pump inhibitors
Nutritional support	Provide early nutritional support Enteral route is preferred over parenteral route
External cooling	Use external cooling to achieve normothermia (36.5–37°C)

Abbreviations: CVP, central venous pressure; CVVH, continuous venovenous hemofiltration; H_2, histamine 2; LMWH, low-molecular-weight heparin; MAP, mean arterial pressure; MDR, multidrug resistant; SBT, spontaneous breathing trial; $Scvo_2$, central venous oxygen saturation; UFH, unfractionated heparin.

Adapted from Dellinger RP, Levy MM, Carlet JM, et al. Surviving Sepsis Campaign: international guidelines for management of severe sepsis and septic shock: 2008. Crit Care Med 2008;36(1): 296–327.

BLOODSTREAM INFECTION
Epidemiology

Most cases of bloodstream infection (BSI) are associated with a vascular access. In 2009, the Centers for Disease Control and Prevention (CDC) reported an estimated 23,000 episodes of central line–associated BSI (CLABSI) in American ICUs with a mortality of 12% to 25%.[44] BSIs are associated with increased length of hospital stay and additional cost.[44–46] **Table 5** summarizes the terminology of the 2 variations of BSI, namely catheter-related BSI (CRBSI) and CLABSI. Host-related risk factors for developing BSI include total parenteral nutrition, granulocytopenia, chemotherapy, burns, infection at different sites, and bone marrow transplantation. The size of the catheter, number of lumens, location, type, function, duration of placement, emergent

Table 5
Terminology and diagnostic criteria used for BSI

Terminology	Meaning	Criteria	Purpose	Problems
CRBSI	Defines the catheter as the cause of the BSI	Presence of bacteremia or fungemia in a patient who has an intravascular catheter At least 1 positive blood culture obtained peripherally Clinical signs of infection (fever, chills, or hypotension) Absence of infection at another site One of the following: a. Positive semiquantitative[a] or quantitative[b] catheter tip culture b. Quantitative blood culture with a ratio >3:1 cfu/mL (catheter vs peripheral) c. Differential time to positivity (blood culture from catheter is detected at least 2 h before detection of peripheral blood culture)	Clinical definition; used when diagnosing or treating patients	Requires microbiologic data that might not be available
CLABSI	Describes a BSI in a patient who had a recent central catheter	Presence of bacteremia or fungemia (a single positive blood culture is required for most organisms, whereas 2 positive blood cultures are required for skin flora organisms) Presence of central line within 48 h Absence of an infection at a different site	Used by NHSN for surveillance	Overestimates the true incidence of CRBSI

Abbreviations: BSI, blood stream infections; cfu, colony forming unit; NHSN, National Healthcare Safety Network.
[a] >15 cfu per catheter segment.
[b] >10^2 cfu per catheter segment.

placement, skill of venipuncturist, failure of providers to wash hands, and nursing/ patient ratio all play a role as well.[47,48]

In a surveillance study of BSI, coagulase-negative *Staphylococcus* (CoNS) species were reported to be the most common pathogens followed by *S aureus*.[49] BSIs with *Candida* species, *Pseudomonas aeruginosa*, and *Enterococcus* species had the higher associated crude mortality. **Table 6** shows the microbiology and associated crude mortality of BSI.

Pathogenesis

Catheters can be infected intraluminally (catheter hub or intravenous solution contamination), extraluminally (transversion of organisms from the skin), or hematogenously (distant source). The intracutaneous tract becomes contaminated at the time of catheter insertion or within the first week. In patients with short-term central venous catheters (CVC), extraluminal acquisition occurs, followed by the release of microorganisms from the biofilm of the implanted portion of the catheter. However, catheters placed for longer periods (>10 days) are more likely to undergo hub manipulation, which can lead to bacterial contamination followed by intraluminal colonization, resulting in BSI.[50]

Diagnosis

Local signs of infection such as phlebitis and inflammation at the catheter insertion site are uncommon. Although fever is frequently seen in bacteremic patients, it is not specific for CRBSI.[48] Before initiating antibiotics in patients with suspected CRBSI, paired peripheral and central blood cultures should be obtained. Because most vascular catheters that are removed for possible CRBSI do not yield positive cultures, certain techniques were investigated for their ability to diagnose CRBSI while the catheter is kept in place.

Quantitative blood cultures that indicate CRBSI require a bacterial colony count from the catheter hub sample that is at least 3-fold to 5-fold higher than that from

Table 6
Incidence rates of most common pathogens isolated from monomicrobial nosocomial BSI and associated crude mortality

Pathogen	BSIs per 10,000 Admissions	BSIs (%) n = 20,978	Crude Mortality (%) Total
CoNS	15.8	31.3	20.7
Staphylococcus aureus[a]	10.3	20.2	25.4
Enterococcus species[b]	4.8	9.4	33.9
Candida species[b]	4.6	9.0	39.2
Escherichia coli	2.8	5.6	22.4
Klebsiella species	2.4	4.8	27.6
Pseudomonas aeruginosa	2.1	4.3	38.7
Enterobacter species	1.9	3.9	26.7
Serratia species[a]	0.90	1.7	27.4
Acinetobacter baumannii	0.6	1.3	34.0

[a] Significantly more frequent in patients without neutropenia.
[b] Significantly more frequent in patients with neutropenia.
Adapted from Wisplinghoff H, Bischoff T, Tallent SM, et al. Nosocomial bloodstream infections in US hospitals: analysis of 24,179 cases from a prospective nationwide surveillance study. Clin Infect Dis 2004;39(3):309–17.

a peripheral blood. This method was reported to have the highest accuracy in diagnosing CRBSI (pooled sensitivity and specificity of 100%) compared with other diagnostic methods.[51] Differential time to positivity refers to a catheter-drawn blood culture turning positive 2 hours or more earlier than the peripheral culture (pooled sensitivity 88% and pooled specificity 87%).[51]

If the catheter is removed because of CRBSI, the catheter tip should be cultured.[52] Quantitative sonication technique ($>10^2$ colony forming units [cfu] per catheter segment) and semiquantitative roll-plating method (>15 cfu per catheter segment) can be performed to aid in the diagnosis.[51] The diagnosis criteria for CRBSI are presented in **Table 5**. Recently investigated PCR-based techniques that target bacterial 16S ribosomal DNA can provide early diagnosis of CRBSI.[53]

Prevention

The Healthcare Infection Control Practices Advisory Committee recently published guidelines for prevention of CRBSI.[54] Adherence to aseptic technique, including hand washing and using maximum sterile barrier precautions (cap, mask, sterile gown, sterile gloves, and a sterile full body drape), is crucial when placing CVC or peripherally inserted central catheters (PICC). The patient's skin is preferably prepared with more than 0.5% chlorhexidine with alcohol before central catheter placement. Femoral vein access should be avoided given the high rate of infection. Ultrasound guidance is recommended if the technology and the expertise are available. Emergently placed catheters should be removed within 48 hours if aseptic technique has not been implemented.[54]

The CVC and PICC should not be routinely replaced as a means of preventing CRBSI nor should they be removed because of fever alone if clinical suspicion of CRBSI is low.[55] The use of antibiotic lock solution to prevent CRBSI is controversial. A meta-analysis showed a marginal benefit of instilling a vancomycin lock solution for preventing CRBSI in patients with cancer.[56] Another meta-analysis that included cancer and hemodialysis patients did not show a difference between antibiotic-containing lock versus just heparin lock solution.[57]

Catheters impregnated with minocycline/rifampin (MR) or chlorhexidine/silver sulfadiazine can be used if they are expected to remain in place for 5 days or longer and if other previously mentioned measures failed to decrease the rate of CRBSI.[54] These 2 types of CVC can result in major cost-savings when kept in place for 2 weeks or longer,[58] more so with the former than the latter because of superior degree of clinical protection.[59] The silver/platinum/carbon-coated catheters can reduce catheter colonization but do not protect against CRBSI.[60,61]

Management

In patients with suspected CRBSI, empiric antibiotic therapy should be started after obtaining blood cultures. Empiric vancomycin is appropriate in most cases. Vancomycin should be replaced by β-lactam antibiotics, for the sake of achieving better efficacy, in patients infected by methicillin-sensitive *S aureus* and who are not allergic to penicillins or cephalosporins. Daptomycin can be used as an alternative agent in institutions in which MRSA has an increased minimum inhibitory concentration (MIC) of vancomycin greater than 2 μg/mL.[52] Linezolid is generally not recommended as an empiric choice.[52,62] Coverage for MDR gram-negative organisms is recommended in severely ill patients, neutropenic patients, and those with a history of colonization by these organisms.[52]

Antifungal coverage with echinocandins should be considered in selected cases (total parenteral nutrition, prolonged use of broad-spectrum antibacterial therapy, hematologic malignancy, solid organ or bone marrow transplantation, or femoral catheterization).[52] Fluconazole can be empirically initiated for treatment of candidemia in the absence of azole exposure in the previous 3 months and if the prevalence of *Candida krusei* or *C glabrata* is low.[52,63] Because echinocandins have a higher minimum antifungal inhibitory concentration for *C parapsilosis* than *C albicans*, it is preferable that it is not used for treatment of the former *Candida* species, which is responsible for about one-third of fungal infections of indwelling devices.[64]

Antibiotics should be adjusted when the results of cultures become available. Duration of treatment of uncomplicated CRBSI is addressed in **Table 7**. In most cases, *S aureus* should be treated for 4 to 6 weeks. A shorter course (minimum of 2 weeks) of antibiotic therapy requires: (1) no evidence of endocarditis on transesophageal echocardiography (TEE), (2) no evidence of thrombophlebitis on ultrasonography, (3) absence of immunosuppression, neutropenia, renal failure requiring hemodialysis, AIDS, and diabetes, (4) removal of the catheter, (5) absence of prosthetic intravascular devices, (6) resolution of fever and bacteremia within 72 hours after initiating appropriate antibiotics, and (7) no evidence of metastatic infections by physical examination or diagnostic tests.[52] In cases of complicated infections, including suppurative thrombophlebitis, endocarditis, osteomyelitis, and persistent bacteremia or fungemia (more than 3 days after initiating appropriate therapy), the catheter should be removed and the antibiotics should be continued for 4 to 6 weeks, and possibly longer (6–8 weeks) in cases of osteomyelitis.[52]

Table 7
Pathogen-specific management of uncomplicated CRBSIs

Organism	Preferred Agents	Treatment Duration	Catheter Removal
CoNS species[a]	Vancomycin if methicillin-resistant Nafcillin if methicillin-sensitive	5–7 d if the catheter is removed 10–14 d if the catheter is retained	Optional
Staphylococcus aureus	Vancomycin if methicillin-resistant Nafcillin if methicillin-sensitive	4–6 wk ≥2 wk in selected cases[b]	Recommended in all cases[c]
Enterococcus species	Ampicillin ± aminoglycosides If ampicillin resistant: vancomycin, linezolid, or daptomycin	7–14-d course	Recommended for short-term catheters Optional for long-term catheters[c]
Gram-negative bacilli	Third-generation or fourth-generation cephalosporins, carbapenems, β-lactam/β-lactamase ± aminoglycosides	7–14-d course	Recommended in all cases[c]
Candida species	Echinocandin or fluconazole	14-d course	Recommended in all cases[d]

[a] *Staphylococcus lugdunensis* should be treated like *S aureus*.
[b] See text for shorter course requirements.
[c] Antibiotic lock therapy should be added in cases of catheter retention.
[d] Limited data for antifungal or ethanol-based lock in cases of catheter retention.

Long-term catheters should be removed in cases of BSI with *S aureus*, *P aeruginosa*, fungi, or mycobacteria regardless of disease severity. Short-term catheters should be removed in most cases of suspected CRBSI when possible. Exceptions include contamination with CoNS species, *Bacillus* species, *Micrococcus* species, or propionibacteria if repeat blood cultures are negative.[52]

When catheter removal is not possible, antibiotic lock therapy (ALT) should be used for 1 to 2 weeks as an adjunct to systematic antimicrobial treatment of management of CRBSI.[52] Not only was ALT able to eradicate biofilm in vitro,[65] but a meta-analysis showed that the addition of culture-guided ALT to systemic antibiotics was superior to systematic antibiotics alone.[66] Given the difficulty of eradicating the biofilm, the antibiotic concentration in the lock solution should be 10 to 1000 higher than the MIC in most cases, and even higher in patients who receive vancomycin-based ALT (>1000 higher than the MIC).[65] In 1 study, daptomycin-containing ALT was superior to vancomycin in the management of CRBSI in patients who have cancer.[67]

Catheter exchange is another option when catheter removal is not performed because of increased risk of mechanical complications.[68] Although a recent study in patients who have cancer showed that exchanging CVC over a wire for MR-impregnated catheters may improve the overall response rate compared with catheter removal,[69] it is important to further assess this issue. Studies are also needed to compare catheter exchange over a wire versus ALT as a salvage therapy in cases in which catheter removal is not possible.[66]

DEVICE-RELATED INFECTIONS

Infections associated with surgically implanted devices have huge clinical impact in terms of morbidity and mortality, and incur tremendous cost. In general, infections of surgical implants are more difficult to manage than CRBSI because they require longer duration of antibiotic therapy and repeated surgical procedures.[70] Biofilm plays an important role in the pathogenesis of device-related infections. Like with CRBSI, biofilm-embedded organisms form sessile communities and are more resistant to antimicrobials compared with planktonic cells.[71] In this review, the diagnosis and management of 3 infections associated with select surgical implants are discussed.

Cardiac Implantable Electronic Devices

The use of permanent pacemakers (PPM) and implantable cardioverter defibrillators (ICDs) continues to escalate.[72,73] In that regard, CIEDs are being implanted more frequently in older patients and in patients with more comorbidities.[74] These 2 factors have led to an increase in infections from cardiac implantable electronic devices (CIEDs),[75] with associated increase in the morbidity, mortality, and financial costs.[70,76] The infection rates of ICD are higher than those of PPM.[75] Several risk factors for CIED infections have been identified, including fever within 24 hours before implantation, lack of antibiotic prophylaxis, operator inexperience, previous CIED infection, recent device manipulation, use of corticosteroid or anticoagulation agents, and other comorbid conditions.[77] CoNS species are the most common causes of CIED infections (42%) followed by *S aureus* (29%).[76] The median time from implantation to CIED infection is 414 days for PPM and 125 days for ICD.[76] Infection of CIED most often presents itself as a generator pocket site infection (localized inflammatory symptoms), and less so as an occult BSI, or lead or valvular vegetation.[76,77] The most common site for valvular vegetation is the tricuspid valve, followed by the pulmonary valve and left-sided valves.[77]

Antimicrobial prophylaxis before CIED implantation is imperative. A single dose of cefazolin or vancomycin before the procedure is acceptable.[78,79] Postoperative antibiotic use is not recommended because of lack of evidence and potential development of antibiotic resistance.[79] In a case series, lower rates of infection were reported when an MR antibacterial envelope was implanted around the CIED generator.[80]

In cases of suspected or documented infections, blood cultures should be obtained before administering antibiotics.[75] The whole CIED system should be removed, even in patients with negative blood cultures or infection limited to the generator pocket, in order to reduce the likelihood that bacteria colonizing the cardiac leads could subsequently result in endocarditis or BSI.[75] A swab culture of drainage, but not swab of open wound without discharge, can be helpful.[77] Percutaneous aspiration of the generator pocket should not be performed. If CIED infection is suspected, TEE should be obtained in bacteremic as well as nonbacteremic patients who had previously received antibiotics. On removal of the CIED, the lead tip should be sent for culture.[75] It has been suggested that the following modalities could be helpful in the diagnosis of CIED infection, including indium-labeled leukocyte scintigraphy, gallium scanning, technetium-labeled leukocyte scintigraphy,[81] and positron emission tomography (PET)/computed tomography.[82]

Antibiotics active against gram-positive organisms should be empirically started, then adjusted after obtaining the results of cultures of blood and cardiac leads. Patients with only pocket infection can be treated for 10 to 14 days after device extraction. In bacteremic patients with a negative TEE and in patients with uncomplicated lead vegetations, a 2-week course of therapy after device removal is recommended in most cases. In cases of *S aureus* bacteremia, a TEE could be repeated after the end of therapy or the duration of antibiotic therapy could be extended to 4 weeks.[75] Patients with complicated lead vegetations, as evident by osteomyelitis, organ or deep abscesses, or septic vein thrombosis, and patients with valvular vegetations should be treated for 4 to 6 weeks.[75] A recent noncontrolled study showed that high-dose daptomycin is a safe and effective treatment of CIED endocarditis.[83]

The optimal time for implanting a new CIED is at least 3 days from first negative blood cultures. Implantation of the new device should be delayed for 2 weeks or so from the first negative blood culture in cases of valve vegetations.[75] If device removal is not possible, long-term suppressive therapy is indicated.[84]

CSF Shunts

CSF shunts are considered as a fundamental therapy for hydrocephalus. Internal devices comprise a proximal portion that is typically placed in the ventricles and a distal portion that can be placed in the peritoneal, pleural, or vascular space (atrium).[85] The reported incidence of shunt infection varies from 1% to 18%.[86] Risk factors for CSF shunt infection include intraventricular or subarachnoid hemorrhage, depressed cranial fracture, CSF leak, duration of catheterization, systemic infection, and catheter manipulation or irrigation.[85,87] Infection of CSF shunts is most commonly caused by CoNS species, followed by *S aureus* and *Propionibacterium acnes*.[88] However, some recent studies reported that gram-negative organisms are the leading cause of infection of CSF shunts.[87]

Patients with CSF shunt infection usually present with nausea, headache, fever, altered mental status, or lethargy. Patients can develop peritonitis or pleuritis if the infection involves the distal portion of the shunt. Bacteremia can be detected up to 80% to 90% of patients with ventriculoatrial shunts but it is rarely seen in patients with ventriculoperitoneal shunts.[85,88] The CDC/National Healthcare Safety Network (NHSN) definition of hospital-acquired meningitis/ventriculitis is presented in **Box 1**.[89]

Antibiotic administration before central nervous system (CNS) shunt placement has been shown to decrease the risk of shunt infection.[85] One meta-analysis showed a possible benefit of antibiotic-impregnated catheters in preventing CSF shunt infection.[90]

Recommended management of CSF shunt infection preferably comprises a 2-stage shunt replacement (including a temporary insertion of an external drainage ventriculostomy catheter followed by insertion of a new CSF shunt) plus intravenous antibiotics.[88] In patients with suspected CSF shunt infection, empiric antibiotic treatment should be started after obtaining blood cultures and CSF studies. Empiric use of vancomycin plus antipseudomonal cephalosporin or carbapenem is an appropriate first-line regimen. Antibiotics should be adjusted subsequently based on the results of relevant cultures.[85]

Intraventricular antibiotics are considered for infections caused by organisms sensitive only to drugs with poor CSF penetration or when the infected shunt remains in place.[91] Patients with rifampin-susceptible CoNS species and P acnes shunt infections can be managed conservatively using intravenous antibiotics plus oral rifampin without the need of shunt removal.[88] If the infection is caused by CoNS species or P acnes, the shunt can be reimplanted after 3 days of antibiotics (if the CSF white cell count, protein and glucose values are normal) or even after 7 days (if any of these CSF parameters is abnormal). In contrast, for infections caused by S aureus or gram-negative organisms, shunt reimplantation can be performed after 10 to 14 days of antimicrobial therapy.[85,87]

Prosthetic Joints

More than 600,000 of primary hip and knee arthroplasty and around 70,000 joint revisions were performed in the United States in 2003, and the number is expected to exceed 4 million procedures by 2026.[92] Risk factors for prosthetic joint infection (PJI) include prolonged surgery, postoperative bleeding, previous PJI, concurrent infection at the time of surgery, steroid use, malignancy, rheumatoid arthritis, diabetes, psoriasis, and obesity.[93]

Box 1
Diagnosis of CSF shunt infections

The diagnosis requires 1 of the 2 following criteria:

1. Positive CSF culture

2. Clinical and laboratory evidence of ventriculitis (requires all of the following):

   a. Presence of fever (>38.0°C), headache, neck stiffness, meningeal signs, cranial nerve signs, or irritability

   b. No other recognized cause

   c. Increased CSF white cells or protein, decreased glucose, presence of organisms on CSF Gram stain, positive blood culture, positive antigen from blood, CSF, or urine, increased IgM titer or 4-fold increase in paired sera IgG for a pathogen

   d. Physician prescribing antibiotics (if the diagnosis is made antemortum)

Data from Horan TC, Andrus M, Dudeck MA. CDC/NHSN surveillance definition of health care-associated infection and criteria for specific types of infections in the acute care setting. Am J Infect Control 2008;36:309–32.

Like infections caused by all other types of devices, biofilm formation plays an essential role in the pathogenesis of PJI. S aureus and CoNS species are responsible for more than half of PJIs, followed by gram-negative bacteria, streptococci, anaerobes, Enterococci, and fungi.[94,95]

Early-onset infections (<3 months) usually manifest with fever, surgical site erythema, wound drainage, joint pain, or joint effusion. Patients with delayed-onset (3–24 months) or late-onset (>24 months) infection are more likely to present with chronic pain without other symptoms.[93] Increased white blood cell count, erythrocyte sedimentation rate, and CRP as well as the imaging findings of plain radiographs, arthrography, magnetic resonance imaging, radioisotopic scans, and PET scans can help establish the diagnosis of PJI.[93,95]

The joint fluid can be aspirated or intraoperative tissue frozen section can be performed when the diagnosis of PJI is unclear. Increased white blood cell (WBC) count in the aspiration fluid (>4200 cells/mm^3), positive culture of aspiration fluid or tissue, and pathologic evidence of inflammation of periprosthetic tissue can confirm the diagnosis of PJI.[94,95] One study indicated that a sonicate culture of the joint fluid is more sensitive than culture of the periprosthetic tissue (75% vs 45%, P<.001).[96]

Antibiotic prophylaxis before prosthesis insertion is an effective method in preventing PJI. Implantation of antibiotic-impregnated cement and the use of filtered laminal airflow system were shown to further decrease the risk of PJI.[95]

Management of PJI requires total removal of the hardware and administration of intravenous antibiotics. In patients who are not septic, antibiotics should be delayed until surgical specimens are collected for microbiologic analysis. A 2-stage surgical replacement is the preferred approach for management of PJI because it has the highest success rate in terms of cure (90%–97%) and functional outcome.[94,95] After completing the 6-week course of preferably intravenous antibiotic therapy, reimplantation is usually performed weeks to months while off antibiotics and having almost normal inflammatory markers.[94,95] In 1 study of patients treated with a 2-stage approach, a vancomycin-loaded spacer was found to be superior to no spacer.[97]

A 1-stage approach, more commonly performed in Europe than in the United States, is often used in older patients and for less virulent infections caused by organisms other than S aureus or gram-negative bacteria.[95] Explanting the hardware and implanting a new prosthesis with an antibiotic-loaded methylmethacrylate cement during the 1-stage approach has an 80% success rate.[98,99] Debridement with retention of device (DRD) can be used in selected cases, including early-onset infections, shorter duration of symptoms, and infections caused by less virulent organisms for which oral antibiotics are available. The DRD approach is not preferred in cases of S aureus or multidrug resistant organisms and is not recommended in patients with unstable prosthesis, sinus tract, or abscesses.

Suppressive antibiotics should be continued for at least 3 to 6 months when infected implants are not completely removed.[93] Rifampin has good biofilm penetration and it should be included in the suppressive regimen whenever possible.[100]

REFERENCES

1. American College of Chest Physicians/Society of Critical Care Medicine Consensus Conference: definitions for sepsis and organ failure and guidelines for the use of innovative therapies in sepsis. Crit Care Med 1992;20:864–74.
2. Levy MM, Fink MP, Marshall JC, et al. 2001 SCCM/ESICM/ACCP/ATS/SIS International Sepsis Definitions Conference. Crit Care Med 2003;31:1250–6.

3. Zhao H, Heard SO, Mullen MT, et al. An evaluation of the diagnostic accuracy of the 1991 American College of Chest Physicians/Society of Critical Care Medicine and the 2001 Society of Critical Care Medicine/European Society of Intensive Care Medicine/American College of Chest Physicians/American Thoracic Society/Surgical Infection Society sepsis definition. Crit Care Med 2012;40:1700–6.

4. Klein Klouwenberg PM, Ong DS, Bonten MJ, et al. Classification of sepsis, severe sepsis and septic shock: the impact of minor variations in data capture and definition of SIRS criteria. Intensive Care Med 2012;38:811–9.

5. Martin GS, Mannino DM, Eaton S, et al. The epidemiology of sepsis in the United States from 1979 through 2000. N Engl J Med 2003;348:1546–54.

6. Sands KE, Bates DW, Lanken PN, et al. Epidemiology of sepsis syndrome in 8 academic medical centers. JAMA 1997;278:234–40.

7. Danai P, Martin GS. Epidemiology of sepsis: recent advances. Curr Infect Dis Rep 2005;7:329–34.

8. Danai PA, Sinha S, Moss M, et al. Seasonal variation in the epidemiology of sepsis. Crit Care Med 2007;35:410–5.

9. Dombrovskiy VY, Martin AA, Sunderram J, et al. Rapid increase in hospitalization and mortality rates for severe sepsis in the United States: a trend analysis from 1993 to 2003. Crit Care Med 2007;35:1244–50.

10. Rangel-Frausto MS, Pittet D, Costigan M, et al. The natural history of the systemic inflammatory response syndrome (SIRS). A prospective study. JAMA 1995;273:117–23.

11. Angus DC, Linde-Zwirble WT, Lidicker J, et al. Epidemiology of severe sepsis in the United States: analysis of incidence, outcome, and associated costs of care. Crit Care Med 2001;29:1303–10.

12. Stearns-Kurosawa DJ, Osuchowski MF, Valentine C, et al. The pathogenesis of sepsis. Annu Rev Pathol 2011;6:19–48.

13. Cinel I, Dellinger RP. Advances in pathogenesis and management of sepsis. Curr Opin Infect Dis 2007;20:345–52.

14. Huttunen R, Aittoniemi J. New concepts in the pathogenesis, diagnosis and treatment of bacteremia and sepsis. J Infect 2011;63:407–19.

15. Vincent JL, Zhang H, Szabo C, et al. Effects of nitric oxide in septic shock. Am J Respir Crit Care Med 2000;16:1781–5.

16. Landry DW, Levin HR, Gallant EM, et al. Vasopressin deficiency contributes to the vasodilation of septic shock. Circulation 1997;95:1122–5.

17. Price S, Anning PB, Mitchell JA, et al. Myocardial dysfunction in sepsis: mechanisms and therapeutic implications. Eur Heart J 1999;20:715–24.

18. Astiz ME, DeGent GE, Lin RY, et al. Microvascular function and rheologic changes in hyperdynamic sepsis. Crit Care Med 1995;23:265–71.

19. Aird WC. The role of the endothelium in severe sepsis and multiple organ dysfunction syndrome. Blood 2003;101:3765–77.

20. Luce JM. Pathogenesis and management of septic shock. Chest 1987;91:883–8.

21. Annane D, Bellissant E, Cavaillon JM. Septic shock. Lancet 2005;365:63–78.

22. Hassoun HT, Kone BC, Mercer DW, et al. Post-injury multiple organ failure: the role of the gut. Shock 2001;15:1–10.

23. Russell JA. Management of sepsis. N Engl J Med 2006;355:1699–713.

24. Lodes U, Bohmeier B, Lippert H, et al. PCR-based rapid sepsis diagnosis effectively guides clinical treatment in patients with new onset of SIRS. Langenbecks Arch Surg 2012;397:447–55.

25. Kudo M, Matsuo Y, Nakasendo A, et al. Potential clinical benefit of the in situ hybridization method for the diagnosis of sepsis. J Infect Chemother 2009;15:23–6.

26. Clec'h C, Fosse JP, Karoubi P, et al. Differential diagnostic value of procalcitonin in surgical and medical patients with septic shock. Crit Care Med 2006;34: 102–7.

27. Tang BM, Eslick GD, Craig JC, et al. Accuracy of procalcitonin for sepsis diagnosis in critically ill patients: systematic review and meta-analysis. Lancet Infect Dis 2007;7:210–7.

28. Schuetz P, Chiappa V, Briel M, et al. Procalcitonin algorithms for antibiotic therapy decisions: a systematic review of randomized controlled trials and recommendations for clinical algorithms. Arch Intern Med 2011;171: 1322–31.

29. Gibot S, Béné MC, Noel R, et al. Combination biomarkers to diagnose sepsis in the critically ill patient. Am J Respir Crit Care Med 2012;186:65–71.

30. Kiehntopf M, Schmerler D, Brunkhorst FM, et al. Mass spectometry-based protein patterns in the diagnosis of sepsis/systemic inflammatory response syndrome. Shock 2011;36:560–9.

31. Dellinger RP, Levy MM, Carlet JM, et al. Surviving Sepsis Campaign: international guidelines for management of severe sepsis and septic shock: 2008. Crit Care Med 2008;36:296–327.

32. Gaieski DF, Mikkelsen ME, Band RA, et al. Impact of time to antibiotics on survival in patients with severe sepsis or septic shock in whom early goal-directed therapy was initiated in the emergency department. Crit Care Med 2010;38:1045–53.

33. Garnacho-Montero J, Garcia-Garmendia JL, Barrero-Almodovar A, et al. Impact of adequate empirical antibiotic therapy on the outcome of patients admitted to the intensive care unit with sepsis. Crit Care Med 2003;31:2742–51.

34. Kumar A, Ellis P, Arabi Y, et al. Initiation of inappropriate antimicrobial therapy results in a fivefold reduction of survival in human septic shock. Chest 2009; 136:1237–48.

35. Grossi P, Gasperina DD. Antimicrobial treatment of sepsis. Surg Infect (Larchmt) 2006;7(Suppl 2):S87–91.

36. Traugott KA, Echevarria K, Maxwell P, et al. Monotherapy or combination therapy? The *Pseudomonas aeruginosa* conundrum. Pharmacotherapy 2011; 31:598–608.

37. Brunkhorst FM, Oppert M, Marx G, et al. Effect of empirical treatment with moxifloxacin and meropenem vs meropenem on sepsis-related organ dysfunction in patients with severe sepsis: a randomized trial. JAMA 2012;13(307):2390–9.

38. Safdar N, Handelsman J, Maki DG. Does combination antimicrobial therapy reduce mortality in gram negative bacteraemia? Lancet Infect Dis 2004;4: 519–27.

39. Paul M, Benuri-Silbiger I, Soares-Weiser K, et al. Beta lactam monotherapy versus beta lactam-aminoglycoside combination therapy for sepsis in immunocompetent patients. BMJ 2004;328:668.

40. Kumar A, Safdar N, Kethireddy S, et al. A survival benefit of combination antibiotic therapy for serious infections associated with sepsis and septic shock is contingent only on the risk of death. Crit Care Med 2010;38:1651–64.

41. Kumar A, Zarychanski R, Light B, et al. Early combination antibiotic therapy yields improved survival compared with monotherapy in septic shock. Crit Care Med 2010;38:1773–85.

42. Seder CW, Villalba MR Jr, Robbins J, et al. Early colectomy may be associated with improved survival in fulminant *Clostridium difficile* colitis: an 8-year experience. Am J Surg 2009;197:302–7.

43. FDA Drug Safety Communication: Voluntary Market Withdrawal of Xigris [Drotre-cogin alfa (activated)] due to failure to show a survival benefit. Available at: http://www.fda.gov/Drugs/DrugSafety/ucm277114.htm. Accessed October 25, 2011.

44. Centers for Disease Control and Prevention (CDC). Vital signs: central line-associated blood stream infections–United States, 2001, 2008, and 2009. MMWR Morb Mortal Wkly Rep 2011;60:243–8.

45. Renaud B, Brun-Buisson C. Outcomes of primary and catheter-related bacter-emia: a cohort and case-control study in critically ill patients. Am J Respir Crit Care Med 2001;163:1584–90.

46. Dimick JB, Pelz RK, Consunji R, et al. Increased resource use associated with catheter-related bloodstream infection in the surgical intensive care unit. Arch Surg 2001;136:229–34.

47. Tokars JI, Cookson ST, McArthur MA, et al. Prospective evaluation of risk factors for bloodstream infection in patients receiving home infusion therapy. Ann Intern Med 1999;131:340–7.

48. Beekmann SE, Henderson DK. Infections caused by percutaneous intravascular devices. In: Mandell GL, Bennett JE, Dolin R, editors. Mandell, Douglas and Bennett's principles and practice of infectious diseases, vol. 2, 7th edition. Phil-adelphia: Elsevier; 2010. p. 3697–715.

49. Wisplinghoff H, Bischoff T, Tallent SM, et al. Nosocomial bloodstream infections in US hospitals: analysis of 24,179 cases from a prospective nationwide surveil-lance study. Clin Infect Dis 2004;39:309–17.

50. Garland JS, Alex CP, Sevallius JM, et al. Cohort study of the pathogenesis and molecular epidemiology of catheter-related bloodstream infection in neonates with peripherally inserted central venous catheters. Infect Control Hosp Epide-miol 2008;29:243–9.

51. Safdar N, Fine JP, Maki DG. Meta-analysis: methods for diagnosing intra-vascular device-related bloodstream infection. Ann Intern Med 2005;142: 451–66.

52. Mermel LA, Allon M, Bouza E, et al. Clinical practice guidelines for the diagnosis and management of intravascular catheter-related infection: 2009 Update by the Infectious Diseases Society of America. Clin Infect Dis 2009;49:1–45.

53. Warwick S, Wilks M, Hennessy E, et al. Use of quantitative 16S ribosomal DNA detection for diagnosis of central vascular catheter-associated bacterial infec-tion. J Clin Microbiol 2004;42:1402–8.

54. O'Grady NP, Alexander M, Burns LA, et al. Guidelines for the prevention of intra-vascular catheter-related infections. Clin Infect Dis 2011;52:e162–93.

55. Uldall PR, Merchant N, Woods F, et al. Changing subclavian haemodialysis cannulas to reduce infection. Lancet 1981;1:1373.

56. Safdar N, Maki DG. Use of vancomycin-containing lock or flush solutions for prevention of bloodstream infection associated with central venous access devices: a meta-analysis of prospective, randomized trials. Clin Infect Dis 2006;43:474–84.

57. Snaterse M, Rüger W, Scholte Op Reimer WJ, et al. Antibiotic-based catheter lock solutions for prevention of catheter-related bloodstream infection: a system-atic review of randomised controlled trials. J Hosp Infect 2010;75:1–11.

58. Raad I, Darouiche R, Dupuis J, et al. Central venous catheters coated with min-ocycline and rifampin for the prevention of catheter-related colonization and bloodstream infections. A randomized, double-blind trial. The Texas Medical Center Catheter Study Group. Ann Intern Med 1997;127:267–74.

59. Marciante KD, Veenstra DL, Lipsky BA, et al. Which antimicrobial impregnated central venous catheter should we use? Modeling the costs and outcomes of antimicrobial catheter use. Am J Infect Control 2003;31:1–8.

60. Darouiche RO, Raad II, Heard SO, et al. A comparison of two antimicrobial-impregnated central venous catheters. Catheter Study Group. N Engl J Med 1999;340:1–8.

61. Ramritu P, Halton K, Collignon P, et al. A systematic review comparing the relative effectiveness of antimicrobial-coated catheters in intensive care units. Am J Infect Control 2008;36:104–17.

62. Wilcox MH, Tack KJ, Bouza E, et al. Complicated skin and skin-structure infections and catheter-related bloodstream infections: noninferiority of linezolid in a phase 3 study. Clin Infect Dis 2009;48:203–12.

63. Blot S, Janssens R, Claeys G, et al. Effect of fluconazole consumption on long-term trends in candidal ecology. J Antimicrob Chemother 2006;58:474–7.

64. Spellberg BJ, Filler SG, Edwards JE Jr. Current treatment strategies for disseminated candidiasis. Clin Infect Dis 2006;42:244–51.

65. Kim EY, Saunders P, Yousefzadeh N. Usefulness of anti-infective lock solutions for catheter-related bloodstream infections. Mt Sinai J Med 2010;77:549–58.

66. O'Horo JC, Silva GL, Safdar N. Anti-infective locks for treatment of central line-associated bloodstream infection: a systematic review and meta-analysis. Am J Nephrol 2011;34:415–22.

67. Chaftari AM, Hachem R, Mulanovich V. Efficacy and safety of daptomycin in the treatment of Gram-positive catheter-related bloodstream infections in cancer patients. Int J Antimicrob Agents 2010;36:182–6.

68. Carlisle EJ, Blake P, McCarthy F, et al. Septicemia in long-term jugular hemodialysis catheters; eradicating infection by changing the catheter over a guidewire. Int J Artif Organs 1991;14:150–3.

69. Chaftari AM, Kassis C, El Issa H, et al. Novel approach using antimicrobial catheters to improve the management of central line-associated bloodstream infections in cancer patients. Cancer 2011;117(11):2551–8.

70. Darouiche RO. Treatment of infections associated with surgical implants. N Engl J Med 2004;350:1422–9.

71. Costerton JW, Stewart PS, Greenberg EP. Bacterial biofilms: a common cause of persistent infections. Science 1999;284:1318–22.

72. Cabell C, Heidenreich P, Chu V, et al. Increasing rates of cardiac device infections among Medicare beneficiaries: 1990–1999. Am Heart J 2004;147:582–6.

73. Zhan C, Baine WB, Sedrakyan A, et al. Cardiac device implantation in the United States from 1997 through 2004: a population-based analysis. J Gen Intern Med 2008;23(Suppl 1):13–9.

74. Mond HG, Irwin M, Morillo C, et al. The world survey of cardiac pacing and cardioverter defibrillators: calendar year 2001. Pacing Clin Electrophysiol 2004;27:955–64.

75. Baddour LM, Epstein AE, Erickson CC, et al. Update on cardiovascular implantable electronic device infections and their management: a scientific statement from the American Heart Association. Circulation 2010;121:458–77.

76. Sohail MR, Ulsan DZ, Khan AH, et al. Management and outcome of permanent pacemaker and implantable cardioverter-defibrillator infections. J Am Coll Cardiol 2007;49:1851–9.

77. Sohail MR, Wilson WR, Baddour LM. Infections of nonvalvular cardiovascular devices. In: Mandell GL, Bennett JE, Dolin R, editors. Mandell, Douglas and

Bennett's principles and practice of infectious diseases, vol. 1, 7th edition. Philadelphia: Elsevier; 2010. p. 1127–42.

78. de Oliveira JC, Martinelli M, Nishioka SA, et al. Efficacy of antibiotic prophylaxis before the implantation of pacemakers and cardioverter-defibrillators: results of a large, prospective, randomized, double-blinded, placebo-controlled trial. Circ Arrhythm Electrophysiol 2009;2:29–34.

79. Gandhi T, Crawford T, Riddell J 4th. Cardiovascular implantable electronic device associated infections. Infect Dis Clin North Am 2012;26:57–76.

80. Bloom HL, Constantin L, Dan D, et al. Implantation success and infection in cardiovascular implantable electronic device procedures utilizing an antibacterial envelope. Pacing Clin Electrophysiol 2011;34:133–42.

81. Howarth DM, Curteis PG, Gibson S. Infected cardiac pacemaker wires demonstrated by Tc-99m labeled white blood cell scintigraphy. Clin Nucl Med 1998;23:74–6.

82. Sarrazin JF, Philippon F, Tessier M, et al. Usefulness of fluorine-18 positron emission tomography/computed tomography for identification of cardiovascular implantable electronic device infections. J Am Coll Cardiol 2012;59:1616–25.

83. Durante-Mangoni E, Casillo R, Bernardo M, et al. High-dose daptomycin for cardiac implantable electronic device-related infective endocarditis. Clin Infect Dis 2012;54:347–54.

84. Baddour LM, Infectious Diseases Society of America's Emerging Infections Network. Long-term suppressive antimicrobial therapy for intravascular device-related infections. Am J Med Sci 2001;322:209–12.

85. Tunkel AR, Drake JM. Cerebrospinal fluid shunt infections. In: Mandell GL, Bennett JE, Dolin R, editors. Mandell, Douglas and Bennett's principles and practice of infectious diseases, vol. 1, 7th edition. Philadelphia: Elsevier; 2010. p. 1231–6.

86. von der Brelie C, Simon A, Gröner A, et al. Evaluation of an institutional guideline for the treatment of cerebrospinal fluid shunt-associated infections. Acta Neurochir (Wien) 2012;154(9):1691–7.

87. Stenehjem E, Armstrong WS. Central nervous system device infections. Infect Dis Clin North Am 2012;26:89–110.

88. Conen A, Walti LN, Merlo A, et al. Characteristics and treatment outcome of cerebrospinal fluid shunt-associated infections in adults: a retrospective analysis over an 11-year period. Clin Infect Dis 2008;47:73–82.

89. Horan TC, Andrus M, Dudeck MA. CDC/NHSN surveillance definition of health care-associated infection and criteria for specific types of infections in the acute care setting. Am J Infect Control 2008;36:309–32.

90. Thomas R, Lee S, Patole S, et al. Antibiotic-impregnated catheters for the prevention of CSF shunt infections: a systematic review and meta-analysis. Br J Neurosurg 2012;26:175–84.

91. Wen DY, Bottini AG, Hall WA, et al. The intraventricular use of antibiotics. Neurosurg Clin N Am 1992;3:343–54.

92. Kurtz S, Ong K, Lau E, et al. Projections of primary and revision hip and knee arthroplasty in the United States from 2005 to 2030. J Bone Joint Surg Am 2007;89:780–5.

93. Shuman EK, Urquhart A, Malani PN. Management and prevention of prosthetic joint infection. Infect Dis Clin North Am 2012;26:29–39.

94. Del Pozo JL, Patel R. Clinical practice. Infection associated with prosthetic joints. N Engl J Med 2009;361:787–94.

95. Brause BD. Infections with prosthesis in bones and joints. In: Mandell GL, Bennett JE, Dolin R, editors. Mandell, Douglas and Bennett's principles and

practice of infectious diseases, vol. 1, 7th edition. Philadelphia: Elsevier; 2010. p. 1469–74.

96. Trampuz A, Piper KE, Jacobson MJ, et al. Sonication of removed hip and knee prostheses for diagnosis of infection. N Engl J Med 2007;357:654–63.

97. Cabrita HB, Croci AT, Camargo OP, et al. Prospective study of the treatment of infected hip arthroplasties with or without the use of an antibiotic-loaded cement spacer. Clinics (Sao Paulo) 2007;62:99–108.

98. Hanssen AD, Rand JA. Evaluation and treatment of infection at the site of a total hip or knee arthroplasty. J Bone Joint Surg Am 1998;80:910–22.

99. Jackson WO, Schmalzried TP. Limited role of direct exchange arthroplasty in the treatment of infected total hip replacements. Clin Orthop 2000;381:101–5.

100. Zimmerli W, Widmer AF, Blatter M, et al. Foreign-Body Infection (FBI) Study Group. Role of rifampin for treatment of orthopedic implant-related staphylococcal infections: a randomized controlled trial. JAMA 1998;279:1537–41.

Infectious Disease Emergencies in Returning Travelers
Special Reference to Malaria, Dengue Fever, and Chikungunya

Chand Wattal, BSc, MBBS, MD*, Neeraj Goel, MBBS, MD

KEYWORDS

- Returning traveler • Dengue • Malaria • Chikungunya • Fever • Break bone fever
- *P knowlesi*

KEY POINTS

- *Plasmodium falciparum* malaria in returning, nonimmune travelers can be a medical emergency.
- Dengue hemorrhagic fever (DHF)/dengue shock syndrome (DSS) occurs mostly in secondary dengue infections and carries a high mortality rate if not diagnosed early and treated expeditiously.
- Detection of nonstructural protein (NS) 1 antigen in serum/blood can be a useful tool for early diagnosis (within the first week of fever) of dengue infection.
- Chikungunya is an essential differential diagnosis for dengue fever (DF) in travelers returning from endemic zones.
- Because no effective vaccine is available for the most common systemic infections in returning travelers, such as malaria, dengue, and chikungunya, pretravel advice, adequate prophylaxis, and prevention of mosquito bite remain the only effective tools in preventing these infections.

INTRODUCTION

The twenty-first century has enabled people to crisscross the globe at an enormous speed, whether trade or curiosity about the planet takes them to various parts of the world. We live in a world of microbes, so likewise the various demographic diseases of the continents have caught up with the travelers going back to their destinations. An estimated more than 800 million travelers worldwide cross international

Funding sources: Nil. Conflict of interest: Nil.
Department of Clinical Microbiology and Immunology, Sir Ganga Ram Hospital, Rajinder Nagar, New Delhi 110060, India
* Corresponding author.
E-mail address: chandwattal@gmail.com

boundaries each year.[1] Whether associated with tourism, humanitarian efforts, globalization of industry, or migrant work, studies suggest only a small number of travelers seek pretravel health advice. In addition, the composition of those traveling continues to become more diverse and medically complex, creating a vastly different perspective on travel-associated medical concerns, preparations, and required medical knowledge.[2] Recent establishment of collaborative sentinel surveillance networks created specifically to monitor disease trends among travelers offers new insight for evaluating travel health issues. These networks can help pretravel and post-travel patient management by providing complementary surveillance information, facilitating communication and collaboration between participating network sites, and enabling new analytical options for travel-related research. Annually, Americans make more than 300 million trips to other countries. An increasing number of these trips are to developing countries, and 30% to 60% of these travelers, estimated at more than 10 million people, become ill as a result of their travel.[3,4]

In a GeoSentinel Surveillance Network report on fever in returned travelers from different destinations spread across 6 continents during the period 1997 to 2006, febrile illness was reported in 28% of travelers as a chief complaint. The most common causes of fever were systemic illness (35%), diarrheal disease (15%), and respiratory illness (14%). Malaria was the most common cause of systemic febrile illness (21%), followed by dengue (6%). Other less common specific causes of systemic fever included enteric fever (2%) and rickettsioses (2%) (**Table 1**).[5]

Although fever in a returning traveler may be benign and due to a self-limiting infection, it must initially be considered a medical emergency. For arriving at a possible diagnosis of fever in returning traveler, a comprehensive history that details places of visit, duration, purpose, activities undertaken, and any medical exposure abroad or chemoprophylaxis taken along with physical examination is essential for initial work-up. Knowledge of incubation period (**Table 2**) and disease risk by geographic area helps in making a differential diagnosis.[6] Systemic febrile illness is most commonly noted in visitors traveling to sub-Saharan Africa and Southeast Asia.[5,7] In systemic febrile illness, malaria is most commonly reported among travelers from Oceania and sub-Saharan Africa and dengue predominates among travelers from Southeast Asia.[5] Acute diarrheal illness is more common in travelers from South Central Asia and dermatologic disorders are reported in a high proportion of travelers

Table 1 Top 5 illnesses in returning travelers	
Diagnosis	**%**
1. Systemic illnesses	35
Malaria	21
Malaria due to *P falciparum*	14
Malaria due to *P vivax*	6
Malaria due to other species	2
Dengue	6
Salmonella enterica serovar Typhi or Paratyphi infection	2
Rickettsia	2
2. Acute diarrhea	15
3. Respiratory illness	14
4. Genitourinary diseases	4
5. Gastrointestinal illnesses (other than diarrhea)	4

Table 2
Incubation periods for diseases

Incubation Period	Diseases
<7 Days	Common: malaria, traveler's diarrhea, dengue, enteric fever, respiratory tract infection Others: rickettsioses, leptospirosis, meningitis, yellow fever, arbovirus, meningococcal
7–21 Days	Common: malaria, enteric fever Others: rickettsioses, viral hepatitis, leptospirosis, HIV, Q fever, brucellosis, African trypanosomiasis
>21 Days	Common: malaria, enteric fever Others: tuberculosis, hepatitis B virus, bacterial endocarditis, HIV, Q fever, brucellosis, amebic liver disease, melioidosis

from sub-Saharan Africa and South Central Asia.[7] Based on this knowledge, comprehensive but judicious laboratory investigations should further help in confirmation of preliminary diagnosis in most of the cases.

There are several life-threatening illnesses that a traveler can acquire but this article discusses only malaria, dengue, and chikungunya, all 3 of which are caused by mosquito bites and, if left undetected or unsuspected, could be life threatening in travelers returning home. Because these diseases are not commonly seen in places far away from endemic areas, they are likely to be ignored or missed by a physician attending to a patient in an emergency department. Much of the illness encountered could be reduced, however, with adequate pretravel education and preparation.

MALARIA
Introduction

Malaria is caused by a protozoan parasite of the genus *Plasmodium* infecting red blood cells and is transmitted to humans by bite of a female anopheline mosquito. The 4 *Plasmodium* species that infect humans are *P falciparum*, *P vivax*, *P ovale*, and *P malariae*. Malaria is a life-threatening illness, caused by the asexual form of the parasitic protozoan *Plasmodium*. The clinical manifestations of malaria vary with geography, epidemiology, immunity, and age. It is an entirely preventable and treatable disease, provided that currently recommended interventions are properly implemented. The 2 most common species of malaria parasite that cause disease across the world are *P falciparum* and *P vivax*.[8] *P vivax* and *P ovale* have the ability to stay dormant or persist in the liver as hypnozoites. These hypnozoites can result in relapse of infection weeks to months after the primary infection. Recrudescence results from a failure to eliminate the parasites, which may occur within days or weeks. This could be due to either failure of the immune system or incomplete therapy, which commonly occurs in *P falciparum* but can happen in all the species of plasmodium.

Epidemiology

An estimated 216 million clinical cases and 655,000 deaths due to malaria were reported in 2010, mostly in children aged less than 5 years living in sub-Saharan Africa.[8] It is estimated that approximately half of the world's population in 100 countries live in areas where malaria is transmitted.[9] Malaria is prevalent in regions of Africa, Asia, the Middle East, Eastern Europe, Central and South America, the Caribbean, and Oceania.[9] The major burden of malarial disease lies in Africa (81%) followed by Southeast Asia (13%) and the Eastern Mediterranean regions (5%).[8]

As for the geographic distribution of specific *Plasmodium* species, falciparum malaria predominates in sub-Saharan Africa and vivax malaria in the Indian subcontinent, Mexico, Central America, and China; both species occur in Southeast Asia and South America. *P malariae* is prevalent at low levels in nearly all malaria endemic areas of the world, and *P ovale* has limited distribution in Africa, New Guinea, and the Philippines.[10]

Malaria in developed and nonendemic countries is mostly imported. A malaria surveillance program in the United States in 2010 showed that among the total 1691 cases reported to Centers for Disease Control and Prevention (CDC), 1688 were classified as imported, 1 was transfusion related, and 2 were cryptic cases. Of these, *P falciparum* was the leading cause of malaria (58.1%), followed by *P vivax* (19.2%), *P malariae* (2.1%), and *P ovale* (1.9%). Of the total imported cases in the United States, 65% were acquired in Africa, 19% in Asia, 15% in the Americas, and 0.3% in Oceania.[9] Travelers who are visiting friends and relatives are at higher risk of malaria compared with other travelers, due to their longer stays, higher-risk destinations, inadequate use of chemoprophylaxis, fewer personal protection measures, and belief that they are already immune.[5]

Clinical Features

Patients remain asymptomatic from the time of the original mosquito bite until approximately a week later. The typical incubation period usually varies between 8 and 17 days for *P falciparum, P vivax,* and *P ovale* and 18 to 40 days for *P malariae*.[11] Therefore, febrile patients presenting within 7 days of entering an endemic area are unlikely to have malaria. The initial symptoms of malaria are nonspecific and similar to the symptoms of a minor systemic viral illness, such as fever, headache, fatigue, muscle and joint pain, nausea, and vomiting. Fever is the common chief complaint in malaria and is present in 78% to 100% of patients.[12] Fever is often characterized by the classic malaria paroxysm of chills and rigors, followed by fever spikes, followed by profuse sweating and fatigue.[13] Paroxysms coincide with the synchronous rupture of blood schizonts and liberation of metabolic waste by-products into the bloodstream. Paroxysms can occur in 48-hour cycles (tertian malaria) in *P falciparum, P vivax,* and *P ovale* infections and 72-hour cycles (quartan malaria) in *P malariae*.[13] Although cyclic paroxysms are suggestive of malaria, they may not be discerned in all cases, especially in early stages of fever.[11] Uncomplicated malaria is defined as a symptomatic malaria characterized by the absence of clinical or laboratory signs of vital organ dysfunction and, therefore, suspected clinically mostly on the basis of fever or nonspecific symptoms. Physical findings may show enlarged spleen/liver, mild jaundice, and increased respiratory rate. Severe malaria or complicated malaria is generally defined as acute malaria with high levels of parasitemia (>5%) and/or major signs of organ dysfunction[10] (listed in **Box 1**). Physical findings may include pallor, petechiae, jaundice, hepatomegaly, and/or splenomegaly. Severe malaria is a life-threatening illness—a high case fatality rate, typically 10% to 20%, is seen in cases receiving treatment—and is fatal in the majority of untreated cases.[10]

The pathogenesis of clinical findings seen in severe malaria essentially involves sequestration of erythrocytes that contain mature forms of the parasite in the deep vascular beds of vital organs. This sequestration is promoted by several processes: the adherence of infected erythrocytes to endothelial cells, rosetting—the binding of infected erythrocytes to noninfected erythrocytes, reduced red cell deformability, and platelet-mediated clumping of infected erythrocytes.[13] This results in causing small infarcts, capillary leakage, and organ dysfunction, producing cerebral malaria, renal failure, hepatic dysfunction, or acute respiratory distress syndrome. Severe

---

Box 1
Clinical features of severe malaria

- Impaired consciousness/coma
- Prostration or sit up with assistance
- Failure to accept feed
- Multiple convulsions—more than 2 episodes in 24 h
- Deep breathing, respiratory distress (acidotic breathing)
- Circulatory collapse/shock, systolic blood pressure <70 mm Hg in adults and <50 mm Hg in children
- Jaundice
- Hemoglobinuria
- Abnormal spontaneous bleeding
- Acute renal failure
- Pulmonary edema (radiologic)

---

anemia and thrombocytopenia that causes bleeding diathesis is produced by hemolysis, reduced cell deformity of parasitized and nonparasitized erythrocytes, increased splenic clearance, reduction of platelet survival, decreased platelet production, and increased splenic uptake of platelets.

Uncomplicated malaria is seen more often with *P vivax, P ovale*, and *P malariae*, whereas *P falciparum* is more commonly associated with severe malaria.[9] *P vivax* is usually considered benign but can be associated with debilitating illness with serious complications.[14,15] In a systematic review on clinical presentation of *P vivax*, a wide spectrum of clinical complications commonly associated with *P falciparum* were observed in *P vivax*, including severe anemia, thrombocytopenia, coagulation disorders, acute respiratory distress syndrome, acute renal failure, and jaundice.[16] *P ovale* and *P malariae* mainly present as uncomplicated malaria. *P ovale* presents with less severe course and usually tends to relapse less frequently compared with *P vivax*.[11] *P malariae* is often characterized by low parasitemia difficult to detect by microscopy.[13] Patients with *P malariae* infection may have a long latency period of many years before presenting with fevers, malaise, and splenomegaly.[13] Patients may experience a spontaneous recovery, or there may be series of recrudescence over many years (>50 years).[11] Chronic infection with *P malariae* may result in proteinuria and may be associated with nephrotic syndrome in young children living in endemic areas. Nephrotic syndrome is caused by immune complex–mediated glomerulonephritis. Nonimmune travelers are at high risk for progression to severe disease, especially if infected with *P falciparum*. For this reason, it is important to consider malaria in the differential diagnosis of all febrile patients with a history of travel to malaria endemic areas.

Diagnosis of Malaria

Clinicians should have high index of suspicion for malaria in travelers presenting with fever and history of travel to malaria endemic regions within the past 1 year and especially in the past 3 months. Apart from fever, patients usually present with nonspecific clinical features in uncomplicated malaria. If the diagnosis of falciparum malaria has been delayed, an apparently well-looking patient may rapidly deteriorate and present with jaundice, confusion, or seizures with high fatality rates. Therefore, accurate and rapid laboratory diagnosis of malaria is essential for proper clinical management of patients. During work-up, malaria should not be ruled out in febrile patients who give history of prophylaxis, because approximately 10% of the travelers can develop P falciparum malaria, in spite of having taken effective chemoprophylaxis.[17] Chemo-prophylaxis may result in delayed onset of symptoms and even obscure microscopic diagnosis.[18] Therefore, all chemoprophylaxis should be stopped while patients are investigated for malaria.

There are many diagnostic modalities available for diagnosis of malaria, but micros-copy and rapid diagnostic tests (RDTs) are the most common diagnostic tools used to arrive at a specific diagnosis of malaria. In all suspected cases, blood examinations by microscopy and/or RDT should be submitted to the laboratory. All positive results ideally should be communicated to the treating physician within 4 hours of the sample reaching the laboratory for early initiation of therapy. Negative microscopy and RDT results should trigger contemplation of an alternative diagnosis, and empiric therapy for malaria should be withheld unless patients with a convincing exposure history demonstrate features of severe malaria.[19] In a scenario where the diagnosis of malaria is suspected but proficient laboratory services are unavailable, empiric treatment of P falciparum malaria should be instituted, pending referral of patient and/or specimen.[12]

Microscopy

Giemsa staining (thick and thin films) Microscopy remains the gold standard for malarial diagnosis and also for endpoint assessment of outcome of therapy and drug trials. When malaria is suspected, both thick and thin Giemsa smear of blood should be prepared immediately. Diagnosis is made by detecting parasites in the thick smear because it concentrates the parasites 40-fold and adds to the sensitivity.[13] Thin smear subsequently helps in determining the malaria species and the level of parasi-temia (the percentage of a patient's red blood cells that are infected with malaria para-sites). Speciation helps in choosing the antimalarial therapy and parasite density can indicate disease severity, which needs be monitored during and after treatment to ensure adequate resolution of the infection.[12] The detection threshold of Giemsa-stained thick blood film has been estimated at 20 to 50 parasites per microliter of blood (0.0004%–0.001% parasitemia).[20] This threshold of microscopy has shown to correspond to sensitivity of 68% to 92% for detection of malaria in field conditions.[21] Exclusion of malaria by microscopy requires 3 separate negative blood smears per-formed and read at 12-hour intervals over a 24-hour to 48-hour period.[19]

A major drawback of light microscopy is that the efficiency of the test depends on the type and quality of the smear, skill of the technician, parasite density, and time spent on examining the smear. In addition, mixed infections with P malariae or P ovale are often missed, because their densities are often low in comparison to that of P fal-ciparum. These problems may occur more frequently in nonendemic areas where malaria microscopy is performed infrequently. Illustrating this point, a Canadian study reported a low sensitivity of microscopy (41%) for the diagnosis of malaria involving 100 patients.[22]

Quantitative buffy coat Quantitative buffy coat (QBC) is fluorescent microscopy based on the principle of concentrating the red blood cell–containing parasites within a narrow zone by centrifugation of blood in capillary tubes and staining of malarial parasite nucleic acid with acridine dyes. The sensitivity of QBC almost equals that of Giemsa-stained films.[23] The advantage of QBC is ease of interpretation and rapidity. Species identification and quantification are difficult, however, with this tech-nique and, therefore, thick and thin blood film examination is still required. Moreover,

QBC requires expensive fluorescent microscope for interpretation of the result, which restricts its widespread use, especially in resource-poor countries.

Antigen detection RDTs detect malaria antigen in blood by immunochromatographic test with monoclonal antibodies directed against the target parasite antigen, which is impregnated on a test strip. The result is usually obtained in 5 to 20 minutes. Currently, different combinations of immunochromatographic tests are commercially available, targeting different genus specific or species-specific antigen for malaria diagnosis. Some of the commonly used antigens in RDTs are HRP-2 (*P falciparum* specific), aldolase (pan-specific), plasmodium lactate dehydrogenase (pLDH) (*P falciparum* specific), pLDH (*P vivax-* specific), and pLDH (panspecific).

RDTs based on different antigens have been shown to vary in their performance in field conditions. In a meta-analysis on diagnosing uncomplicated *P falciparum* malaria by RDTs, the overall sensitivity and specificity for histidine-rich protein 2 (HRP-2)–based RDTs were 95.0% and 95.2%, respectively, and for pLDH-based RDTs, 93.2% and 98.5%, respectively. HRP-2–based tests tended to be more sensitive but less specific than pLDH-based tests.[24] RDTs based on aldolase have shown inadequate detection thresholds, possibly because of the low concentrations of this target antigen in parasites.[25] Several RDTs are commercially available. Among these assays, BinaxNOW Malaria (Binax, Inc, Inverness Medical Professional Diagnostics, Scarborough, Maine) received US Food and Drug Administration (FDA) approval in 2007 for diagnosis of symptomatic malaria. This assay is based on the combination of detection of *P falciparum*–specific HRP-2 and pan-specific aldolase.

The BinaxNOW Malaria test has shown a superior sensitivity (97%) and negative predictive value (NPV) (99.6%) compared with microscopy (sensitivity 85% and NPV 99.6%).[25] Antigenemia level is associated with parasite density, so the apparent sensitivity of the BinaxNOW test may vary with differing levels of parasitemia. Its sensitivity varies in *P falciparum* and *P vivax* between 99% and 93% (for parasitemia in excess of 5000 parasites/µL) to 54% and 6% (for parasitemia of 0–100 parasites/µL of blood), with an overall specificity of 94% and 99%, respectively.[26] Because nonimmune travelers generally tend to have high parasitemia (10,000 parasites/µL),[26] the excellent sensitivity and NPV of RDTs, particularly for *P falciparum*, make it a valuable tool in making a rapid diagnosis of malaria in the ED.

The limitation of the BinaxNOW Malaria test is its low sensitivity (60%) for detection of *P ovale* infection, probably due to its lower production of the aldolase and/or low parasite density.[25,27] This test also has limited use in quantifying the parasite load and monitoring the antimalarial treatment because HRP-2 can persist in blood after successful treatment,[28] although aldolase and pLDH fall rapidly after initiation of effective therapy but can subsequently become positive on appearance of gametocytes, because not all therapeutic regimens are gametocidal.[26] Moreover, false-negative reactions up to 40% have been noted in *P falciparum* in some parts of South America due to HRP-2 gene deletions.[28]

In conclusion, RDTs for malaria are rapid tests and are helpful in making a quick diagnosis of malaria in emergency departments, especially at odd hours when expert microscopic advice may not be available. RDTs are almost as sensitive as malaria microscopy for falciparum malaria but less sensitive for nonfalciparum malaria and cannot give additional information, such as parasite count and maturity. Therefore, RDT must be accompanied or followed by confirmatory blood smears for quantification of parasitemia and determination of the species.

Serology Detection of antibodies against malaria parasites, using either indirect immunofluorescence assay or ELISA, does not indicate current infection but rather measures past exposure. Therefore, it has no role in diagnosis of acute infections. Serology may be used to screen donors to prevent transfusion-related malaria, however, and to confirm the diagnosis of malaria in recently treated cases in which the diagnosis could not be confirmed previously.[29]

Molecular methods Molecular technologies have been developed to improve the diagnosis of malaria by detecting specific parasite nucleic acid. The advantage of molecular methods is their exquisite sensitivity down to the level of 5 parasites/µL or 0.0001% parasitemia.[30]

Molecular methods are also useful in confirming *Plasmodium* species, when in doubt or when it is not possible by other methods. Real-time assays may also help in quantification of parasitemia.[31] Molecular methods, however, find limited use in routine diagnosis of acute cases because of high cost, need for specialized infrastructure, and longer turnaround time.

In addition to ordering the malaria-specific diagnostic tests, a baseline complete blood count and a chemistry panel should be requested. In the event of a positive malaria test, these additional tests aid in determining whether a patient has uncomplicated or severe manifestations of the malaria infection. Although nonspecific, fever accompanied by thrombocytopenia, a low white blood cell count, and signs of hemolysis, such as an elevated bilirubin level, are predictive clues to the presence of malaria.[12] Some of key laboratory findings in severe malaria[10] are listed in **Box 2**.

Treatment

The choice of treatment of malaria is guided by the infecting species of plasmodium, the probable drug susceptibility as determined by the region of acquisition of infection, the severity of infection, the clinical status of the person, and any previous use of antimalarials.

Uncomplicated malaria

Appropriately treated, uncomplicated malaria has a good prognosis, with a case fatality rate of approximately 0.1%.[32] Uncomplicated malaria caused by *P ovale, P vivax*, and *P malariae* can usually be managed with oral drugs on an outpatient basis, unless a patient has other comorbidities or is unable to take drugs orally. *P falciparum* infections in travelers can rapidly progress, however, to severe illness or death in as few as 1 to 2 days, due to little immunity against these infections. Therefore, all patients diagnosed with *P falciparum* or mixed infections or infections with unconfirmed species should be admitted to a hospital[12] and treated for multidrug-resistant *P falciparum* for at least 48 hours to ensure adequate response to therapy, regardless of how well they appear at presentation.

Box 2
Laboratory findings of severe malaria

- Hypoglycemia (blood glucose <2.2 mmol/L or <40 mg/dL)
- Metabolic acidosis (plasma bicarbonate <15 mmol/L)
- Severe normocytic anemia (hemoglobin <7 g/dL)
- Hemoglobinuria
- Hyperparasitemia (>5%)
- Hyperlactatemia (lactate >5 mmol/L)
- Renal impairment (serum creatinine >265 µmol/L)

Chloroquine is the treatment of choice for malaria, when it is sensitive, but emergence of resistance has been noted from various regions. Chloroquine resistance in *P vivax* is confined largely to Indonesia, Papua New Guinea, Timor-Leste, and other parts of Oceania.[10] Rare cases of chloroquine-resistant *P vivax* have also been documented in Myanmar, India, and Central and South America. *P ovale* and *P malariae* continue to remain sensitive to chloroquine throughout the world. Chloroquine resistance in *P falciparum* is prevalent throughout the world except for regions of Haiti, the Dominican Republic, most regions of the Middle East, and Central America west of the Panama Canal.[33] If chloroquine-resistant *P falciparum* is anticipated, then artemisinin combination therapy (ACT) is preferred for treatment of uncomplicated falciparum malaria.[10] ACT consists of an artemisinin derivative (artesunate, artemether, and artemotil) combined with a long-acting antimalarial (amodiaquine, lumefantrine, mefloquine, or sulfadoxine-pyrimethamine). Alternative treatment options for uncomplicated malaria by various plasmodium species are listed in **Table 3**.[10,33] Relapse has been reported in 25% of cases of vivax malaria when treated with chloroquine or other drugs,[34] because these antimalarials do not eliminate liver stages of parasite. Primaquine is required additionally for radical cure and to prevent relapse. Antimalarial drugs and their dosing are outlined in **Table 4**.[32,33]

Severe malaria

Severe malaria is a medical emergency. After rapid clinical assessment and diagnosis of severe falciparum malaria, full doses of parenteral antimalarial treatment should be started without delay (see **Table 3**). There are 2 major classes of drugs available for parenteral treatment of severe malaria: the cinchona alkaloids (quinine and quinidine) and the artemisinin derivatives. Artesunate is recommended by the World Health Organization (WHO) in preference to quinidine for the treatment of severe malaria. Various randomized trials comparing artesunate and quinine have shown evidence of benefit with artesunate over quinine in adults and children.[10,35] Intravenous artesunate of reliable quality is not yet available in many countries; in these areas, quinine remains the treatment of choice. Artesunate was unavailable in the United States until 2007, when the Food and Drug Administration approved it as an investigational new drug for treatment of severe malaria. Parenteral quinine was replaced with quinidine for the treatment of severe falciparum malaria by the CDC, because quinidine was found more potent and effective in severe *P falciparum* infections. When intravenous therapy cannot be given immediately, options include intramuscular administration of quinine or an artemisinin or rectal administration of artesunate. Although the WHO has strongly recommended artesunate as the first line of therapy for severe malaria, CDC guidelines state that if both quinidine and artesunate can be obtained in similar time frames, the treating physician may choose either option. The CDC recommends artesunate in treatment of severe malaria if quinidine is unavailable, in patients with adverse effects or contraindications to quinidine, or in patients with a parasitemia greater than 10% of baseline at 48 hours after initiation of intravenous quinidine.

Management of patients with severe malaria also presents a broad array of clinical challenges given the complex pathophysiology of the infection involving multiple organ systems. **Box 3** outlines the intensive care management of severe malaria.[10,12]

Treatment of malaria in pregnancy

Malaria in pregnancy is associated with high rate of maternal and perinatal mortality.[12] Pregnant women are more likely to develop severe *P falciparum* malaria than other adults because of physiologic immunosupression that occurs during gestation and

Table 3
Guidelines for treatment of malaria

Diagnosis	Chloroquine Sensitive/Resistance	Treatment
Uncomplicated malaria		
P malariae	All regions	Chloroquine phosphate or hydroxychloroquine
P vivax or P ovale	Sensitive region	Chloroquine phosphate or hydroxychloroquine plus primaquine phosphate
P vivax	Resistant region	Atovaquone/proguanil or mefloquine or oral quinine sulfate plus doxycycline or tetracycline or clindamycin plus primaquine phosphate
P falciparum	Sensitive region	Chloroquine phosphate or hydroxychloroquine
P falciparum or species not yet identified	Resistant region	Artemether-lumefantrine or any ACT effective in region or atovaquone/proguanil or oral quinine sulfate plus doxycycline or tetracycline or clindamycin or mefloquine
Severe malaria		
Any species	All regions	Intravenous quinidine gluconate plus tetracycline, doxycycline, or clindamycin or intravenous artesunate[a] followed by one of the following: atovaquone/proguanil, doxycycline, clindamycin, or mefloquine
Malaria during pregnancy		
Uncomplicated malaria any species	Sensitive region	Chloroquine phosphate or hydroxychloroquine
P falciparum/P vivax	Resistant region	Quinine sulfate plus clindamcyin or mefloquine
Severe malaria	Resistant region	Quinine sulfate plus clindamycin or artesunate plus clindamycin

If a person develops malaria despite taking chemoprophylaxis, that particular medicine should not be used as a part of the treatment regimen. Use any one of the other options. If a patient cannot tolerate oral therapy, parenteral formulations of antimalarial drugs are recommended.

There is no evidence that there is clinical difference between currently available various ACTs.

Treatment with mefloquine is not recommended in persons who have acquired infections from Southeast Asia due to drug resistance. Because of a higher rate of severe neuropsychiatric reactions seen at treatment doses, mefloquine is not recommended unless the other options cannot be used.

For P vivax or P ovale infections, primaquine phosphate for radical treatment of hypnozoites should not be given during pregnancy. Pregnant patients with P vivax or P ovale infections should be maintained on chloroquine prophylaxis for the duration of their pregnancy. After delivery, pregnant patients who do not have G6PD deficiency should be treated with primaquine.

[a] Artesunate is an investigational new drug (contact CDC for information).

Data from Centers for Disease Control and Prevention (CDC). Treatment of malaria: guidelines for clinicians (United States). 2011. Available at: http://www.cdc.gov/malaria/resources/pdf/treatmenttable.pdf. Accessed July 14, 2012; and World Health Organization. Guidelines for the treatment of malaria. 2nd edition. 2010. Available at: http://whqlibdoc.who.int/publications/2010/9789241547925_eng.pdf. Accessed July 1, 2012.

the accumulation of erythrocytes infected with P falciparum in the placenta through cytoadherence mechanisms. Complications, such as hypoglycemia and pulmonary edema, are more common than in nonpregnant individuals.[19] Prompt antimalarial therapy (**Table 3**) should be administered in addition to supportive care. For severe malaria, parenteral artesunate is preferred over quinine in the second and third trimesters because quinine is associated with recurrent hypoglycemia and artemisinins are

Table 4
Doses of antimalarial drugs

Drug	Adult Dose	Pediatric Dose	Comments
Artesunate	2.4 mg/kg IV push at 0, 12, 24, and 48 h	2.4 mg/kg IV push at 0, 12, 24, and 48 h	
Atovaquone-proguanil	4 Adult tabs (each adult tab contains 250 mg atovaquone and 100 mg proguanil) PO as a single dai y dose for 3 consecutive days	Dosage is based on weight. Each ped tab contains 62.5 mg atovaquone and 25 mg proguanil. Daily dose to be taken for 3 consecutive days: 5–8 kg: 2 ped tabs 9–10 kg: 3 ped tabs 11–20 kg: 1 adult tab 21–30 kg: 2 adult tabs 31–40 kg: 3 adult tabs ≥41 kg: 4 adult tabs	Not indicated for use in pregnant women
Artemether-lumefantrine	1 Tablet = 20 mg artemether and 120 mg lumefantrine A 3-d treatment schedule with a total of 6 oral doses is recommended for both adult and pediatric patients based on weight. The patient should receive the initial dose, followed by the second dose 8 h later, then 1 dose PO bid for the following 2 d. 5 To <15 kg: 1 tab per dose 15 To <25 kg: 2 tabs per dose 25 To <35 kg: 3 tabs per dose ≥35 kg: 4 tabs per dose		Lumefantrine absorption is enhanced by coadministration with fat, so should be taken after fatty meal. If patient vomits within 30 minutes of taking dose, then repeat the dose.
Chloroquine phosphate	600 mg Base (= 1 g salt) PO, then 300 mg base (= 500 mg salt) and 6, 24, and 48 h	10 mg Base/kg PO, then 5 mg base/kg at 6, 24, and 48 h	Use with caution in impaired liver functions because the drug is concentrated in liver.
Clindamycin, oral	20 mg Base/kg/d PO divided tid × 7 d	20 mg Base/kg/d PO divided tid × 7 d	
Clindamycin, parenteral	10 mg Base/kg IV followed by 5 mg base/kg IV q8h Switch to oral clindamycin as soon as patient is able to complete 7-d course	10 mg Base/kg IV followed by 5 mg base/kg IV q8h Switch to oral clindamycin as soon as patient is able to complete 7-d course	Safe in children and pregnant women

(continued on next page)

Table 4
(continued)

Drug	Adult Dose	Pediatric Dose	Comments
Doxycycline	100 mg PO or IV bid × 7 d	2.2 mg/kg PO or IV bid × 7 d	Contraindicated in children <8 y, pregnant women
Mefloquine	750 mg Salt (= 684 mg base) PO followed by 500 mg salt (= 456 mg base) PO 6–12 h after the initial dose	15 mg Salt/kg (= 13.7 mg base/kg) PO followed by 10 mg salt/kg (= 9.1 mg base/kg) PO 6–12 h after the initial dose	Contraindicated in children with epilepsy, other seizure disorders, and persons allergic to mefloquine, with psychiatric disorders, or with cardiac conduction abnormalities
Primaquine phosphate	30 mg Base PO qd × 14 d	0.5 mg Base/kg PO qd × 14 d	Primaquine can cause hemolytic anemia in G6PD-deficient persons. G6PD screening must occur before starting treatment with primaquine. Primaquine should not be used during pregnancy and children less than 4 y old.
Quinidine gluconate	6.25 mg Base/kg (= 10 mg salt/kg) loading dose IV over 1–2 h, then 0.0125 mg base/kg/min (= 0.02 mg salt/kg/min) continuous infusion for at least 24 h. Once parasite density is <1% and patient can take oral medication, complete treatment with oralquinine.	6.25 mg Base/kg (=10 mg salt/kg) loading dose IV over 1–2 h, then 0.0125 mg base/kg/min (= 0.02 mg salt/kg/min) continuous infusion for at least 24 h. Once parasite density is <1% and patient can take oral medication, complete treatment with oralquinine.	Associated with cinchonism, tachycardia, prolongation of QRS and QTc intervals, flattening of T waves, hypotension, and hypoglycemia. Contraindicated in history of blackwater fever or thrombocytopenia purpura. Cardiac and glucose monitoring required during its administration.
Quinine sulfate (Qualaquin)	650 mg Salt (= 542 mg base) PO tid = 3 or 7 d (× 7 d if acquired in Southeast Asia)	10 mg Salt/kg = 8.3 mg base/kg) PO tid = 3 d (× 7 d if acquired in Southeast Asia)	Associated with cinchonism, sinus arrythmia, ventricular tachycardia, atrioventricular block, and prolongation of QT intervals (these are rare compared with quinidine)
Tetracycline	250 mg PO qid × 7 d	25 mg/kg/d PO divided qid × 7 d	Contraindicated in children <8 y, pregnant women

Abbreviations: G6PD, Glucose-6-phosphate dehydrogenase; ped, pediatrics; tab, tablet.
Data from Mace KE, Lynch MF. Malaria. In: Bope E, Kellerman R, editors. Conn's current therapy. 1st edition. Saunders; 2012. p. 122–32; and Centers for Disease Control and Prevention (CDC). Treatment of malaria: guidelines for clinicians. 2011. Available at: http://www.cdc.gov/malaria/resources/pdf/treatmenttable.pdf. Accessed July 14, 2012.

Box 3
Intensive care management of severe malaria

- Medication (diazepam or paraldehyde) for convulsions
- Management of fluid balance to optimize oxygen delivery and reduce acidosis
- Propping patients at angle of 45°C; intubation or diuretics to manage acute pulmonary edema
- Careful monitoring and correction of hypoglycemia
- Dialysis for oliguric acute renal failure or control of electrolyte imbalance/acidosis
- Broad-spectrum antibiotics to manage shock or secondary bacterial infection
- Exchange transfusion considered if parasite density >10% or there is spontaneous bleeding

---

superior in reducing the risk of death due to severe malaria.[10] In the first trimester, however, risk of hypoglycemia is lower with quinine and there is greater uncertainty on the safety of artemisinins; therefore, both artesunate and quinine may be considered options until more data is available.[10]

Prevention

When visiting endemic regions, travelers should prevent mosquito bites by using adequate body covering clothing, bed nets, and repellents. Up to 50% DEET (chemical name, *N,N*-diethyl-*meta*-toluamide) is recommended as an effective repellent for all individuals over the age of 2 months, including pregnant women. The decision to use chemoprophylaxis depends on the benefit of chemoprophylaxis against the risk of possible adverse drug reactions. It is proposed that there is no need for chemoprophylaxis in areas where the annual incidence of malaria is below 10 cases per 1000 individuals.[36] Various regimens for chemoprophylaxis are outlined in **Table 5**.[37] For effective prophylaxis, all regimens should be taken before, during, and after travel to an area with malaria.[37,38]

Table 5
Chemoprophylaxis of malaria

Drug	Dose	Duration
Chloroquine-resistant regions		
Atovaquone-proguanil	1 Tablet (250 atovaquone and 100 mg), daily	Begin 1–2 d before travel and for 7 d after leaving malarious areas
Mefloquine	250 mg, Once a week	Begin ≥2 wk before travel and for 4 wk after leaving malarious areas
Doxycycline	100 mg, Daily	Begin 1–2 d before travel and for 4 wk after leaving malarious areas
Primaquine	52.6 Salt, daily	Begin 1–2 d before travel and for 7 d after leaving malarious areas
Chloroquine-sensitive regions		
Chloroquine phosphate	500 mg (Salt), once a week	Begin 1–2 wk before travel and for 4 wk after leaving malarious areas

Data from Centers for Disease Control and Prevention (CDC). Chapter 3 Infectious diseases related to travel. In: Malaria. Available at: http://wwwnc.cdc.gov/travel/yellowbook/2012/chapter-3-infectious-diseases-related-to-travel/malaria.htm. Accessed August 4, 2012.

Vaccine

The most important step in potential eradication of malaria is the development of an efficacious vaccine. This goal has remained elusive, partly because of the problems of selecting appropriate targets and the lack of reliable and predictive animal models for plasmodium. Because most of the morbidity and mortality (over 90%) due to malaria is caused by *P falciparum*, the primary focus has been on the development of an effective *P falciparum* vaccine. After failure of many candidate vaccines, the most promising candidate on the horizon is the RTS,S/AS01E vaccine, the only malaria vaccine in phase 3 evaluation. It is a pre-erythrocytic malaria vaccine that targets the circumsporozoite protein in combination with the adjuvant AS01. The hypothesized mode of action of this vaccine is to induce circulating antibodies to circumsporozoite that would prevent the load of sporozoites from reaching the liver and in addition stimulate T-cell response to promote the destruction of infected liver cells to further impede intracellular parasite development. This could lead to a significant decrease in infection in vaccines. It could also decrease load of parasites emerging from the liver with a subsequent impact on disease rate and severity. The clinical efficacy of this vaccine is predicted to be between 25% and 60% in different malaria endemic settings.[39] Depending on the full trial results expected in 2014, WHO recommendation for use may become available in 2015.

Zoonotic malaria

Recently, a fifth malarial species, known as *P knowlesi*, has been reported from forested regions of Southeast Asia. *P knowlesi* was originally believed restricted to macaques in Southeast Asia but now have been shown to cause naturally acquired human infections.[40] Significantly, *P knowlesi* infections are known to result in result in severe malaria and are commonly associated with complications, such as respiratory distress, acute renal failure, and shock, with high mortality. In a 2-year case series from Sabah, Malaysia, severe malaria was seen in 39% of the patients with *P knowlesi* infections at a tertiary care referral hospital. Severe malaria was also associated with high parasite (2%–4%) count and case fatality rate of 27%, comparable to that of *P falciparum*. *P knowlesi* may have been underreported previously because it is indistinguishable from *P malariae* on blood smear examination and needs molecular methods for definite diagnosis.[41] Because *P malariae* infections are associated with low parasitemia, *P malariae* parasitemia on microscopy should arouse suspicion for *P knowlesi* and treatment should be given for severe *P knowlesi*, if molecular tools are not available for confirmation of diagnosis.

Chloroquine is recommended by the CDC for treatment of *P knowlesi* infections, whereas WHO[10] malaria treatment guideline has not given any recommendations for the same. Recently, in a 2-year retrospective case study of 56 patients in Malaysia, the group receiving artemether-lumefantrine had faster parasite clearance compared with other regimens. Also, a lower case fatality rate (17%) was noted with intravenous artesunate than for those who received quinine (31%) for *P knowlesi*. Therefore, oral artemether-lumefantrine for uncomplicated knowlesi malaria and intravenous artesunate therapy for severe knowlesi malaria was more efficacious in this particular study.[42]

DENGUE FEVER

DF is one of the most significant arboviral diseases in terms of mortality and morbidity, affecting the tropical and subtropical regions of the world. According to a WHO estimate, its incidence has increased by a factor of 30 over the past 50 years.[43]

Dengue virus (DENV) belongs to the genus *Flavivirus* of the family *Flaviviridae*. It is an enveloped, single-stranded, positive-sense RNA virus. The genome is approximately

11 kilobases long and encodes for 3 structural proteins and 7 NSs. NS1 is a highly conserved glycoprotein that seems to be essential for virus viability but has no established biologic activity.[44] Unusually for a viral glycoprotein, NS1 is produced in both membrane-associated and secreted forms.

DF is caused by any of 4 closely related viruses or serotypes: dengue 1–4. Infection with one serotype does not protect against the others, and sequential infections with heterologous DENV strains put people at greater risk for DHF and DSS.[45]

Epidemiology and Transmission of the Dengue Virus

Dengue is transmitted between people by the mosquitoes *Aedes aegypti* and *A albopictus*, found throughout the world. Symptoms of infection usually begin 4 to 7 days after a mosquito bite and typically last 3 to 10 days. In order for transmission to occur, the mosquito must feed on a person during the 5-day period when viral burden in the blood is high; this period usually begins a little before a person becomes symptomatic. After entering the mosquito through the blood meal, the virus requires an additional 8 to 12 days before it can be transmitted to another human. The mosquito remains infected for the remainder of its life, which may be days or a few weeks.

In rare cases, dengue can be transmitted by organ transplants or blood transfusions from infected donors, and there is evidence of vertical transmission.[46] But in the vast majority of infections, a mosquito bite is responsible.

In many parts of the tropics and subtropics, dengue is endemic, that is, it occurs every year, usually during a season when *Aedes* mosquito populations are high, often when rainfall is optimal for breeding. These areas are at periodic risk for epidemic dengue, when large numbers of people become infected during a short period. Dengue epidemics require a concurrence of large number of vector mosquitoes, a large number of people with no immunity to 1 of the 4 virus types (DENV 1, DENV 2, DENV 3, and DENV 4), and the opportunity for contact.

The 4 DENVs originated in monkeys and independently jumped to humans in Africa or Southeast Asia between 100 and 800 years ago. Dengue remained a minor, geographically restricted disease until the middle of the twentieth century. The disruption of World War II—in particular the coincidental transport of *Aedes* mosquitoes around the world in cargo—is thought to have played a crucial role in the dissemination of this virus. DHF was first documented in the 1950s during epidemics in the Philippines and Thailand. It was not until 1981 that large number of DHF cases began to appear in the Caribbean and Latin America, where highly effective *Aedes* control programs had been in place until the early 1970s.

Today approximately 2.5 billion people, or 40% of the world's population, live in areas with risk of dengue transmission. Dengue is endemic in at least 100 countries in Asia, the Pacific, the Americas, Africa, and the Caribbean.[43] Estimates suggest that annually 100 million cases of DF and half a million cases of DHF occur in the world, with a case fatality in Asian countries of 0.5% to 3.5%. The first epidemic of DHF in Southeast Asia occurred in 1954 in Manila, Philippines. The incidence of DHF has increased dramatically since 1950. However, in recent years since 1980, the incidence of DHF has increased approximately 5 times.

Most of the dengue infections (89%) among US residents occur in returning travelers from endemic areas. Travel to the Caribbean (43%); Mexico, Central America, or South America (34%); and Asia and the Pacific (21%) are the leading regions for imported dengue infection in United States.[47] Because contact between *Aedes* and people is infrequent in the continental United States, these imported cases rarely result in secondary transmission. DF epidemics have occurred occasionally in the continental United States since the end of World War II. The last reported continental dengue outbreak was in south Texas in 2005.[48] Most dengue cases in US citizens occur in inhabitants of Puerto Rico, the US Virgin Islands, Samoa, and Guam, which are endemic for the virus. The most recent island-wide epidemic occurred in 2007, when more than 10,000 cases were diagnosed.[49]

Clinical Presentation

Patients usually presents with a history of high-grade fever, rash, and severe headache for 2 days associated with body aches. Rash first appears on the trunk and spreads to the limbs. Patients subsequently may develop altered sensorium.

The symptoms of dengue infection usually start after 3 to 7 days of mosquito bite but may extend up to 14 days. So DF should be considered in all febrile travelers who give a brief history of travel to a dengue endemic area within the past 2 weeks.[49] DENV infections present with wide variety of clinical manifestations, ranging from asymptomatic infection to mild febrile illness to severe disease.[50]

The majority (75%) of DENV infections are asymptomatic or may present as undifferentiated febrile illness, often only with a maculopapular rash. Classic DF is an acute febrile illness with headaches noted in 63%, musculoskeletal pain in 52%, and rash in 34% of cases.[51] The onset is sudden with high fever, severe headache (especially in the retro-orbital area), and intense arthralgia, myalgia, and deep bone pain. Therefore, DF is also often called "break bone fever."[52,53] After 3 to 4 days of fever, an indistinct macular rash can develop, sparing the palms and soles. As the rash fades or desquamates in 1 to 5 days,[45] localized clusters of petechiae on the extensor surfaces of the limbs may remain (**Fig. 1**). Moderate leukopenia and thrombocytopenia can be seen in 47% of patients and are useful diagnostic features.[54–56] Raised lactate dehydrogenase, aspartate aminotransferase, and alanine aminotransferase levels may be seen in more than half of the cases.[45] Hemorrhagic manifestations are uncommon in DF but in rare cases can be life threatening. The main bleeding sites, apart from petechiae in skin, may present as epistaxis and less commonly as gastrointestinal bleeding. Case fatality rate of DF is less than 1% and recovery from DF is usually uneventful.[57] Sometimes, convalescence may be prolonged as generalized weakness, lasting several weeks, especially in adults.

DHF and DSS are the serious and life-threatening manifestations of dengue. DHF/DHS is an acute immunopathologic disease that is usually seen in secondary infection, in approximately 90% of cases, after exposure to heterologous DENV serotype. DHF may occur after primary infection in infants due to prior presence of maternal anti-dengue antibodies.[45]

The case definition of DHF includes 4 features: fever, a positive tourniquet test, thrombocytopenia ($<100 \times 10^9$/L), and hemoconcentration (>20% above normal level).[57] DHF is characterized by sudden onset of fever, which usually lasts for 2 to 7 days and is followed by a fall in temperature to normal or subnormal levels. A maculopapular rash similar to that seen in DF is also seen in many patients. The period of defervescence is the critical stage in DHF[58] and coincides with severe thrombocytopenia and elevation of aminotransferases.[59] Plasma leakage due to increased vascular permeability[60] begins during this stage and can be a life-threatening feature. Plasma leakage is manifested as tachycardia, hypotension, pleural effusions, ascites, pericardial effusion, hemoconcentration, and hypoproteinemia. Tender hepatomegaly is observed in almost all patients and splenomegaly may be seen in some.

Hemorrhagic manifestations usually occur once the fever has settled.[61] The cause of hemorrhage is thrombocytopenia and associated platelet dysfunction or disseminated intravascular coagulation seen in DHF.[57] In DHF, bleeding may occur from any site and does not correlate with the platelet counts.[61] Spontaneous petechiae

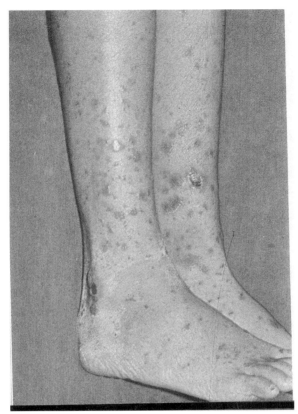

Fig. 1. Rash of DF. (*Reproduced from* Wattal C, Gupta PS, Datta S. Dengue fever and encephalitis. In: Khardori NM, Wattal C, editors. Emergencies in infectious disease. From head to toe. Delhi [India]: Byword Books Private Limited; 2010. p. 41–8.)

or ecchymoses may be noted in approximately one-half of patients with DHF and manifest as positive tourniquet test, easy bruising, and bleeding at a venipuncture site. Gastrointestinal bleeding (15%–30%), metorrhagia (40%), and epistaxis (10%) are also seen in some cases.[62] Convalescence in DHF is usually short and uneventful with overall case fatality of 1% to 5%.[45]

The term, DSS, is used when shock is present along with the 4 criteria.[57] DSS is characterized by rapid weak pulse with narrowing of pulse pressure (ie, the difference between the systolic and diastolic pressures) less than or equal to 20 mm Hg or signs of poor capillary perfusion (cold extremities, delayed capillary refill, or rapid pulse rate).[57] Severe abdominal pain, persistent lethargy, and change from fever to hypothermia on days 2 through 7 are usually the warning signs for impending DSS.[63] Other complications associated with DSS are liver failure, disseminated intravascular coagulation, encephalopathy, myocarditis, acute renal failure, and hemolytic uraemic syndrome.[61,64] Patients presenting with DSS are a medical emergency, because they may deteriorate rapidly and die within 12 to 24 hours.[57] Early diagnosis and aggressive treatment are critical in the outcome of DSS, because a high mortality rate of 25% to 50% associated with it can be reduced to 0.5% to 1.0% with appropriate treatment.[45]

These criteria for classification of dengue, especially that of DHF/DSS, in the past have resulted in diagnostic dilemmas. There were difficulties in applying the criteria for DHF in a clinical situation, together with reports of missing of severe cases, because they did not fulfill the strict criteria of DHF. For these reasons, the WHO published a revised set of guidelines to help in arriving at more specific diagnosis and disease classification of dengue for case management.[60] According to this revised classification, dengue has been divided into 2 broad categories—dengue (with or without warning signs) and severe dengue (summarized in **Fig. 2**). These revised guidelines of WHO are currently being evaluated for performance in practical settings.

Differential Diagnosis

The following are usually the alternate diagnoses:

1. Other hemorrhagic arboviral disease
2. Chickengunya viral infections
3. Meningitis
4. Measles
5. Typhoid fever

Evaluating patients who present with fever and rash can be challenging because the differential diagnosis is extensive and includes minor and life-threatening illnesses. For patients presenting with fever and rash, 4 concerns must be addressed immediately: first, whether the patient is well enough to provide a history or whether cardiorespiratory support is urgently required; second, if the nature of the rash requires patient isolation; third, whether skin lesions require urgent institution of antimicrobial therapy, as in meningococcal rash; and finally, consideration must be given to the possibility that the patient has an exotic disease acquired during travel.

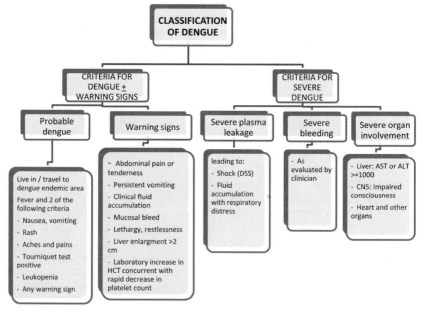

Fig. 2. Dengue classification for diagnosis and assessing levels severity. ALT, alanine aminotransferase; AST, aspartate aminotransferase; CNS: central nervous system; HCT: hematocrit.

Key points in arriving at a presumptive diagnosis include determination of the primary types of skin lesions present, the distribution and progression of the rash, and the timing of the onset of the rash relative to the onset of fever and other signs of systemic illness.

The differential diagnosis of the rash in DF is provided in **Table 6**.[64]

Diagnosis

In view of the high mortality rate in untreated complicated dengue cases[45] and to reduce the disease burden, it is imperative to have a rapid and accurate diagnosis of dengue infection.

History of travel to dengue endemic area in the past 2 weeks in a febrile traveler is the first clue towards a diagnosis of DF. A complete blood cell count at the first visit and thorough physical examination for signs of deranged hemodynamic status, plasma leakages, and hemorrhages should alert a clinician to possible diagnosis of dengue and its complications. A rapid decrease in platelet count associated with a rising hematocrit compared with the baseline is suggestive of progress to the plasma leakage/critical phase of disease and a requirement for hospitalization. In all suspected cases of dengue infection, tests for specific diagnosis of dengue should be performed to confirm its diagnosis.

The major diagnostic methods currently available are based on detection of the virus, antibodies, antigens, or a combination of these techniques.

Diagnosis of dengue infection can be established by testing acute-phase serum samples during the first 5 days of symptoms. This detection coincides with the febrile phase of illness and detection of viremia. Convalescent-phase serum (more than 5 days of symptoms) is usually associated with defervescence and the detection of IgM/IgG antidengue antibodies.

Table 6
Different types of rashes and their causative organisms

Rash	Causative Organisms
Maculopapular rash	Viral illness (DF, measles, rubella, cocksackie, echo, cytomegalo, hepatitis B virus, hepatitis C virus, herpes simplex virus, West Nile fever, human parvovirus B19) Bacteria (chronic meningococcemia, bacterial endocarditis, secondary syphilis, staphylococcal scalded skin syndrome, staphylococcal toxic shock syndrome, *Mycoplasma pneumoniae*, salmonella)
Nodular lesions	Bacteria (nocardia, atypical mycobacteria, pseudomonal sepsis) Fungi (candidal sepsis, blastomycosis, histoplasmosis, coccidioidomycosis, sporotrichosis)
Diffuse erythema	Scarlet fever, toxic shock syndrome, staphylococcal scalded skin syndrome
Vesiculobullous eruptions	Varicella, disseminated herpes simplex virus, echo, cocksackie, poxvirus
Petechial and purpuric eruptions	Bacteria (*Neisseria meningitidis*, rickettsiae, listeria, staphylococci) Viruses (viral hemorrhagic fevers—dengue cocksackie A9, echovirus 9, cytomegalovirus, Epstein-Barr virus)

Reproduced from Wattal C, Gupta PS, Datta S. Dengue fever and encephalitis. In: Khardori NM, Wattal C, editors. Emergencies in infectious disease. From head to toe. Delhi [India]: Byword Books Private Limited; 2010. p. 41–8.

Virus detection

Acute infection with DENV is confirmed when the virus is isolated from serum or autopsy tissue specimens or the specific DENV genome is identified by reverse transcription–polymerase chain reaction from serum or plasma, cerebrospinal fluid, or autopsy tissue specimens during an acute febrile illness.

Cell culture Owing to the availability of freely circulating viable virus particles in the blood for the initial 5 days after onset of the disease, virus isolation by cell culture and subsequent detection by immunofluorescence is the gold standard for diagnosis of DENV infection in the acute phase.[65] But due to its low sensitivity, laborious procedure, and time consumption (a minimum incubation period of 7 days is required), it has gradually been replaced by PCR.[66,67]

Molecular methods Molecular methods have become a primary tool to detect virus early in the course of illness because PCR can detect DENV in the blood (serum) from patients approximately in the first 5 days of the appearance of symptoms, when antibodies are usually not detectable. A positive PCR result is a definite proof of current infection and usually confirms the infecting serotype as well. A negative result, however, is interpreted as indeterminate. Current tests are between 80% and 90% sensitive and more than 95% specific.[68] Currently, several PCR tests, such as 1-step, real-time PCR (RT-PCR) or nested RT-PCR, are used to detect the viral genome in acute-phase serum. Several RT-PCR assays have been developed and automated, but none of these tests is commercially available yet. RT-PCR developed by CDC, called CDC DENV-1-4 Real-Time RT-PCR Assay, diagnoses dengue within the first 7 days after symptoms of the illness appear, which is when most people are likely to see a health care professional. The test can identify all the 4 serotypes. The CDC has developed this assay using the Applied Biosystems 7500 Fast Dx Real-Time PCR Instrument, used also for influenza testing.

The requirement of a highly trained staff and the need for sophisticated equipment as well as the cost involved associated with molecular methods have limited their application as a routine diagnostic assay.

Serology

The acquired immune response after a DENV infection consists of the production of IgM and IgG antibodies directed against primarily the virus envelope proteins. A primary dengue infection is characterized by a slow and low titer antibody response. IgM antibodies first appear on days 3 to 5 of illness, peak in approximately 2 weeks, and then decline to undetectable levels in 2 to 3 months.[60,69,70] It is estimated that 80% of all dengue cases have detectable IgM antibody by day 5 of illness, 93% to 99% by days 6 to 10 days of illness, and subsequently may remain detectable for several months.[60,68]

Antidengue IgG is detectable at low titers at the end of the first week of illness, which slowly increases and is detectable for several months thereafter.[60] In contrast, during a secondary infection, the kinetics of the IgM response is more variable. Although IgM levels may also peak at approximately 2 weeks, their levels are significantly lower in secondary dengue infections. Therefore, some antidengue IgM false-negative reactions are observed during secondary infections.[60] IgG antibodies in secondary dengue infection appear early, before, or simultaneously with IgM and rise dramatically over the proceeding 2 weeks. The IgG antibodies may persist for up to 10 months or a lifetime. These IgG antibodies are nonspecific and react broadly with many flaviviruses, including West Nile virus, St. Louis encephalitis virus, Japanese encephalitis virus (JEV), and yellow fever virus (YFV).[50,60]

IgM ELISA (MAC-ELISA) The IgM antibody capture ELISA (MAC-ELISA) is based on capturing human IgM antibodies on a microtiter plate using antihuman-IgM antibody followed by the addition of dengue viral antigen (DENV 1–4). The antigens used for this assay are derived from the envelope protein of the virus. This test is most commonly used in diagnostic laboratories because of its automation and high sensitivity and specificity (90% and 98%, respectively) when used in convalescent-phase sera.[66] High specificity of MAC-ELISA is due to its detection of non–cross-reacting anti-dengue IgM antibodies with other flaviviruses. The major limitation of MAC-ELISA is that it is often not useful in early diagnosis of acute dengue because IgM antibodies appear after 5 to 10 days in primary and 4 to 5 days in secondary infections.[44] MAC-ELISA is more sensitive in detecting primary than secondary infections,[71] and it may be negative in up to 30% of secondary infections.[69,72]

IgG ELISA IgG ELISA used for the detection of a past dengue infection uses the same viral antigens as the MAC-ELISA. This assay correlates with the hemagglutination assay previously used. In general IgG ELISA lacks specificity within the flavivirus sero-complex groups and, therefore, is less specific than IgM ELISA.[50,60] It can also make interpretation difficult in assessing dengue infection in travelers previously immunized with JEV and YFV vaccines. In a study of DF among Israeli travelers to Thailand, IgG tests showed false-positive results in 11% to 17% and 15% to 14% of healthy individuals vaccinated against JEV and YFV, respectively.[73]

Interpretation of serology assays A single positive MAC-ELISA indicates a probable recent dengue infection.[66,68] This is because IgM antibodies for dengue may remain elevated for 2 to 3 months after the illness and, therefore, cannot differentiate between acute and recent dengue infections.[60] A single positive IgG test is unreliable because of its cross-reactivity with other flaviviruses. Therefore, to confirm diagnosis of acute dengue, paired serum samples are required to demonstration seroconversion of IgG/IgM antibody or rising titer ($\geq$4-fold) of IgG antidengue antibodies (**Table 7**).[57,66] The optimal time interval for collecting paired sera is 7 to 10 days. Paired serum samples can also be useful in differentiating primary and secondary dengue infections. Samples with a negative IgG in the acute phase and a positive IgG in the convalescent phase of the infection are considered primary dengue infections,[68] whereas samples with a positive IgG in the acute phase and a 4-fold rise in IgG titer in the convalescent phase are considered secondary dengue infection. Ratio of IgM and IgG antibodies in a single serum sample can also be used to differentiate primary from secondary infection ($\geq$1.2 for primary and $\leq$1.2 for secondary dengue infections).[66]

Table 7 Interpretation of serologic assays	
Diagnosis of Dengue	**Serology Results**
Highly suggestive	Positive IgM in single serum sample Positive IgG in a single sample with an HI titer of $\geq$1280
Confirmed diagnosis	IgM seroconversion in paired sera IgG seroconversion in paired sera or $\geq$4-fold IgG titer in paired sera
Primary infection	Negative IgG in the acute-phase serum and a positive IgG in the convalescent-phase serum Ratio of IgM and IgG in single serum sample $\geq$1.2
Secondary infection	Positive IgG in the acute-phase serum and a 4-fold rise in IgG titer in the convalescent-phase serum sample Ratio of IgM and IgG in single serum sample $\leq$1.2

In a study among 1035 febrile returning travelers, the diagnostic value of IgG and IgM testing on single serum sample, had high false-positivity rate (42.5%) with positive predictive value of 50%.[74] But, combinations of thrombocytopenia or both leukopenia and thrombocytopenia and positive ELISA results greatly improved the positive predictive value value of the test to 88.5% and 90.5%, respectively.

Antigen (NS1) detection

The NS1 of the dengue viral genome has been shown a useful tool for the diagnosis of acute dengue infections. NS1 antigen can be detected as early as the first day after the onset of fever up to day 9, once the clinical phase of the disease is over.[75] Dengue NS1 antigen has been detected in high concentrations in the sera of DENV-infected patients during the early phase of the disease.[44] NS1 Ag levels are similar in both the primary and secondary dengue infection (range 0.01–2 µg/mL).[75,76]

ELISA-based NS1 antigen assay is commercially available and many investigators have evaluated its sensitivity and specificity. In a study at the authors' center,[77] for early diagnosis of dengue infection, acute-phase serum and convalescent-phase serum were investigated using IgM capture ELISA and NS1. The positivity rate of NS1 in acute-phase sera was 71.4% whereas IgM capture ELISA remained 6.4%. During convalescence period, NS1 sensitivity fell to 28.6% whereas IgM capture ELISA improved to 93.6%. Higher detection rate by NS1 Ag in acute area and by IgM in convalescent sera has been observed by other investigators also.[78,79] This is because of early appearance and waning of NS1 compared with IgM.[75] The specificity of NS1 assay was 100%.[77] Due to its highly conserved region, NS1 Ag circulates uniformly in all serotypes of DENV and does not cross-react with other flaviviruses, rendering it highly specific for dengue infection. This results in its higher specificity of 98% to 100%.[80]

Therefore, NS1 assay complements the shortcomings of serology and is useful in early detection (within first 5 days) and provides specific diagnosis of dengue infection without the requirement of paired sera. The method using simple equipment and large number of samples can be processed at a time. Its cost-effectiveness in comparison to the cell culture and molecular methods makes it the test of choice in resource poor settings. At the authors' center, both MAC-ELISA and NS1 assay are used on a single scrum sample to improve the diagnostic algorithm for dengue infection.

Treatment

Management of dengue infections is mainly symptomatic and with antipyretics (aspirin should be avoided to avert development of Reye syndrome) and fluid resuscitation is the mainstay of treatment. Intensive supportive care of patients with suspected DHF-DSS is lifesaving. Blood component transfusions, especially platelets, are used only for risk of bleeding rather than a certain level of thrombocytopenia.

Prevention by way of use of mosquito nets and repellents is effective. Mosquito breeding sites can be eliminated by avoiding stagnant water bodies. Other antimosquito measures are discussed later.

CHIKUNGUNYA FEVER
Introduction

Chikungunya fever (CHIKF) is a viral illness caused by an RNA virus that belongs to the *Alphavirus* genus in the family *Togaviridae* and is transmitted by the *Aedes* mosquitoes. The name is derived from the Makonde dialect, which means, *that which bends up*, referring to the posture of an affected patient acquired due to excruciating pain in the joints. Chikungunya virus (CHIKV) is geographically distributed in Africa, Southeast

Asia, and India.[81] CHIKV is believed to have originated in Africa where it is maintained in nature by a sylvatic cycle involving wild primates and forest-dwelling mosquitoes, such as *A furcifer, A luteocephalus,* or *A taylori.* It was subsequently introduced in Asia where it is transmitted from human to human mainly by *A aegypti* and, to a lesser extent, by *A albopictus* through an urban transmission cycle.[81] CHIKV has been divided into 3 genotypes based on phylogenetic studies. These genotypes, based on the gene sequences of an envelope protein (E1), are Asian, East/Central/South African, and West African.[82–84] Unlike DF, CHIKF results in greater and prolonged morbidity than mortality.

Epidemiology

The disease was documented first time in the form of an outbreak in Tanzania.[85] After the initial identification of CHIKV, sporadic outbreaks continued to occur in Central and Southern Africa, but little activity was reported after the mid-1980s.[86] In 2004, however, an outbreak originating on the coast of Kenya subsequently spread for the first time outside the continental Africa to Comoros and La Réunion. From the spring of 2004 to the summer of 2006, an estimated 500,000 had occurred in La Réunion.[87] This rapid spread of this outbreak was attributed to a mutation of alanine at position 226 with valine (E1-A226V) in CHICKV,[88] which enabled an increase in infectivity to a second vector, *A albopictus*, compared with its infectivity of *A aegypti*.[89] *A albopictus* has wider distribution in temperate regions, making it possible for the spread CHIKV to European regions.[86,87,89] In the following 2 years, CHICKV spread to several other Indian Ocean islands and other parts of the world. The epidemic also spread from the Indian Ocean islands to India, where large outbreaks occurred in 2006.[87] The outbreak in India continued into 2010, resulting in millions of cases[90] with new cases appearing in areas that had not been affected early. The persistence of cases of infection in India is presumably attributable to a vast number of immunologically naive people who help sustain viral transmission.[91] The disease is now reported from almost 40 countries from various WHO regions, including Southeast Asia.[92] The first outbreak of CHIKF in Europe was reported from Italy.[93] In 2010, imported cases also were identified in Taiwan, France, and the United States. These cases were due to the infected viremic travelers returning from Indonesia, La Réunion, and India, respectively. Between 2006 and 2010, 106 laboratory-confirmed or probable cases of CHIKV were detected among travelers returning to the United States compared with only 3 cases reported between 1995 and 2005.[87]

Clinical Symptoms

The incubation period for CHIKV after the bite of Aedes mosquito is 3 to 7 days (range 1–12 days).[87] Not all individuals infected with virus develop symptoms and it is estimated that 3% to 28% of infections are asymptomatic.[87]

CHIKV can manifest as acute, subacute, or chronic disease.[07] In the acute stage, a case is suspected when a patient presents with acute onset of fever greater than 38.5°C (101.3°F) and severe arthralgia or arthritis not explained by other medical conditions or by a patient who has resided in or visited epidemic or endemic areas within 2 weeks before the onset of symptoms. The fever can be continuous or intermittent; defervescence is not associated with worsening of symptoms,[87] in contrast to dengue infections. The fever typically last from several days up to 2 weeks.[87,92] Shortly after the onset of fever, the majority of infected persons develop severe, often debilitating, and migrating polyarthralgias.[91,92] The joint pains are usually symmetric and occur most commonly in wrists, elbows, fingers, knees, and ankles but can also affect more proximal joints.[91] The joint pain may show saddleback patterns and tends to be worse in the morning and relieved by mild exercise.[92] Swelling of joints due to tenosynovitis can be seen in some cases. Arthralgias are often incapacitating due to pain, tenderness, swelling, and stiffness.[87] The lower extremity arthralgia can be severely disabling, resulting in a slow, broad-based, halting gait, which can persist for months.[91]

Transient maculopapular rash usually occurs 2 to 5 days after onset of fever in approximately 50% of patients.[87,92] It is typically maculopapular, involving the trunk and extremities but can also include palms, soles, and face.[87] Other skin lesions recognized during recent outbreaks include vesiculobullous lesions with desquamation, aphthous-like ulcers, and vasculitic lesions.[94,95] Common features in patients presenting with CHICKF are given in **Box 4**.

There has also been infrequent documentation of hemorrhagic manifestations, including hematemesis and melena due to CHIKV infection in Southeast Asia, although some of these cases also exhibited concomitant rising titers of dengue antibodies.[96,97] Other infrequent signs and symptoms reported include headache, retro-orbital pain, nausea, vomiting, meningeal syndrome, conjunctivitis, uveitis, retinitis, and acute encephalopathy.[91,92,98] The acute phase of CHIKF usually lasts for 3 to 10 days.[87]

Subacute CHIK disease is most common 2 to 3 months after infection and is characterized by reappearance of distal polyarthritis after improvement and development of transient vascular disorders (such as Raynaud syndrome).[87] In addition to physical symptoms, the majority of patients complain of depressive symptoms, general fatigue, and weakness.[87]

Chronic CHIK disease is persistence of arthralgias for more than 3 months. It may be associated with destructive arthropathy/arthritis resembling rheumatoid or psoriatic arthritis, in some cases.[87] It is estimated that 80% to 93%, 57%, and 47% of patients with CHIKV infection complain of persistent symptoms after 3 months, 15 months, and even 2 years, respectively.[99,100]

Risk factors for protracted disease are older age (>45 years), pre-existing joint disorders, and more severe acute disease.[99,101]

Pregnant women with CHIKV infections do not have different clinical outcomes.[91] During pregnancy CHIKV infections do not seem to result in transmission of the virus to the fetus but in up to 49% of cases vertical transmission can occur if pregnant woman is viremic at the time of delivery.[102] Intrapartum transmission resulting in neonatal complications, including neurologic disease, hemorrhage, and myocardial disease, has been reported.[91]

Clinical and epidemiologic similarities of infection due to CHIKV, DENV, and *Plasmodium* can make the differential diagnosis difficult in a febrile traveler. Few differentiating features may give clinicians an early clue to the possible diagnosis. In chickengunya infection, fever occurs early in the course of the illness and is of shorter duration than with dengue. A terminal maculopapular rash, conjunctival injection, myalgia, and arthralgia or arthritis is seen more often with chikungunya. DF is

---

Box 4
Common features seen in CHIKF

Common

Fever (76%–100%), polyarthralgia (71%–100%), backache (34%–50%), headache (7%–74%)

Infrequent

Rash (28%–77%), stomatitis (25%), oral ulcers (15%), hyperpigmentation (20%), exfoliative dermatitis (5%)

suggested by severe backpain with features of bleeding and plasma leakage like purpura, malena, and shock. Periodicity of fever and alteration of consciousness/ seizures should prompt a diagnosis of malaria. Confirmation by laboratory diagnosis is essential to arrive at a specific diagnosis.

Diagnosis

Infections with CHIKV are diagnosed in the laboratory by virus isolation RT-PCR, and serology.[87,91]

Virus isolation

Virus isolation being the gold standard, is possible from acute serum specimens ($\leq$8 days)[87,91] by inoculating into a susceptible cell line or suckling mouse. CHIKV produces typical cytopathic effects within 3 days after inoculation in a variety of cell lines. The cytopathic effects must be confirmed by CHIKV specific antiserum and the results can take 1 to 2 weeks.[103] Virus isolation must only be performed in biosafety level 3 laboratories to reduce the risk of viral transmission.[87] Virus isolation, although the gold standard, is infrequently used for the diagnosis of CHIKV infection due to time-consuming laborious procedure and risk of laboratory transmission.

RT-PCR

RT-PCR is currently the most sensitive and rapid method for detecting CHIKV mRNA[87] and, therefore, more commonly used for the diagnosis and confirmation of CHIKV infection. RT-PCR can detect CHIKV from sera within first week of infection.[104,105] Real-time PCR demonstrates high sensitivity of less than 1 plaque-forming unit or 50 genome copies and results can be available from within 1 to 2 days.

Serologic tests

For serologic diagnosis, an acute-phase serum must be collected immediately after clinical onset and a convalescent-phase sera after 10 to 14 days after the onset of the disease. Serologic diagnosis can be made by demonstration of a 4-fold increase in CHIK IgG antibody in acute and convalescent sera. Getting paired sera is, however, usually not practical. Alternatively, the demonstration of IgM antibodies (MAC-ELISA) specific for CHIKV in acute-phase sera is used when paired sera cannot be obtained. Results of MAC-ELISA can be available within 2 to 3 days. Cross-reaction with other flavivirus antibodies, such as o'nyong-nyong and Semliki Forest, occurs in the MAC-ELISA; however, the latter viruses are rare in Southeast Asia but if further confirmation is required, it can be done by neutralization tests and hemagglutination inhibition assay.[103]

Treatment

There is no specific antiviral therapy available for CHIKV and treatment is mostly supportive, bed rest, fluids, and symptomatic treatment of fever and pain.[07,92] Paracetamol is the drug of choice with use of other analgesics, if paracetamol does not provide relief. Aspirin is preferably avoided for fear of gastrointestinal and other side effects, such as Reye syndrome. Nonsteroidal anti-inflammatory drugs, narcotics (eg, morphine) or short-term corticosteroids may be tried for recalcitrant pains, after evaluating the risk-benefit of these treatments.

Prevention

Because currently there is no vaccine available for CHIKV, protection against the mosquito remains the best way to prevent infection. The best way to control mosquito-borne disease is an integrated approach that includes antilarval and antiadult methods and protection against mosquito bites. In antilarval methods, source reduction where the mosquitoes lay eggs should be eliminated, such as flower vases, discarded tires, and water storage tanks for air coolers. Chemical larvicides include use of fenthion, chlorpyrifos, whereas biologic larvicides, such as *Gambusia affinis* fish, can be used in stagnant ponds or sewage oxidation ponds. Antiadult measures include spraying or fogging of insecticides, such as Pyrethrum, or residual spray, such as DDT, Lindane, and Malathion. Protection against mosquito bites includes use of mosquito nets, mosquito repellant, such as DEETn and adequate body covering by light clothing. Individuals acutely infected with CHIKV can also contribute to the spread of the disease through infected vectors[87]; therefore, they are also advised to take mosquito protection measures.

REFERENCES

1. Reed CM. Travel recommendations for older adults. Clin Geriatr Med 2007; 23(3):687–713, ix.
2. Leder K. Travelers as a sentinel population: use of sentinel networks to inform pretravel and posttravel evaluation. Curr Infect Dis Rep 2009;11(1):51–8.
3. Bhadelia N, Klotman M, Caplivski D. The HIV-positive traveler. Am J Med 2007; 120(7):574–80.
4. Jong EC, Sanford CA. Travel and tropical medicine manual. 4th edition. WB Saunders Co; 2008.
5. Wilson ME, Weld LH, Boggild A, et al, GeoSentinel Surveillance Network. Fever in returned travelers: results from the GeoSentinel Surveillance Network. Clin Infect Dis 2007;44:1560–8.
6. Public Health Agency of Canada. Canada Communicable Disease Report. Available at: http://www.phac-aspc.gc.ca/publicat/ccdr-rmtc/11vol37/acs-3/index-eng.php. Accessed July 14, 2012.
7. Freedman DO, Weld LH, Kozarsky PE, et al, GeoSentinel Surveillance Network. Spectrum of disease and relation to place among ill returned travelers. N Engl J Med 2006;354(2):119–30.
8. World Health Organization. World Malaria Report. 2011. Available at: http://www.who.int/entity/malaria/world_malaria_report_2011/9789241564403_eng.pdf. Accessed July 1, 2012.
9. Mali S, Kachur SP, Arguin PM, Division of Parasitic Diseases and Malaria, Center for Global Health; Centers for Disease Control and Prevention (CDC). Malaria surveillance–United States, 2010. MMWR Surveill Summ 2012;61(2):1–17.
10. World Health Organization. Guidelines for the treatment of malaria. 2nd edition. 2010. Available at: http://whqlibdoc.who.int/publications/2010/9789241547925_eng.pdf. Accessed July 1, 2012.
11. Garcia LS. Malaria. Clin Lab Med 2010;30(1):93–129.
12. Griffith KS, Lewis LS, Mali S, et al. Treatment of malaria in the United States: a systematic review. JAMA 2007;297:2264–77.
13. Fairhurst RM, Wellems TE. *Plasmodium* Species (Malaria). In: Mandell GL, Bennett JE, Dolin R, editors. Bennett's principles and practice of infectious diseases. 7th edition. PA: Elsevier Churchill Livingstone; 2009. p. 3437–62.
14. Kochar DK, Saxena V, Singh N, et al. Plasmodium vivax malaria. Emerg Infect Dis 2005;11(1):132–4.
15. Mirdha RB, Wattal C. Sepsis syndrome. In: Khardori NM, Wattal C, editors. Emergencies in infectious disease. From head to toe. Delhi (India): Byword Books Private Limited; 2010. p. 241–6.

16. Lacerda MV, Mourão MP, Alexandre MA, et al. Understanding the clinical spectrum of complicated Plasmodium vivax malaria: a systematic review on the contributions of the Brazilian literature. Malar J 2012;11:12.

17. Schwartz E, Parise M, Kozarsky P, et al. Delayed onset of malaria—implications for chemoprophylaxis in travelers. N Engl J Med 2003;349(16):1510–6.

18. Reyburn H, Behrens RH, Warhurst D, et al. The effect of chemoprophylaxis on the timing of onset of falciparum malaria. Trop Med Int Health 1998;3(4):281–5.

19. Lalloo DG, Shingadia D, Pasvol G, et al, HPA Advisory Committee on Malaria Prevention in UK Travellers. UK malaria treatment guidelines. J Infect 2007; 54(2):111–21.

20. Guerin PJ, Olliaro P, Nosten F, et al. Malaria: current status of control, diagnosis, treatment, and a proposed agenda for research and development. Lancet Infect Dis 2002;2:564–73.

21. Pöschl B, Waneesorn J, Thekisoe O, et al. Comparative diagnosis of malaria infections by microscopy, nested PCR, and LAMP in northern Thailand. Am J Trop Med Hyg 2010;83:56–60.

22. Kain KC, Harrington MA, Tennyson S, et al. Imported malaria: prospective analysis of problems in diagnosis and management. Clin Infect Dis 1998;27:142–9.

23. Fagbenro-Beyioku AF, Ojuromi OT, Orenaike IK. Qualitative comparison of qualitative buffy coat and light microscopy in malaria diagnosis. Trop Doct 2007; 37(1):60–1.

24. Abba K, Deeks JJ, Olliaro PL, et al. Rapid diagnostic tests for diagnosing uncomplicated P. falciparum malaria in endemic countries. Cochrane Database Syst Rev 2011;(7):CD008122.

25. Stauffer WM, Cartwright CP, Olson DA, et al. Diagnostic performance of rapid diagnostic tests versus blood smears for malaria in US clinical practice. Clin Infect Dis 2009;49(6):908–13.

26. Murray CK, Gasser RA Jr, Magill AJ, et al. Update on rapid diagnostic testing for malaria. Clin Microbiol Rev 2008;21(1):97–110.

27. Bigaillon C, Fontan E, Cavallo JD, et al. Ineffectiveness of the Binax NOW malaria test for diagnosis of Plasmodium ovale malaria. J Clin Microbiol 2005;43(2):1011.

28. Gamboa D, Ho MF, Bendezu J, et al. A large proportion of P. falciparum isolates in the Amazon region of Peru lack pfhrp2 and pfhrp3: implications for malaria rapid diagnostic tests. PLoS One 2010;5(1):e8091.

29. Centers for Disease Control and Prevention (CDC). Malaria Diagnosis (U.S.) Serology. Available at: http://www.cdc.gov/malaria/diagnosis_treatment/diagnosis. html. Accessed July 1, 2012.

30. Zalis MG, Ferreira-da-Cruz MF, Balthazar-Guedes HC, et al. Malaria diagnosis: standardization of a polymerase chain reaction for the detection of Plasmodium falciparum parasites in individuals with low-grade parasitemia. Parasitol Res 1996;82(7):612–6.

31. Elsayed S, Plewes K, Church D, et al. Use of molecular beacon probes for real-time PCR detection of Plasmodium falciparum and other plasmodium species in peripheral blood specimens. J Clin Microbiol 2006;44:622–4.

32. Mace KE, Lynch MF. Malaria. In: Bope E, Kellerman R, editors. Conn's current therapy. 1st edition. Saunders; 2012. p. 122–32.

33. Centers for Disease Control and Prevention (CDC). Treatment of malaria: guidelines for clinicians (United States). 2011. Available at: http://www.cdc.gov/malaria/resources/pdf/treatmenttable.pdf. Accessed July 14, 2012.

34. Baird JK, Hoffman SL. Primaquine therapy for malaria. Clin Infect Dis 2004; 39(9):1336–45.

35. Dondorp AM, Fanello CI, Hendriksen IC, et al. Artesunate versus quinine in the treatment of severe falciparum malaria in African children (AQUAMAT): an open-label, randomised trial. Lancet 2010;376(9753):1647–57.

36. Schlagenhauf P, Petersen E. Malaria chemoprophylaxis: strategies for risk groups. Clin Microbiol Rev 2008;21(3):466–72.

37. Centers for Disease Control and Prevention (CDC). Chapter 3 infectious diseases related to travel. In: malaria. Available at: http://wwwnc.cdc.gov/travel/yellowbook/2012/chapter-3-infectious-diseases-related-to-travel/malaria.htm. Accessed August 4, 2012.

38. Swales CA, Chiodini PL, Bannister BA, Health Protection Agency Advisory Committee on Malaria Prevention in UK Travellers. New guidelines on malaria prevention: a summary. J Infect 2007;54(2):107–10.

39. Schwartz L, Brown GV, Genton B, et al. A review of malaria vaccine clinical projects based on the WHO rainbow table. Malar J 2012;11:11.

40. Lee KS, Divis PC, Zakaria SK, et al. Plasmodium knowlesi: reservoir hosts and tracking the emergence in humans and macaques. PLoS Pathog 2011;7(4):e1002015.

41. Singh B, Sung LK, Matusop A, et al. A large focus of naturally acquired *Plasmodium knowlesi* infections in human beings. Lancet 2004;363:1017–24.

42. William T, Menon J, Rajahram G, et al. Severe *Plasmodium knowlesi* malaria in a tertiary care hospital, Sabah, Malaysia. Emerg Infect Dis 2011;17(7):1248–55.

43. World Health Organization. Global alert and response (GAR). Available at: http://www.who.int/csr/disease/dengue/impact/en/. Accessed July 10, 2012.

44. Dussart P, Labeau B, Lagathu G, et al. Evaluation of an Enzyme Immunoassay for Detection of Dengue Virus NS1 Antigen in Human Serum. Clin Vaccine Immunol 2006;13:1185–9.

45. Petersen LR, Barrett AD. Arthropod-borne flaviviruses. In: Richman DD, Whitley RJ, Hayden FG, editors. Clinical Virology. 3rd edition. Washington, DC: ASM Press; 2009. p. 1173–214.

46. Vaughan DW, Barrett A, Solomon T. Flaviviruses (yellow fever, dengue, dengue hemorrhagic fever, Japanese encephalitis, West Nile encephalitis, St. Louis encephalitis, Tick-borne encephalitis). In: Mandell GL, Bennett JE, Dolin R, editors. Bennett's principles and practice of infectious diseases. 7th edition. PA: Elsevier Churchill Livingstone; 2009. p. 2133–56.

47. Centers for Disease Control and Prevention (CDC). Travel associated Dengue surveillance - United States, 2006-2008. MMWR Morb Mortal Wkly Rep 2010;59(23):715–9.

48. Centers for Disease Control and Prevention (CDC). Dengue hemorrhagic fever—U.S.-Mexico border, 2005. MMWR Morb Mortal Wkly Rep 2007;56(31):785–9 [Erratum appears in MMWR Morb Mortal Wkly Rep 2007;56(32):822].

49. Centers for Disease Control and Prevention (CDC). Entomology & ecology. Available at: http://www.cdc.gov/Dengue/entomologyEcology/index.html. Accessed June 11, 2012.

50. Simmons CP, Farrar JJ, Nguyen vV, et al. Dengue. N Engl J Med 2012;366(15):1423–32.

51. Wichmann O, Mühlberger N, Jelinek T. Dengue—the underestimated risk in travellers. Dengue Bull 2003;27:126–37.

52. Ahmed FU, Mahmood CB, Sharma JD, et al. Dengue fever and dengue haemorrhagic fever in chidren the 2000 out break in Chittatong, Bangladesh. Dengue Bull 2001;25:33–9.

53. Hongsiriwon S. Dengue hemorrhagic fever in infants. Southeast Asian J Trop Med Public Health 2002;33:49–55.

54. Trofa AF, DeFraites RF, Smoak BL, et al. Dengue fever in US military personnel in Haiti. JAMA 1997;277:1546.

55. Halstead SB. Dengue. Lancet 2007;370:1644.

56. Shirtcliffe P, Cameron E, Nicholson KG, et al. Don't forget dengue! Clinical features of dengue fever in returning travellers. J R Coll Physicians Lond 1998;32(3):235–7.

57. WHO. Dengue haemorrhagic fever: diagnosis, treatment, prevention and control. 2nd edition. Geneva (Switzerland): World Health Organization; 1997.

58. Anonymous. Dengue hemorrhagic fever, diagnosis, treatment and control. Geneva (Switzerland): World Health Organization; 1986.

59. Kalayanarooj S, Vaughn DW, Nimmannitya S, et al. Early clinical and laboratory indicators of acute dengue illness. J Infect Dis 1997;176:313.

60. WHO. Dengue: Guidelines for Diagnosis, Treatment Prevention and Control. In: Organization WHO, editor. World health Organization. New edition. Geneva (Switzerland): World Health Organization; 2009.

61. Malavige GN, Fernando S, Fernando DJ, et al. Dengue viral infections. Postgrad Med J 2004;80(948):588–601.

62. Guzmán MG, Kourí G, Martínez E, et al. Clinical and serologic study of Cuban children with dengue hemorrhagic fever/dengue shock syndrome (DHF/DSS). Bull Pan Am Health Organ 1987;21:270.

63. Rigau-Pérez JG, Laufer MK. Dengue-related deaths in Puerto Rico, 1992-1996: diagnosis and clinical alarm signals. Clin Infect Dis 2006;42:1241.

64. Wattal C, Gupta PS, Datta S. Dengue fever and encephalitis. In: Khardori NM, Wattal C, editors. Emergencies in infectious disease. From head to toe. Delhi (India): Byword Books Private Limited; 2010. p. 41–8.

65. Chakravarti A, Kumaria R, Batra VV, et al. Improved detection of dengue virus serotypes from serum samples—evaluation of single-tube multiplex RT-PCR with cell culture. Dengue Bull 2006;30:133–40.

66. Shu PY, Huang JH. Current advances in dengue diagnosis. Clin Diagn Lab Immunol 2004;11(4):642–50.

67. Sekaran SD, Lan EC, Mahesawarappa KB, et al. Evaluation of a dengue NS1 capture ELISA assay for the rapid detection of dengue. J Infect Dev Ctries 2007;1(2):182–8.

68. Centers for Disease Control and Prevention (CDC). Laboratory guidance and diagnostic testing. Available at: http://www.cdc.gov/dengue/clinicalLab/laboratory.html. Accessed July 10, 2012.

69. Innis BL, Nisalak A, Nimmannitya S, et al. An enzyme-linked immunosorbent assay to characterize dengue infections where dengue and Japanese encephalitis co-circulate. Am J Trop Med Hyg 1989;40(4):418–27.

70. Koraka P, Burghoorn-Maas CP, Falconar A, et al. Detection of immune-complex-dissociated nonstructural-1 antigen in patients with acute dengue virus infections. J Clin Microbiol 2003;41(9):4154–9.

71. Chanama S, Anantapreecha S, Neugoonpipat A, et al. Analysis of specific IgM responses in secondary dengue virus infections: levels and positive rates in comparison with primary infections. J Clin Virol 2004;31(3):185–9.

72. Sa-Ngasang A, Anantapreecha S, A-Nuegoonpipat A, et al. Specific IgM and IgG responses in primary and secondary dengue virus infections determined by enzyme-linked immunosorbent assay. Epidemiol Infect 2006;134(4):820–5.

73. Schwartz E. Study of dengue fever among Israeli travellers to Thailand. Dengue Bull 2002;26:162–6.

74. Wichmann O, Stark K, Shu PY, et al. Clinical features and pitfalls in the laboratory diagnosis of dengue in travellers. BMC Infect Dis 2006;6:120.

75. Alcon S, Talarmin A, Debruyne M, et al. Enzyme-linked immunosorbent assay specific to dengue virus type 1 nonstructural protein NS1 reveals circulation of the antigen in the blood during the acute phase of disease in patients experiencing primary or secondary infections. J Clin Microbiol 2002;40(2): 376–81.

76. Young PR, Hilditch PA, Bletchly C, et al. An antigen capture enzyme-linked immunosorbent assay reveals high levels of dengue virus protein NS1 in the sera of infected patients. J Clin Microbiol 2000;38(3):1053–7.

77. Datta S, Wattal C. Dengue NS1 antigen detection: a useful tool in early diagnosis of dengue virus infection. Indian J Med Microbiol 2010;28(2):107–10.

78. Schilling S, Ludolfs D, Le VA, et al. Laboratory diagnosis of Primary and secondary dengue infections. J Clin Virol 2004;31(3):179–84.

79. Ampaiwan C, Wathanee C, Viroj P, et al. The use of Nonstructural protein 1 antigen for the early diagnosis during the febrile stage in patients with dengue infection. Pediatr Infect Dis J 2008;27(1):43–8.

80. Bessoff K, Phoutrides E, Delorey M, et al. Utility of a commercial nonstructural protein 1 antigen capture kit as a dengue virus diagnostic tool. Clin Vaccine Immunol 2010;17(6):949–53.

81. Lahariya C, Pradhan SK. Emergence of chikungunya virus in Indian subcontinent after 32 years: a review. J Vector Borne Dis 2006;43(4):151–60.

82. Kumar NP, Joseph R, Kamaraj T, et al. A226V mutation in virus during the 2007 chikungunya outbreak in Kerala, India. J Gen Virol 2008;89:1945–8.

83. Cherian SS, Walimbe AM, Jadhav SM, et al. Evolutionary rates and timescale comparison of Chikungunya viruses inferred from the whole genome/E1 gene with special reference to the 2005–07 outbreak in the Indian subcontinent. Infect Genet Evol 2009;9:16–23.

84. Tsetsarkin KA, Vanlandingham DL, McGee CE, et al. A single mutation in chikungunya virus affects vector specificity and epidemic potential. PLoS Pathog 2007;3:e201. http://dx.doi.org/10.1371/journal.ppat.0030201.

85. Lumsden WH. An epidemic of virus disease in Southern Province, Tanganyika Territory, in 1952-53: II. General description and epidemiology. Trans R Soc Trop Med Hyg 1955;49(1):33–57.

86. Cavrini F, Gaibani P, Pierro AM, et al. Chikungunya: an emerging and spreading arthropod-borne viral disease. J Infect Dev Ctries 2009;3(10):744–5.

87. Centers for Disease Control and Prevention (CDC). Preparedness and response for introduction in the Americas chikungunya virus. Available at: http://www.cdc.gov/chikungunya/. Accessed August 8, 2012.

88. Vazeille M, Moutailler S, Coudrier D. Two Chikungunya isolates from the outbreak of La Reunion (Indian Ocean) exhibit different patterns of infection in the mosquito, Aedes albopictus. PLoS One 2007;2(11):e1168.

89. Thiboutot MM, Kannan S, Kawalekar OU, et al. Chikungunya: a potentially emerging epidemic? PLoS Negl Trop Dis 2010;4(4):e623.

90. World Health Organization. Outbreak and spread of chikungunya. Wkly Epidemiol Rec 2007;82:409–15.

91. Staples JE, Breiman RF, Powers AM. Chikungunya fever: an epidemiological review of a re-emerging infectious disease. Clin Infect Dis 2009;49(6): 942–8.

92. World Health Organization (WHO). Guidelines on clinical management of chikungunya fever. Available at: http://www.wpro.who.int/mvp/topics/ntd/Clinical_Mgnt_Chikungunya_WHO_SEARO.pdf. Accessed August 08, 2012.

93. Rezza G, Nicoletti L, Angelini R, et al, CHIKV study group. Infection with chikungunya virus in Italy: an outbreak in a temperate region. Lancet 2007;370: 1805–6.

94. Borgherini G, Poubeau P, Staikowsky F, et al. Outbreak of chikungunya on Reunion Island: early clinical and laboratory features in 157 adult patients. Clin Infect Dis 2007;44:1401–7.

95. Inamadar AC, Palit A, Sampagavi VV, et al. Cutaneous manifestations of chikungunya fever: observations made during a recent outbreak in south India. Int J Dermatol 2008;47:154–9.

96. Shah KV, Gibbs CJ Jr, Banerjee G. Virological investigation of the epidemic of haemorrhage fever in Calcutta: isolation of three strains of chikungunya virus. Indian J Med Res 1964;52:676–83.

97. Powers AM, Logue CH. Changing patterns of chikungunya virus: re-emergence of a zoonotic arbovirus. J Gen Virol 2007;88(Pt 9):2363–77.

98. Schuffenecker I, Iteman I, Michault A, et al. Genome microevolution of chikungunya viruses causing the Indian Ocean outbreak. PLoS Med 2006;3(7):e263.

99. Sissoko D, Malvy D, Ezzedine K, et al. Post-epidemic chikungunya disease on Réunion Island: course of rheumatic manifestations and associated factors over a 15-month period. PLoS Negl Trop Dis 2009;3(3):e389.

100. Soumahoro MK, Gerardin P, Boelle PY, et al. Impact of chikungunya virus infection on health status and quality of life: a retrospective cohort study. PLoS One 2009;4(11):e7800.

101. Hoarau JJ, Jaffar Bandjee MC, Trotot PK, et al. Persistent chronic inflammation and infection by Chikungunya arthritogenic alphavirus in spite of a robust host immune response. J Immunol 2010;184(10):5914–27.

102. Robillard PY, Boumahni B, Gerardin P, et al. Vertical maternal fetal transmission of the chikungunya virus. Ten cases among 84 pregnant women. Presse Med 2006;35(5 Pt 1):785–8.

103. World Health Organization (WHO). Laboratory diagnosis of chikungunya fevers. Available at: http://www.searo.who.int/en/Section10/Section2246_12902.htm. Accessed August 8, 2012.

104. Lanciotti RS, Kosoy OL, Laven JJ, et al. Chikungunya virus in US travelers returning from India 2006. Emerg Infect Dis 2007;13:764–7.

105. Panning M, Grywna K, van Esbroeck M, et al. Chikungunya fever in travelers returning to Europe from the Indian Ocean region, 2006. Emerg Infect Dis 2008;14:416–22.

Index

Note: Page numbers of article titles are in **boldface** type.

A

Abscess(es)
    brain. *See* Brain abscess.
    intra-abdominal, 1049–1050, 1085–1087
    intraperitoneal, 1176–1177, 1180
    liver, 1180–1181
    lung, 1082–1084, 1137–1140
    periappendiceal, 1177
    pericholecystic, 1177
    perinephric, 1086–1087, 1177, 1180
    retropharyngeal, 1117–1120
    spleen, 1181
    visceral, 1180–1181
Acalculous cholecystitis, 1181
Acinetobacter infections, acute respiratory distress in, 1136
Adrenal gland dysfunction, in sepsis, 1096–1098
Adult respiratory distress syndrome, antibiotics for, 1083–1084
Aeromonas hydrophila infections, 1054, 1197–1198
Airway obstruction, 1041–1042, 1080–1081, **1117–1120**
Allostasis, in stress, 1096
Amebiasis, 1179, 1184
American Thoracic Society, pneumonia guidelines of, 1130
Aneurysm
    aortic, 1046–1047
    mycotic, 1152
Animal bite wounds, infection of, 1056–1058
Antibiotic(s), **1079–1094**. *See also specific infections.*
    for adult respiratory distress syndrome, 1083–1084
    for airway obstruction, 1119–1120
    for bloodstream infections, 1089, 1212–1214
    for brain abscess, 1080–1081
    for cardiac infections, 1084–1085
    for cholangitis, 1178
    for cholecystitis, 1178
    for colitis, 1179
    for device-related infections, 1215–1216
    for empyema, 1143
    for encephalitis, 1080–1081, 1113
    for endocarditis, 1084, 1155–1160
    for epiglottitis, 1080, 1082
    for head and neck infections, 1080–1082
    for intra-abdominal abscess, 1085–1087

Med Clin N Am 96 (2012) 1257–1272
http://dx.doi.org/10.1016/S0025-7125(12)00181-2
0025-7125/12/$ – see front matter © 2012 Elsevier Inc. All rights reserved.

United States Postal Service

Statement of Ownership, Management, and Circulation
(All Periodicals Publications Except Requestor Publications)

1. Publication Title	2. Publication Number	3. Filing Date
Medical Clinics of North America	3 3 7 - 3 4 0	9/14/12

4. Issue Frequency	5. Number of Issues Published Annually	6. Annual Subscription Price
Jan, Mar, May, Jul, Sep, Nov	6	$232.00

7. Complete Mailing Address of Known Office of Publication *(Not printer) (Street, city, county, state, and ZIP+4®)*

Elsevier Inc.
360 Park Avenue South
New York, NY 10010-1710

Contact Person
Stephen Bushing

Telephone *(Include area code)*
215-239-3688

8. Complete Mailing Address of Headquarters or General Business Office of Publisher *(Not printer)*

Elsevier Inc., 360 Park Avenue South, New York, NY 10010-1710

9. Full Names and Complete Mailing Addresses of Publisher, Editor, and Managing Editor *(Do not leave blank)*

Publisher *(Name and complete mailing address)*

Kim Murphy, Elsevier, Inc., 1600 John F. Kennedy Blvd. Suite 1800, Philadelphia, PA 19103-2899

Editor *(Name and complete mailing address)*

Pamela Hetherington, Elsevier, Inc., 1600 John F. Kennedy Blvd. Suite 1800, Philadelphia, PA 19103-2899

Managing Editor *(Name and complete mailing address)*

Adrienne Brigido, Elsevier, Inc., 1600 John F. Kennedy Blvd. Suite 1800, Philadelphia, PA 19103-2899

10. Owner *(Do not leave blank. If the publication is owned by a corporation, give the name and address of the corporation immediately followed by the names and addresses of all stockholders owning or holding 1 percent or more of the total amount of stock. If not owned by a corporation, give the names and addresses of the individual owners. If owned by a partnership or other unincorporated firm, give its name and address as well as those of each individual owner. If the publication is published by a nonprofit organization, give its name and address.)*

Full Name	Complete Mailing Address
Wholly owned subsidiary of	1600 John F. Kennedy Blvd., Ste. 1800
Reed/Elsevier, US holdings	Philadelphia, PA 19103-2899

11. Known Bondholders, Mortgagees, and Other Security Holders Owning or Holding 1 Percent or More of Total Amount of Bonds, Mortgages, or Other Securities. If none, check box ☐ **None**

Full Name	Complete Mailing Address
N/A	

12. Tax Status *(For completion by nonprofit organizations authorized to mail at nonprofit rates) (Check one)*

The purpose, function, and nonprofit status of this organization and the exempt status for federal income tax purposes:

☐ Has Not Changed During Preceding 12 Months
☐ Has Changed During Preceding 12 Months *(Publisher must submit explanation of change with this statement)*

PS Form 3526, September 2007 (Page 1 of 3 (Instructions Page 3)) PSN 7530-01-000-9931 **PRIVACY NOTICE:** See our Privacy policy in www.usps.com

---

13. Publication Title	14. Issue Date for Circulation Data Below
Medical Clinics of North America	July 2012

15. Extent and Nature of Circulation		Average No. Copies Each Issue During Preceding 12 Months	No. Copies of Single Issue Published Nearest to Filing Date
a. Total Number of Copies *(Net press run)*		2173	1881
b. Paid Circulation (By Mail and Outside the Mail)	(1) Mailed Outside-County Paid Subscriptions Stated on PS Form 3541. *(Include paid distribution above nominal rate, advertiser's proof copies, and exchange copies)*	1083	978
	(2) Mailed In-County Paid Subscriptions Stated on PS Form 3541 *(Include paid distribution above nominal rate, advertiser's proof copies, and exchange copies)*		
	(3) Paid Distribution Outside the Mails Including Sales Through Dealers and Carriers, Street Vendors, Counter Sales, and Other Paid Distribution Outside USPS®	564	590
	(4) Paid Distribution by Other Classes Mailed Through the USPS (e.g. First-Class Mail®)		
c. Total Paid Distribution *(Sum of 15b (1), (2), (3), and (4))*	▶	1647	1568
d. Free or Nominal Rate Distribution (By Mail and Outside the Mail)	(1) Free or Nominal Rate Outside-County Copies Included on PS Form 3541	97	100
	(2) Free or Nominal Rate In-County Copies Included on PS Form 3541		
	(3) Free or Nominal Rate Copies Mailed at Other Classes Through the USPS (e.g. First-Class Mail)		
	(4) Free or Nominal Rate Distribution Outside the Mail (Carriers or other means)		
e. Total Free or Nominal Rate Distribution *(Sum of 15d (1), (2), (3) and (4))*	▶	97	100
f. Total Distribution *(Sum of 15c and 15e)*	▶	1744	1668
g. Copies not Distributed *(See instructions to publishers #4 (page #3))*	▶	429	213
h. Total *(Sum of 15f and g)*	▶	2173	1881
i. Percent Paid (15c divided by 15f times 100)		94.44%	94.00%

16. Publication of Statement of Ownership

If the publication is a general publication, publication of this statement is required. Will be printed in the **November 2012** issue of this publication.

☐ Publication not required

17. Signature and Title of Editor, Publisher, Business Manager, or Owner

[signature] Stephen R. Bushing

Stephen R. Bushing –Inventory Distribution Coordinator

Date: September 14, 2012

I certify that all information furnished on this form is true and complete. I understand that anyone who furnishes false or misleading information on this form or who omits material or information requested on the form may be subject to criminal sanctions (including fines and imprisonment) and/or civil sanctions (including civil penalties).

PS Form 3526, September 2007 (Page 2 of 3)

Moving?

Make sure your subscription moves with you!

To notify us of your new address, find your **Clinics Account Number** (located on your mailing label above your name), and contact customer service at:

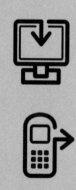

Email: journalscustomerservice-usa@elsevier.com

800-654-2452 (subscribers in the U.S. & Canada)
314-447-8871 (subscribers outside of the U.S. & Canada)

Fax number: 314-447-8029

Elsevier Health Sciences Division
Subscription Customer Service
3251 Riverport Lane
Maryland Heights, MO 63043

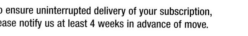

*To ensure uninterrupted delivery of your subscription, please notify us at least 4 weeks in advance of move.

ELSEVIER